ACROMEGALY

A Century of
Scientific and
Clinical Progress

SERONO SYMPOSIA, USA

Series Editor: James Posillico

SOMATOSTATIN: Basic and Clinical Status
Edited by Seymour Reichlin

ACROMEGALY: A Century of Scientific and Clinical Progress
Edited by Richard J. Robbins and Shlomo Melmed

A Continuation Order Plan is available for this series. A continuation order will bring delivery of each new volume immediately upon publication. Volumes are billed only upon actual shipment. For further information please contact the publisher.

ACROMEGALY

A Century of Scientific and Clinical Progress

Edited by

Richard J. Robbins

Yale University
New Haven, Connecticut

and

Shlomo Melmed

Cedars Sinai Medical Center
UCLA School of Medical Science
Los Angeles, California

PLENUM PRESS • NEW YORK AND LONDON

Library of Congress Cataloging in Publication Data

Acromegaly Centennial Symposium (1986: San Francisco, Calif.)
  Acromegaly: a century of scientific and clinical progress.

  ''Proceedings of the Acromegaly Centennial Symposium, sponsored by Serono Symposia, USA and
the University of California, held June 29–July 1, 1986, in San Francisco, California''—T.p. verso.
  Bibliography: p.
  Includes indexes.
  1. Acromegaly—Congresses. I. Robbins, Richard J., 1948–   . II. Melmed, Shlomo. III. Serono
Symposia, USA. IV. University of California, San Francisco. V. Title.
  RC658.3.A27 1986   616.4'7   87-13016
  ISBN-13: 978-1-4612-9064-3   e-ISBN-13: 978-1-4613-1913-9
  DOI: 10.1007/978-1-4613-1913-9

The views expressed in this volume are the responsibility of the named authors. Great care has been
taken to maintain the accuracy of the information contained in the volume. However, neither Plenum
Press, Serono Symposia, U.S.A., nor the editors can be held responsible for errors or any consequences
arising from the use of information contained herein.

Some of the names of products referred to in this book may be registered trademarks or proprietary
names, although specific references to this fact may not be made; however, the use of a name without
designations is not to be construed as a representation by the publisher or editors that it is in the public
domain. In addition, the mention of specific companies or if their products or proprietary names does not
imply any endorsement or recommendation on the part of the publisher or editors.

Proceedings of the Acromegaly Centennial Symposium, sponsored by Serono Symposia, USA, and
the University of California, held June 29–July 1, 1986, in San Francisco, California

© 1987 Plenum Press, New York
Softcover reprint of the hardcover 1st edition 1987
A Division of Plenum Publishing Corporation
233 Spring Street, New York, N.Y. 10013

SCIENTIFIC COMMITTEE

Richard J. Robbins, M.D., Co-Chairman
Yale University
New Haven, CT

Shlomo Melmed, M.D., Co-Chairman
Cedars Sinai Medical Center
Los Angeles, CA

Mark E. Molitch, M.D.
Northwestern University
Chicago, IL

Maurice F. Scanlon, M.D.
Welsh National School of Medicine
Cardiff, Wales

Wylie W. Vale, Ph.D.
Salk Institute
San Diego, CA

Charles B. Wilson, M.D.
University of California
San Francisco, CA

ORGANIZING SECRETARIES

Ching Lau, Ph.D.
James T. Posillico, Ph.D.
Serono Symposia, USA
Randolph, MA

PREFACE

The manuscripts in this volume were contributed by the speakers invited to the Acromegaly Centennial Symposium held in San Francisco, California in July 1986. The meeting was organized to commemorate the description of acromegaly by the French physician Pierre Marie, in 1886. The members of the Scientific Committee spent many hours assisting us in ensuring an outstanding meeting. The support of Serono Symposia, USA in all phases of the planning and execution of the meeting was sincerely appreciated and was highly professional.

Special recognition must be extended to Professor Roger Guillemin of the Salk Institute, whose interest in medical history led him to devote a great deal of time and personal expense in obtaining information about the life of Pierre Marie. Dr. Guillemin's presentation on the life and times of Marie was an extraordinary overview of the cultural, social, and scientific backgrounds in which Marie came to describe the disease, acromegaly. Dr. Guillemin's findings, which were presented at the main banquet in a splendid audiovisual presentation, were clearly the highlight of the meeting and will long be remembered by the attendees.

We were also honored by the presence of Dr. Martine Pierre Marie Granier, the great-granddaughter of Pierre Marie. In her address at the banquet, Dr. Granier provided several delightful and intimate vignettes concerning Pierre Marie, using old family records and photographs. The Scientific Committee wishes to extend its gratitude to Dr. Granier for adding immeasurably to the historical atmosphere of the meeting.

Pierre Marie was a young physician studying in the clinic of Dr. Charcot at the Salpetriere Hospital in Paris. Historically, Marie is more well known for his many significant contributions to clinical neurology concerning cerebrovascular disease, peripheral muscular atrophy, and aphasia. His name, however, is immortalized in endocrinology for the insightfulness to recognize that a collection of reports about mysterious and grotesque patients were in fact describing a discrete medical syndrome. He named the condition "acromegalie" because the enlargement of the hands and feet in these patients was the most consistent and prominent feature. A number of physicians since the time of Marie have attempted to change the name of the disease because it did not address many of the important clinical features. However, Marie's malady has retained the simple and euphonious name which he originally gave to it.

In his initial description, Marie provided a careful and complete differential diagnosis of this condition in which he pointed out that he originally thought it to be a variant of osteitis deformans (Paget's disease). He also clearly distinguished his disease from similar features seen in myxedema, rheumatoid arthritis, and leontiasis ossea of Virchow. Although Marie was uncertain as to the etiology of this condition, a number of putative etiologic factors had been suggested by others prior to 1900, including: blows to the head, abnormal brain function (suggested by Magendie and von Recklinhausen), infections, the thymus, fright, and atavism. The earliest treatments for this condition included: iodine, high dose thyroid, low glucose diets, arsenic, mercury, strychnine, rhubarb and caffeine. Headache, which was a prominent feature of this condition, was relieved by a number of different remedies including codeine and notably ergot derivatives, which reportedly improved the overall condition according to Dr. Claus (1) in France, and Dr. Warda (2) in Germany. This is ironic as, until recently, the only medical therapy partially effective for acromegaly was the ergot derivative, bromergocriptine.

Surgical attempts to remove the enlarged pituitary began in the early 1890s and were perfected by neurosurgeons such as Harvey Cushing who by 1910 had reported many cures of acromegaly and postulated that the disease was due to an overactivity of the pituitary. In 1909, Beclere (3) reported that four acromegalics improved after roentgen ray therapy to the pituitary area. In summary, therefore, by 1910 physicians were aware of virtually all the clinical features of the disease, and patients had been successfully treated by medical, radiation, and transsphenoidal surgical approaches.

The major historical developments in our understanding of growth hormone synthesis, secretion, action, and gene structure which have occurred over the past 100 years are reviewed in this monograph by Dr. Seymour Reichlin. Similarly, Dr. William Daughaday has summarized the major advances in the clinical aspects of this fascinating disease from a historical perspective. It is clear that a number of major problems in this disease need to be resolved: Is this condition due to a hypothalamic or a pituitary etiology? Secondly, how can we selectively destroy neoplastic somatotrophs while leaving adjacent pituitary cells intact? Finally, what are the pathophysiologic mechanisms involved in the adverse cardiovascular and arthritic complications of this condition, which often advanced despite resolution of the growth hormone excess.

Future developments in the understanding of growth hormone gene expression will undoubtedly elucidate the etiology of this disease, and provide physicians and scientists of the future with a rational basis for more effective therapy. We anticipate that the 200th anniversary meeting of the description of acromegaly, in 2086, will be reviewing much more effective and selective modes of therapy as well as diagnostic tests which will detect the condition much earlier. We also anticipate that, at such a meeting, arguments will still persist about the etiology and the optimal therapy of this enigmatic disease.

R.J. Robbins
S. Melmed

REFERENCES

1. Claus A. Un cas d'acromegalie. Ann et Bull de la Soc de Med de Gand 1890; 59:281.
2. Warda W. Ueber Akromegalie. Deutsch. Zeitschr f Nervenheilk (Leipzig) 1901; 19:358.
3. Beclere A. Le traitment medical des tumeurs hypophysaires du gigantisme et de l'acromegalie par la radio-therapie. Bull et Mem Soc Med d'Hop de Paris 1909; 27:274.

CONTENTS

III. DIAGNOSIS OF ACROMEGALY

IV. TREATMENTS FOR ACROMEGALY

THE LIFE OF DOCTOR PIERRE MARIE:

A GREAT-GRANDDAUGHTER'S VIEW

Ladies and Gentlemen, Dear Colleagues: I speak to you today about my great-grandfather, Dr. Pierre Marie, whom I always admired. I am delighted to honor with you tonight the memory of this humble man. But first I would like to thank Dr. Richard Robbins and Prof. Roger Guillemin for their kind invitation. Since I met Prof. Guillemin last year, we have established an exchange of information and documents concerning my great-grandfather.

I do not know if it is heredity or the fact that I have been raised in keeping his memory alive, but the brilliant career of Pierre Marie certainly guided the career of his son, Andre, as well as my own, toward medicine. My father also started to study medicine, but he was interrupted by the war. Since I do not pretend to be able to clarify any scientific aspect of my great-grandfather's work to you who are experts in Acromegaly, I will speak only about the man and will try to make him "alive" again tonight.

Born in Paris in 1852 as the only son, Pierre Marie began his studies in a boarding school in Vanves when he was seven years old. There he received the rigorous training of that time and learned the discipline which was to mark his life. He acquired a very good classical education, speaking and writing fluently in Latin and Greek. He was interested in medicine at an early age but first had to study law because of his father's wish. Once he obtained his law degree, he was able to enter Paris' School of Medicine. After receiving training in Germany and England, Pierre Marie returned to France and, while an intern in Paris' hospitals in 1878, met Prof. Charcot who became his mentor and introduced him to neurology, the field in which he later acquired worldwide recognition.

When Pierre Marie became a professor, the chair in neurology at the Salpetriere was not available. Reluctantly, he instead accepted the position of Physician-in-Chief of Bicetre Hospital for the elderly. He was not upset for very long because he quickly discovered how to make the best out of this situation and continue his research in neurology. With the help of his students, he conducted a thorough clinical examination of all his patients and verified his clinical findings in subsequent post-mortem studies. He was able to find the anatomical lesions corresponding to the pathologies he had discovered clinically. His extensive anatomic-pathologic studies enabled him to demonstrate the role of the pituitary gland and thus to participate in the birth of endocrinology.

He finally obtained his chair at the Salpetriere in 1916 where physicians and students from all over the world came to study. He guarded his private life very carefully. The elected few among his colleagues who were allowed to see him outside of the work environment remembered those times with fond memories.

Until his daughter Juliette's death, he had a happy, balanced life. He enjoyed a number of different hobbies. At a very young age, he showed an interest in learning about the history of religion and developed a taste for art works, which he looked for with delight. He collected sculptures, tapestries, furniture and paintings, most of which are now displayed in our national museums (Petit Palais, Louvre). He practiced sports on occasion, fencing, golf, but most of all, hunting, where he excelled.

He had a unique gift of perception and discernment. When he used this gift in medicine, he could diagnose with incredible accuracy illnesses that he studied but which were still very much undefined. While in the street, he sometimes would ask his chauffeur to stop in order to advise somebody passing by to seek treatment.

His wife, Blanche Savard, had been raised in a wealthy Parisian family. Her intellectual capabilities were enhanced by her elegance and charm. She made great efforts to ensure that her husband's life was without worries. They had two children, Juliette and Andre, and lived a very happy life in their mansion on rue de Lille, their house in Normandie, and their third house on the Riveria in the Pradet.

Everything fell apart when Juliette died from acute appendicitis; she was ten years old. Mrs. Pierre Marie, unable to recover from the death of her daughter, died a few years later, and was followed by her son, Andre, who died as a hero in July 1929 with the courage and tenacity that characterized him. He was 38 years old at the time of his death which was caused by the botulogenic bacteria that he had just isolated at the Pasteur Institute. Pierre Marie said, "Out of all of them, I should have died first."

He then retired and lived many more years, getting involved in the education of his three grandchildren, Francoise, Juliette and Alain. He loved to teach mythology to his grandchildren, especially during meals. One of my aunts does not have particularly fond memories of these sessions, however.

He lived the latter part of his life in the South of France with very few contacts from his earlier life in Paris. He would only rarely entertain a few friends and loyal students. He did not want to linger in the past, as so many retired people do. In order to maintain his intellectual acuity, he used to follow the political scene very closely and manage his fortune wisely in the stock markets in Paris, New York and Amsterdam. As time went by, he had more and more difficulty walking but his intellectual capacity remained unchanged. His last comments on aphasia preceded his death by only a few months.

This proud, scholarly, extraordinary, generous man died in 1940 at the age of 88 in atrocious suffering which the intervention of DeMartel was not able to alleviate. He died at the beginning of the Second World War, having survived the previous two wars in 1870 and 1914.

This, then, is a very brief summary of the life of my great-grandfather, Pierre Marie, whose work contributed to the development of neurology and to the fame of the School of the Salpetriere.

At this time I would like to thank you again for enabling me to share my memories with you tonight and to pay homage to my great-grandfather, Pierre Marie.

Dr. Martine Pierre Marie Granier

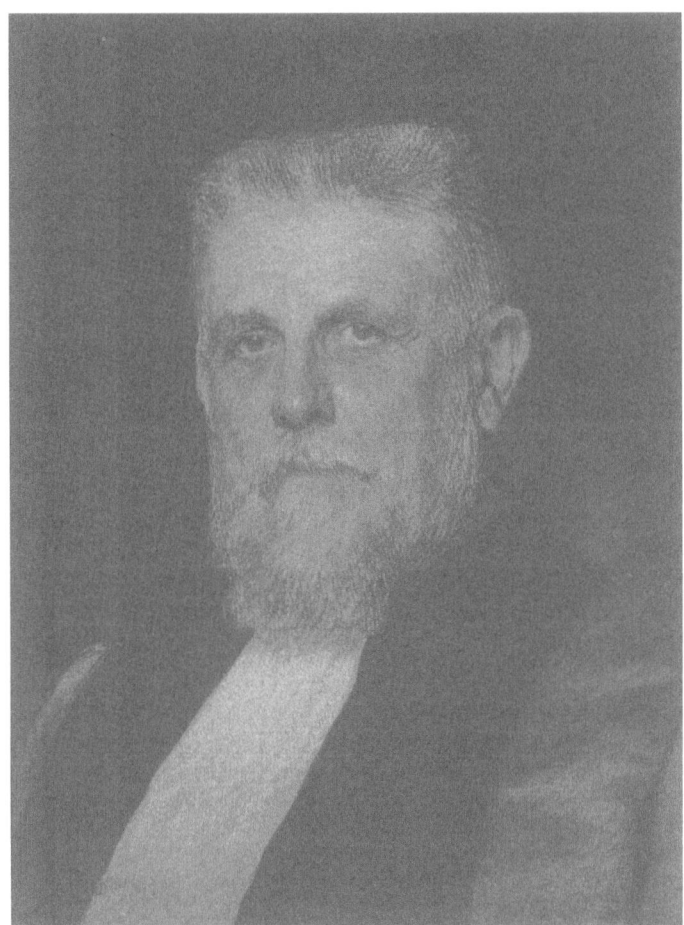

Doctor Pierre Marie

ACKNOWLEDGMENTS

The editors gratefully acknowledge the expert and generous assistance of Michèle Bony, Serono Laboratories, Inc., in translating Dr. Granier's address for this publication. We also thank Dr. Granier for graciously sharing with us the picture of her great-grandfather, Dr. Pierre Marie.

The Editors

I. MOLECULAR BIOLOGY AND PHYSIOLOGY OF GH ACTION

ETIOLOGY OF ACROMEGALY FROM THE NEUROENDOCRINE POINT OF VIEW: A HISTORICAL PERSPECTIVE

Seymour Reichlin, M.D., Ph.D.

Tufts-New England Medical Center

Boston, MA 02111

As we attain the one hundredth anniversary of the report by Pierre Marie of a patient with acromegaly (1), it is not unreasonable to ask how the wealth of physiological study of the mechanism of regulation of growth hormone (GH) secretion carried out particularly since 1960 has illuminated the pathogenesis of the disorder and added to our abilities to diagnose and manage the disease. The object of this chapter is to outline historical aspects of our current understanding of the mechanisms by which GH secretion is normally regulated, and how these may be abnormal in acromegaly. This anniversary report comes at a particularly propitious time because the chemical structures of the two principal hypothalamic factors responsible for GH regulation, growth hormone-releasing factor (GRF) (2,3) and somatostatin (4), and of growth hormone (GH) (5) itself have all been elucidated, and the molecular structure of the gene encoding for GH determined (6). The structures of the genes coding for somatostatin (7,8), and the structure of preproGRF have also been elucidated (9,10). It has, therefore, become possible to define the mechanisms controlling synthesis and secretion in molecular terms. Several reviews of this topic have been published (11-24).

Our current position has not been won easily. GH secretion was the last of the major anterior pituitary functions to be recognized as being under the control of the nervous system. From our current vantage point, it is not surprising to consider that GH secretion should be under the control of the hypothalamus because all of the other anterior pituitary secretions are so regulated. It was not until 1960 that the growth failure in rats with certain hypothalamic lesions was interpreted to be due to GH deficiency (25), and later in 1963, that hypothalamic extracts were shown to possess GH-releasing activity (26). Much of the initial difficulty in the study of regulation of GH secretion was the lack of bioassays of sufficient sensitivity and specificity to adequately measure blood GH. For this reason, the introduction of radioimmunoassay in 1963 by Roth, Glick, Yalow and Berson (27) marks a watershed in our knowledge of GH regulation (28,29). In addition to demonstrating that plasma GH was highly variable from time to time, these workers demonstrated that GH release was triggered by hypoglycemia, and that the hypoglycemia-induced response was abolished by pituitary stalk section (27). Soon thereafter, it was shown by Quabbe and colleagues (30), and Takahashi and colleagues (31), that GH secretion was subject to spontaneous fluctuations, and related to a defined period of sleep. These data, in the aggregate, made it a certainty that GH secretion was under the control of the brain, and that there had to be a GRF (by analogy with the other hypothalamic releasing factors).

Using the newly developed radioimmunoassays in man and rats, the following important insights were gained in the decade ending in 1973 (11-32). GH was shown to be stimulated (in primates) by emotional and physical stress, by amino acid infusion, and by certain centrally acting neurotransmitters. In the primate, at the central level, L-dopa, dopamine and serotonin are excitatory to GH release. Epinephrine is also an important central neurotransmitter controlling GH release (in rats) (14) as is acetylcholine (33). A large variety of neuropeptides are also involved in central regulation of GH secretion (34). Also in rats, it was shown by Martin and collaborators that GH is secreted in a predictable episodic fashion, with a peak at approximately 3½-hour intervals (32), and that this is probably due to episodic release of GRF (35). Unlike the human and other primates, stress suppresses GH secretion in the rat, an effect now known to be due to release of somatostatin since the inhibitory effect is abolished by pretreatment with antisomatostatin (36,37). Lesion studies in the monkey (28) and in the rat (32) established the principal neural pathways through which GH is regulated. This pathway involved the ventromedial and arcuate nuclei and the anterior median eminence as the final common pathway with important afferents from the hippocampus and amygdala. The latter connections with the limbic system provide the anatomical connections through which stress and circadian rhythms can modify GH secretion. Current histological study of GRF-immunostained neural pathways support the earlier physiological work (39).

The clear-cut physiological evidence that the brain must control GH secretion led a number of workers to attempt to isolate GRF from hypothalamic extracts. The laboratories of Guillemin, Schally, McCann, Knobil, and my own group all had active programs, the results of which were summarized in 1968 on the occasion of the International Congress of Endocrinology (40). By 1972 (and subsequently) we were able to demonstrate GRF activity in hypothalamic extracts using in vivo release methods plus radioimmunoassay (41,42). Schally's group had been misled by the so-called depletion assay to identify a fragment of porcine hemoglobin as the GRF (43), and Guillemin's group was unconvinced that GRF could be demonstrated. In 1968 McCann's group (Krulich, McCann and Dhariwal) had found GRF activity in certain regions of rat hypothalamus, and in addition had extracted a material inhibitory to GH secretion (44). Based on the finding of both excitatory and inhibitory compounds, they postulated that GH secretion was under dual control. The inhibitory compound, of course, later proved to be somatostatin.

In 1971, Guillemin's group again made a concerted effort to identify GRF, this time using as an assay dispersed rat pituitary cells, and the side fractions from their LRF isolation program. However, by 1972 they were no closer to identifying GRF and, instead, they decided to isolate and sequence the GH release inhibitory material that they had found in the extract (45). In a surprisingly short time, somatostatin, a 14 amino acid-containing peptide, was isolated, sequenced, and synthesized and shown to possess potent GH release inhibitory activity (4,45). The field of somatostatin research has been extensively reviewed (cf. 11,12,21,22, 24,46).

Immunocytochemical study delineated the somatostatinergic tubero-infundibular pathway (cf. 47,48), and immunoneutralization studies showed that somatostatin exerted a tonic suppressive effect on GH secretion in the rat (49), and was also responsible for stress- (36) and starvation- (37) induced GH suppression. Following the demonstration that direct injection of GH into the hypothalamus inhibited GH secretion (50,51), and that exposure of hypothalamic blocks to GH caused an increase in somatostatin secretion (52), it has become evident that the short-loop feedback control of GH secretion, postulated for many years, involved changes in somatostatin secretion.

From 1973 until 1982, little was accomplished in the endeavor to identify GRF. The most important event in this fallow period was the elucidation of the syndrome of ectopic GRF secretion in a few cases of acromegaly by Frohman and his colleagues who were the first to show that tumor extracts contained a bioactive GRF (53,54). This observation inspired Thorner and his colleagues in their efforts to characterize a GRF-active substance isolated from a patient with pancreatic adenoma (19,23,55) which in turn led to Guillemin's and his group's successful effort to isolate, sequence and synthesize a 44 amino acid peptide from a similar case (2). Rivier et al. isolated a 40 amino acid peptide from the Thorner case (3). Human pancreatic GRF has been shown to be identical with human hypothalamic GRF (56), its prohormone sequence deduced by recombinant technology (7,8), and its anatomical localization shown to correspond to the classical tuberoinfundibular distribution predicted from earlier lesion studies (29,57). The major new physiological insight gained from the availability of human GRF was that somatomedin-C (a peptide secreted under the influence of GH) had a direct inhibitory effect on the pituitary (58), and that it also stimulated somatostatin release (52). Thus, the physiological facts have been assembled to provide an accurate model of the hypothalamic-pituitary-somatomedin axis for regulation of GH (Fig. 1), complete except for our ignorance as to the factors, both neural and hormonal, that regulate the secretion of GRF. At the molecular level, it has been shown that GRF stimulates the transcription of the GH gene in the pituitary, and that this effect is blocked by somatostatin (59). Evidence for an ultrashort-loop feedback control of somatostatin has also been reported. Intraventricular injection of somatostatin brings about an increase in GH secretion (60), but this effect may be indirect (61).

What, then, are the insights into the mechanisms of GH regulation in man, and the nature of the defects of GH secretion regulation that explain the pathogenesis of acromegaly? Although somatotroph hyperplasia is the usual finding in ectopic GRF syndrome, adenomas have also been reported (54). However, screening of 177 acromegalic patients by Thorner, Frohman, and their colleagues has revealed an overall prevalence of elevated serum GRF levels in only 2, both of whom had previously been diagnosed as having ectopic GRF secretion (62). Hence, this syndrome is extremely rare and unlikely to be the cause of the disease very often. Although a relatively high proportion of patients with APUDomas have immunohistochemical evidence of GRF in their tumors (63-65), secretion rarely is sufficient to cause clinical evidence of acromegaly; detailed studies of GH secretion in such cases have not been carried out as yet.

The only fully established examples of hypersecretion of hypothalamic GRF as a cause of acromegaly are the handful of cases reported as being due to gangliocytomas of the hypothalamus in whom GRF has been identified in neurons (66). Both hyperplasia and adenomas have been described. Somatotroph hyperplasia also occurs in acromegaly associated with polyostotic fibrous dysplasia of bone (67; Rodman et al., in preparation). In Rodman's case, GH secretory responses, typical of acromegaly, were observed, i.e., paradoxical response to TRH and glucose ingestion.

Beside these rare examples of acromegaly unequivocally due to GRF excess, what is the role of GRF in the pathogenesis of the majority of cases? The use of GRF has not proven to be illuminating. Responses vary

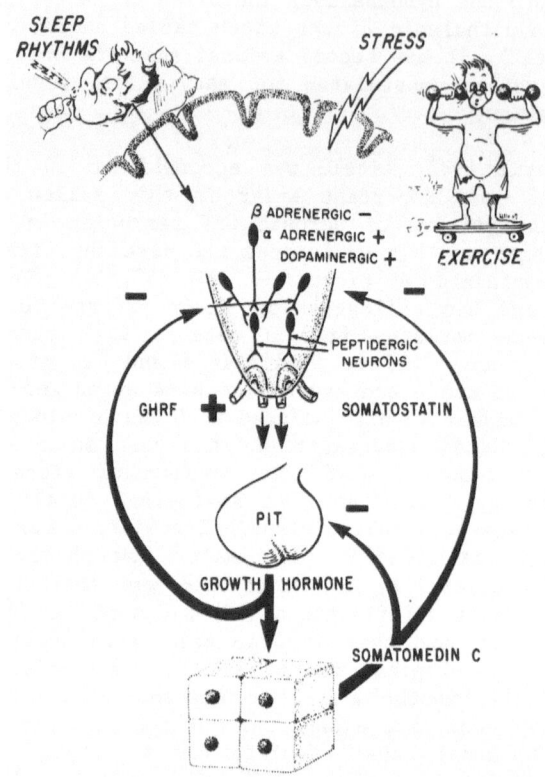

Fig. 1. Hypothalamic-growth hormone-somato-
medin-C axis. This diagram summarizes the
factors that regulate the secretion of
growth hormone. The growth hormone-releasing factor stimulates, and somatostatin
inhibits GH release. GH, acting on the
liver, regulates the production of somatomedin-C which exerts a feedback effect on
both the hypothalamus and the pituitary. At
the pituitary level, it inhibits the response to GHRF, whereas at the level of the
hypothalamus it stimulates the secretion of
somatostatin. In addition, GH exerts a
feedback effect on the hypothalamus by
stimulating the release of somatostatin.
The secretions of both GHRF and somatostatin
are regulated at the hypothalamic level by
neurotransmitters and neuropeptides. Only
the neurotransmitters are illustrated in
this diagram. Dopamine, and alpha-adrener-
gic impulses are stimulatory, while beta-
adrenergic impulses are inhibitory. Among
the neuropeptides which influence GH release, either directly by acting on the
pituitary, or indirectly through the hypothalamus, are the following: stimulatory,
enkephalin, GABA, beta-endorphin, galanin,
motilin CCK, VIP, vasopressin, TRH, neuro-
peptide Y. The principal central inhibitory
regulator is acetylcholine.

widely from exuberant reactions to flat responses (68,69), indicating that the tumors are functionally heterogeneous.

The typical paradoxical GH responses to TRH and to glucose administration observed in acromegaly can be brought about by chronic exposure to GRF as was shown in the case reported by Thorner et al. (55) which was due to ectopic GRF secretion, and which returned to normal following removal of the source of ectopic GRF secretion. This important finding indicates that the paradoxical responses (typical of more than half of acromegalics) can be induced by a GRF. For these reasons, one cannot completely exclude at this moment that some patients with acromegaly have primary hypersecretion of GRF.

We are left to consider the more classical arguments that favor an intrinsic pituitary disorder as the cause of acromegaly (70-73); hyperplasia is rarely the principal finding in acromegalic pituitaries (70-74), physiological responses following successful removal of a tumor usually return to normal (70-73), somatotrophs in the vicinity of the adenoma are usually normal and almost never hyperplastic (74), and somatotroph tumors often are associated with other types of pituitary cell abnormalities including lactotroph hyperplasia and, not infrequently, GH and PRL within the same cell (70-74).

Although the neuroendocrine approach to the study of the pathogenesis of acromegaly has been extensively pursued, has led to the elucidation of normal physiological functioning of this system, to the discovery of GRF, and to the identification of a few rare cases of GRF hypersecretion, it has not led us to the elucidation of the etiology of most forms of acromegalic disease. In my view, the etiology of most cases will more likely be found in the genetic analysis of clonal tumors that encode chromosomal growth factors, an insight we have gained from the study of oncogene pathogenesis of cancer (75).

ACKNOWLEDGMENTS

Work from the author's laboratory was supported by USPHS Grant No. 16684, Clinical Study Unit Grant No. 5 MO1 RR0005.

REFERENCES

1. Marie P. Sur deux cas d'acromegalie: hypertrophie singuliere, non congenitale, des extremites superieures, inferieures et cephalique. Rev Med 1886; 6:297-333.
2. Guillemin R, Brazeau P, Bohlen P, Esch F, Ling N, Wehrenberg WB. Growth hormone-releasing factor from a human pancreatic tumor that caused acromegaly. Science 1982; 218:585-7.
3. Rivier J, Spiess J, Thorner M, Vale W. Characterization of a growth hormone-releasing factor from a·human pancreatic islet tumor. Nature 1982; 300:276-8.
4. Brazeau P, Vale W, Burgus R, et al. Hypothalamic polypeptide that inhibits the secretion of immunoreactive pituitary growth hormone. Science 1973; 179:77-9.
5. Niall HD, Hogan ML, Tregear GW, Segre GV, Huang P, Friesen H. The chemistry of growth hormone and the lactogenic hormones. Recent Prog Horm Res 1973; 29:387-404.
6. Miller WL, Eberhardt NL. Structure and evolution of the growth hormone gene family. Endocr Rev 1983; 4:97-130.
7. Montminy MR, Goodman RH, Horovitch SJ, Habener J. Primary structure of the gene encoding rat preprosomatostatin. Proc Natl Acad Sci USA

1984; 81:3337-40.

8. Shen LP, Rutter WJ. Sequence of the human somatostatin I gene. Science 1984; 224:168-71.

9. Gubler U, Monoghan JJ, Lomedico PT, et al. Cloning and sequence analysis of cDNA for the precursor of human growth hormone-releasing factor, somatocrinin. Proc Natl Acad Sci USA 1983; 80:4311-4.

10. Mayo KE, Vale W, Rivier J, Rosenfeld MG, Evans RM. Expression-cloning and sequence of a cDNA encoding human growth hormone-releasing factor. Nature 1983; 306:86-8.

11. Reichlin S. Somatostatin. N Engl J Med 1983; 309:1495-501; 1556-63.

12. Reichlin S. Somatostatin. In: Krieger DT, Brownstein MJ, Martin JB, eds. Brain peptides. New York: John Wiley & Sons, 1983:711-52.

13. Martin JB. Hypothalamic regulation of growth hormone secretion. In: Black PMcL, Zervas NT, Ridgeway EC, Martin JB, eds. Secretory tumors of the pituitary gland. New York: Raven Press, 1983:109-34.

14. Terry LC. Neuropharmacologic regulation of anterior pituitary hormone secretion in man. In: Givens JR, ed. Hormone-secreting pituitary tumors. Chicago: Year Book Medical Publishers Inc., 1982:27-44.

15. Martin JB. Regulation of growth hormone secretion. In: Raiti S, Tolman RA, eds. Human growth hormone. New York: Plenum Medical Book Company, 1986:303-25.

16. Raiti S, Tolman RA, eds. Human growth hormone. New York: Plenum Medical Book Company, 1986.

17. Vale W, Vaughan J, Sawchenko P, et al. Chemical anatomical and physiological studies on human pancreatic and rat hypothalamic growth hormone-releasing factor. In: Raiti S, Tolman RA, eds. Human growth hormone. New York: Plenum Medical Book Company, 1986:325-36.

18. Brazeau P, Bohlen P, Esch F, et al. Growth hormone-releasing factor: isolation characterization, and physiology. In: Raiti S, Tolman RA, eds. New York: Plenum Medical Book Company, 1986:337-46.

19. Thorner MO, Evans WS, Vance ML, et al. Growth hormone-releasing factor. In: Raiti S, Tolman RA, eds. Human growth hormone. New York: Plenum Medical Book Company, 1986:361-72.

20. Sassolas G, Chatelain P. Acromegaly related to tumoral secretion of growth hormone-releasing factor. In: Raiti S, Tolman RA, eds. Human growth hormone. New York: Plenum Medical Book Company, 1986:373-86.

21. Reichlin S. Somatostatin: historical aspects. Scand J Gastroenterol 1986; 21(suppl 119):1-10.

22. Bloom SR, Greenwood C. Proceedings of somatostatin '85. Scand J Gastroenterol 1986; 21(suppl 119):1-274.

23. Thorner MO, Vance ML, Evans WS, et al. Physiological and clinical studies of GRF and GH. Recent Prog Horm Res 1986; 42:589-632.

24. Epelbaum J. Somatostatin in the central nervous system: physiology and pathological modifications. Prog Neurobiol 1986; 27:63-100.

25. Reichlin S. Growth and the hypothalamus. Endocrinology 1960; 67:760-73.

26. Deuben RR, Meites J. Stimulation of pituitary growth hormone release by a hypothalamic extract in vitro. Endocrinology 1964; 74:408-9.

27. Roth J, Glick SM, Yalow RS, Berson SA. Stimulation of pituitary growth hormone release by a hypothalamic extract in vitro. Science 1963; 140:987-8.

28. Reichlin S. The physiology of growth hormone regulation pre- and postimmunoassay eras. Metabolism 1973; 22:987-94.

29. Reichlin S. Regulation of somatotrophic hormone secretion. In: Knobil E, Sawyer WH, eds. Handbook of physiology. Sect 7, Vol IV, Part 2, 1974; 405-48.

30. Quabbe HJ, Schilling E, Helge H. Pattern of growth hormone secretion during a 24-hour fast in normal adults. J Clin Endocrinol Metab 1966; 26:1173-7.

31. Takahashi Y, Kipnis DM, Daughaday WH. Growth hormone secretion during sleep. J Clin Invest 1968; 47:2079-90.

32. Martin JB, Brazeau P, Tannenbaum GS, et al. Neuroendocrine organization of growth hormone regulation. In: Reichlin S, Baldessarini R, Martin JB, eds. The hypothalamus. New York: Raven Press, 1978: 329-57.

33. Casanueva FF, Villanueva L, Cabranaes JA, Cabezas-Cerrato J, Fernando-Cruz A. Cholinergic mediation of growth hormone secretion elicited by arginine, clonidine, and physical exercise in man. J Clin Endocrinol Metab 1984; 59:526-30.

34. Jacobowitz DM. CSN localization of stress-related neurochemicals. In: Chrousos GP, Loriaux DL, Gold PW, eds. Stress. New York: Plenum Press (in press).

35. Tannenbaum GS, Ling N. The interrelationship of growth hormone (GH)-releasing factor and somatostatin in generation of the ultradian rhythm of GH secretion. Endocrinology 1984; 115:1952-7.

36. Terry LC, Willoughby JO, Brazeau P, Martin JB, Patel Y. Antiserum to somatostatin prevents stress-induced inhibition of growth hormone secretion in the rat. Science 1976; 192:565-7.

37. Tannenbaum GS, Epelbaum J, Colle E, Brazeau P, Martin JB. Antiserum to somatostatin reverses starvation-induced inhibition of growth hormone but not insulin secretion. Endocrinology 1978; 102:1909-14.

38. Brown GM, Schalch DS, Reichlin S. Hypothalamic mediation of growth hormone and cortisol responses to psychological stress in the squirrel monkey. Endocrinology 1971; 89:694-703.

39. Lechan RM, Lin HD, Ling N, Jackson IMD, Jacobson S, Reichlin S. Immunocytochemical evidence that GRF(1-44)NH$_2$ is localized in the tuberoinfundibular system of rhesus monkey hypothalamus. Brain Res 1984; 309:55-61.

40. Reichlin S, Schalch DS. Growth hormone releasing factor. In: Gual C, ed. Progress in endocrinology. Amsterdam: Excerpta Medica Foundation, 1969:584-94.

41. Malacara JM, Valverde C, Reichlin S. Elevation of plasma radio-immunoassayable growth hormone in the rat induced by porcine hypothalamic extract. Endocrinology 1972; 91:1189-98.

42. Boyd AE III, Sanchez-Franco F, Spencer E, Patel YC, Jackson IMD, Reichlin S. Characterization of hypophysiotropic hormones in porcine hypothalamic extracts. Endocrinology 1978; 103:1075-83.

43. Veber DF, Bennett CD, Milkowski JD, Gal G, Denkewalter RG, Hirschman R. Synthesis of a proposed growth hormone releasing factor. Biochem Biophys Res Commun 1971; 45:235-9.

44. Krulich L, Dhariwal AP, McCann SM. Stimulatory and inhibitory effects of purified hypothalamic extracts on growth hormone release from rat pituitary in vitro. Endocrinology 1978; 83:783-90.

45. Brazeau P. Dr. Paul Brazeau's Pimstone prize acceptance speech. In: Raptis S, Rosenthal J, Gerich JE, eds. Second international symposium on somatostatin. Germany: Attempto Verlag, Tubingen GMBH, 1984:9-15.

46. Gottesman IS, Mandarino LJ, Gerich JE. Somatostatin. In: Cohen M, Foa P, eds. Special topics in endocrinology and metabolism; vol 4. New York: Alan R. Liss, 1982:177-243.

47. Krisch B. Hypothalamic and extrahypothalamic distribution of somato-statin-immunoreactive elements in the rat brain. Cell Tissue Res 1978; 195:499-513.

48. Bennett-Clarke C, Romagnano MA, Joseph SA. Distribution of somato-statin in the rat brain telencephalon and diencephalon. Brain Res 1980; 188:473-86.

49. Arimura A, Smith W, Schally A. Blockade of the stress-induced decrease in blood GH by anti-somatostatin serum in rats. Endocrinology 1976; 98:540-3.

50. Tannenbaum G. Evidence for autoregulation of growth hormone secre-

tion via the central nervous system. Endocrinology 1980; 107:2117-20.

51. Abe H, Molitch M, Van Wyk JJ, Underwood LE. Human growth hormone and somatomedin C suppress the spontaneous release of growth hormone in unanesthetized rats. Endocrinology 1983; 113:1319-24.
52. Berelowitz M, Szabo M, Frohman LA, Firestone S, Chu L, Hintz RL. Somatomedin-C mediates growth hormone negative feedback by effects on both the hypothalamus and the pituitary. Science 1981; 212(4500): 1279-81.
53. Frohman LA, Szabo M, Berelowitz M, Stachura ME. Partial purification and characterization of a peptide with growth hormone-releasing activity from extrapituitary tumors in patients with acromegaly. J Clin Invest 1980; 65:43-54.
54. Frohman LA, Thominet JL, Szabo M. Ectopic growth hormone-releasing factor syndromes. In: Raiti S, Tolman RA, eds. Human growth hormone. New York: Plenum Medical Book Company, 1986; 347-61.
55. Thorner MO, Perryman RL, Cronin MJ, et al. Somatotroph hyperplasia. Successful treatment of acromegaly by removal of a pancreatic islet tumor secreting a growth hormone-releasing factor. J Clin Invest 1982; 70:965-77.
56. Bohlen P, Brazeau P, Bloch B, Ling N, Gaillard R, Guillemin R. Human hypothalamic growth hormone releasing factor (GRF): evidence for two forms identical to tumor derived GRF-44-NH2 and GRF-40. Biochem Biophys Res Commun 1983; 114:930-6.
57. Merchenthaler I, Vigh S, Schally AV, Petrusz P. Immunocytochemical localization of growth hormone-releasing factor in the rat hypothalamus. Endocrinology 1984; 114:1082-5.
58. Brazeau P, Guillemin R, Ling N, Van Wyk J, Humbel R. Inhibition par les somatomedines de la secretion de l'hormone de croissance stimulee par le facteur hypothalamique somatocrinine (GRF) ou le peptide de synthese hpGRF. C R Seances Acad Sci (III) 1982; 295:651-4.
59. Barinaga M, Yamanoto G, Rivier C, Evans R, Rosenfeld MG. Transcriptional regulation of growth hormone gene expression by growth hormone-releasing factor. Nature 1983; 306:84-5.
60. Lumpkin MD, Negro-Vilar A, McCann SM. Paradoxical elevation of growth hormone by intraventricular somatostatin; possible ultrashort-loop feedback. Science 1981; 211:1072-4.
61. Tannenbaum GS, Patel YC. On the fate of centrally administered somatostatin in the rat: massive hypersomatostatinemia resulting from leakage into the peripheral circulation has effects on growth hormone secretion and glucoregulation. Endocrinology 1986; 118: 2137-43.
62. Thorner MO, Frohman LA, Leong DA, et al. Extrahypothalamic growth hormone-releasing factor (GRF) secretion is a rare cause of acromegaly: plasma GRF levels in 177 acromegalic patients. J Clin Endocrinol Metab 1984; 59:846-9.
63. Dayal Y, Lin HD, Tallbert K, Reichlin S, Delellis RA, Wolfe HJ. Immunocytochemical demonstration of growth hormone releasing factor in gastrointestinal and pancreatic endocrine tumors. Am J CLin Pathol 1985; 85:13-20.
64. Bostwick DG, Quan R, Hoffman AR, Webber RJ, Chang JK, Nensch KG. Growth hormone-releasing factor immunoreactivity in human endocrine tumors. Am J Pathol 1984; 117:167-70.
65. Asa SL, Kovacs K, Thorner MO, Leong DA, Rivier J, Vale W. Immunohistological localization of growth hormone releasing hormone in human tumors. J Clin Endocrinol Metab 1985; 60:423-27.
66. Asa SL, Scheithauer BW, Bilbao JM, et al. A case for hypothalamic acromegaly: a clinicopathological study of six patients with hypothalamic gangliocytomas producing growth hormone-releasing factor. J Clin Endocrinol Metab 1984; 58:796-803.
67. Kovacs K, Horvath E, Thorner MO, Rogal AS. Mammosomatotroph hyper-

plasia associated with acromegaly and hyperprolactinemia in a patient with the McCune-Albright syndrome. A histologic, immunocytologic and ultrastructural study of the surgically-removed adenohypophysis. Virchows Arch [A] 1984; 403:77-86.

68. Shibasaki T, Shizume K, Masuda A, et al. Studies on the response of growth hormone (GH) secretion to GH-releasing hormone, thyrotropin-releasing hormone, gonadotropin-releasing hormone, and somatostatin in acromegaly. J Clin Endocrinol Metab 1986; 63:167-73.

69. Gelato MC, Merriam GR, Vance ML, et al. Effects of growth hormone-releasing factor on growth hormone secretion in acromegaly. J Clin Endocrinol Metab 1985; 60:251-7.

70. Melmed S, Braunstein GD, Horvath E, Ezrin C, Kovacs K. Pathophysiology of acromegaly. Endocr Rev 1983; 4:271-90.

71. Reichlin S, Molitch M. Neuroendocrine aspect of pituitary adenoma. In: Camanni P, Muller EE, eds. Pituitary hyperfunction. New York: Raven Press, 1984; 47-70.

72. Kobberling J, Mayer G. A CNS versus a pituitary component in the overproduction of growth hormone. In: Cammani P, Muller EE, eds. New York: Raven Press, 1984; 209-14.

73. Molitch ME. Growth hormone secretory states. In: Raiti S, Tolman RA, eds. Human growth hormone. New York: Plenum Medical Book Company, 1986:29-50.

74. Saeger W. Pathology of the pituitary gland. In: Belchetz PE, ed. Management of pituitary disease. New York: John Wiley & Sons, 1984; 253-89.

75. Varmush H, Bishop JM, eds. Cancer surveys (vol 5). 1986:153-434.

2

HUMAN GROWTH HORMONE GENE REGULATION IN SOMATOTROPH

CELL CULTURES

Shlomo Melmed, Shunichi Yamashita, and Sara Pixley

Department of Medicine
Division of Endocrinology and Metabolism
Cedars-Sinai Medical Center—UCLA School of Medicine
Los Angeles, CA

INTRODUCTION

The somatotroph tumor cell is an ideal model for studying the chain of polypeptide gene expression from gene structure through transcription, processing, translation, protein structure and secretion. Studies in rat GH cells are examples of how these studies have led to important insights into the biology of pituitary tumors (1).

Because of the limited amount of functional tissue available, relatively scant progress has been made in studying gene regulation in human somatotroph cells. Regulation of in vitro human growth hormone (GH) secretion and synthesis will be reviewed. Recently, the availability of cDNA probes have also enabled us to measure human GH mRNA regulation in phenotypic somatotroph cells. The results of these experiments will also be reported.

CELL GROWTH CHARACTERISTICS

Human pituitary tumor cells usually grow well in culture with a plating efficiency of 20-30%. Typically, they appear as rounded or hexagonal colony-forming cells with well-defined nuclei and nucleoli. The degree of initial adherence of the cells to the plates appears to depend on the concentration of serum in the medium (2).

Nevertheless, fibroblast overgrowth invariably occurs by 2 weeks. This has prevented the successful cloning of a functional human GH-secreting cell line. The paucity of long-term functional cell cultures has hampered the application of molecular techniques to studying human GH gene expression and regulation in phenotypic somatotroph cells.

IN VITRO GH EXPRESSION BY SOMATOTROPH CELLS

The first successful serial propagation of heterogenous functional human pituitary tumor cells secreting somatotropin was reported in 1959 by Thompson et al. (3). Using the tibial epiphyseal width bioassay, they detected GH in the medium of cultured pituitary cells. In 1962, Reusser

17

et al. (4), using both fluorescin labeled specific human GH antibody and a modified Ouchterlony technique, failed to demonstrate the in vitro production of somatotropin by human anterior pituitary cells. Immunoassay of in vitro GH by a complement fixation method was first reported by Brauman in 1964, when they measured GH production by cultured fetal pituitary cells (5).

Kohler and colleagues (6) were the first to systematically study in vitro GH secretion by primary human pituitary explants and dispersed monolayers. They used specific RIAs to measure hormone secretion and showed that adenomas from patients with acromegaly secreted GH at higher levels and for at least twice as long as cultured normal human pituitary tissue. They also detected low levels of TSH and LH secretion in some of their cultures of acromegalic adenomas, providing the first direct in vitro evidence for the concepts of "mixed" tumors. These workers also established rigid criteria for confirming the viability of hormone-secreting adenoma cell cultures. These included the observation that lethal heat shock completely inhibited GH accumulation in the medium, cycloheximide (1 µg/ml) inhibited incorporation of labeled amino acids into protein and also blocked GH secretion within 48 hours. Furthermore, the amount of GH secreted in vitro was always more than double that extracted from an equivalent amount of pituitary tissue after surgery. Since then, several laboratories have measured in vitro GH secretion by GH cell pituitary adenomas and attempted to correlate in vitro secretory characteristics with clinical and pathological features of acromegaly.

The first systematic in vitro study of acromegalic pituitary cell cultures was reported by Batzdorf et al. in 1971 (7). These workers showed that high GH levels were secreted in vitro by all of 6 adenomas removed from acromegalic patients. Interestingly, 2 of these 6 acromegalic patients were diagnosed as harboring a "mixed" adenoma and a chromophobe adenoma respectively. In contrast, in vitro GH secretion was undetectable in 6 of 8 pituitary tumor cell cultures derived from patients with hypopituitarism.

GH SECRETION

GH secretion by monolayer cultures of both normal and neoplastic somatotroph cells is usually sustained for 2-3 weeks (8). The GH secretory rates in normal pituitary tissue and pituitary cells derived from somatotroph adenomas were similar at 1 and 4 weeks (8).

De novo GH synthesis in vitro was shown by Ishibashi (9) to be continuous for at least 48 hours. Adenoma cells from acromegalic patients were incubated with labeled leucine and incorporation into immunoprecipitable GH was linear under their conditions.

NORTHERN ANALYSIS OF HUMAN PITUITARY GH mRNA

We have studied the expression of GH mRNA transcripts in phenotypic somatotroph cells (10). Total RNA was extracted from a GH-cell adenoma removed at surgery. The RNA was denatured, electrophoresed on 1.0% agarose gel in 6% formaldehyde and transferred to Zeta probe nylon membrane paper. The predominant GH mRNA species identified by hybridization with ^{32}p-GH cDNA was about 1 kb in size (Fig. 1) (10). This is similar to the previously reported size of the GH mRNA in transfected mouse fibroblasts (11), as well as the size of ectopic GH mRNA extracted from a pancreatic tumor (12).

IN SITU MESSENGER RIBONUCLEIC ACID HYBRIDIZATION

Because of the difficulty in obtaining sufficient human tissue for gene expression studies, we have used an in situ mRNA hybridization technique to study GH gene expression at the level of the single cell (13). A radiolabeled human growth hormone cDNA probe kindly provided by Dr. John Baxter (14) was used to identify growth hormone mRNA sequences in pituitary adenoma cells derived from a patient with a growth hormone-secreting pituitary adenoma. Figure 2 shows how the tritiated growth hormone cDNA probe can be used to identify and visualize growth hormone mRNA sequences by in situ hybridization (15). Since human GH specific mRNA can be localized in single cells, this technique may therefore overcome some of the limitations of tissue availability in studying human GH gene regulation.

STIMULATORY REGULATION OF GH EXPRESSION

Growth Hormone-Releasing Hormone (GHRH)

The elucidation of the structure of growth hormone-releasing hormone (GHRH) (16,17) was followed by in vitro testing of the various GH-releasing peptides on human GH-cell tumor tissue. Ectopic GHRH extracted from an hepatic carcinoid tumor was shown to directly stimulate the release of GH during a 4-hour incubation of human GH-secreting adenoma cells (18). These studies showed the direct action of GHRH on GH-adenoma cell function and implicated GHRH in the pathogenesis of the increased secretion of GH by these tumors. Furthermore, the response to GHRH suggested the presence of GHRH receptors on the adenomatous somatotroph cell.

Since then, the stimulatory effects of GHRH on in vitro GH secretion have been studied by several groups (10,19-21). Maximal (200%) stimulation of GH release by monolayers of tumor cells during 4 hours was

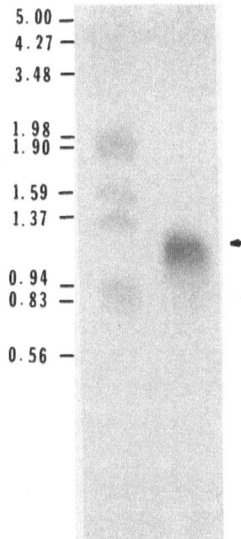

Fig. 1. Northern analysis of human GH mRNA in acromegalic tumor tissue. Arrow = 1 kb. (From reference 10, with permission.)

achieved with 10 nM human GHRH 1-40. This stimulation was blocked by somatostatin (SRIF) (10 nM). Interestingly, long-term culture of tumor cells for 4 days in the presence of dexamethasone (5 nM) resulted in a synergistic response to an acute exposure to GHRH, with GH release increasing tenfold.

Ishibashi et al. (20), using GHRH 1-44, showed that the stimulation of GH was linear for 20 hours. Once again, maximal stimulation with 10 nM peptide resulted in a doubling of GH secretion. The effects of GHRH were blocked by SRIF and dopamine and were also abolished in the absence of added exogenous calcium. Using 100 nM GHRH 1-44, Ceda et al. (21) showed a maximal doubling of the 4-hour release of GH. During 24-hour incubation, D-Ala^2-GHRH$_{1-29}$ also doubled GH release. A purified somatomedin-C preparation inhibited both basal as well as GHRH-stimulated GH release from 3 of 4 GH-cell adenomas cultured in vitro. We have also recently shown that GHRH stimulates the GH mRNA content in acromegalic tumor cells (10).

Vasoactive Intestinal Polypeptide (VIP)

Vasoactive intestinal polypeptide (VIP), originally isolated from porcine duodenum, has been found in hypothalamic nerve endings and high levels of the peptide have been measured in hypophyseal portal blood (22). VIP (50 nM) was shown to acutely stimulate the release of GH by superfused GH-secreting pituitary adenoma cells (23,24). Dopamine, bromocriptine and somatostatin blocked the stimulatory effect of VIP on GH release. Interestingly, VIP shares homologous amino acid sequences with growth hormone-releasing hormone, especially rat GHRH. The observed stimulatory effects of VIP on GH release by acromegalic tumor tissue preceded the isolation and full characterization of authentic GHRH.

Thyrotropin-Releasing Hormone (TRH)

TRH stimulated the secretion of GH by adenomatous pituitary cells in culture (25). Maximal (180-240%) stimulation was achieved with 10 nM TRH (25,9), and this was blocked by simultaneous treatment of the cells with

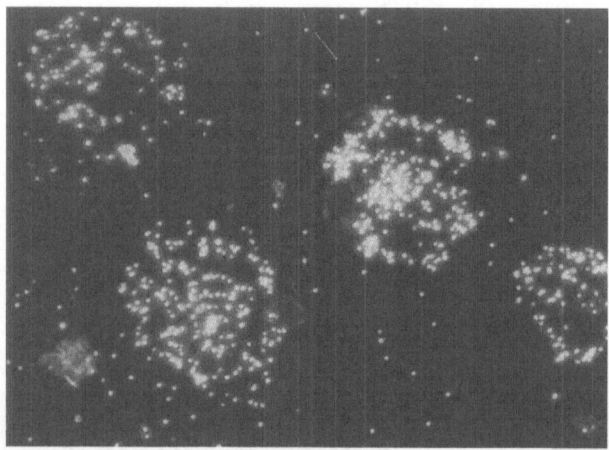

Fig. 2. In situ hybridization of GH mRNA in cultured somatotroph adenoma cells. (From reference 15, with permission.)

dopamine. Normal nontumorous somatotroph cells were unaffected by TRH (9), and in one study GH release was actually inhibited by TRH (26). These data may explain, at least in part, the aberrant response of GH to TRH in acromegalic patients.

Corticotropin-Releasing Factor (CRF)

Ovine corticotropin-releasing factor (CRF) was shown to stimulate acute GH release by 3 out of 7 GH-cell adenomas grown in monolayer culture (28). Maximal stimulation of GH release by about 60% was achieved with 100 nM CRF. Interestingly, this stimulatory effect of CRF was partially blocked by hydrocortisone (1 μM). These results suggest a direct effect of CRF and hydrocortisone on the tumorous somatotroph. The significance of these findings and their extrapolation to the clinical situation is presently unclear.

INHIBITORY REGULATION OF GH EXPRESSION

Dopamine

Adrenergic and dopaminergic agonists were shown to directly inhibit in vivo GH secretion by normal cultured pituitary cells (8,9,25,26,28, 29,30). As dopamine is a powerful in vivo stimulator of normal GH secretion in man, these observations indicate that dopamine probably mediates GH secretion at a suprapituitary level.

Somatostatin (SRIF)

SRIF has been shown to acutely inhibit basal and stimulated GH secretion in vitro from both tumorous and normal human pituitary cell cultures (9,19,20,25,26). Furthermore, specific binding sites for SRIF have been described on adenoma cell membranes (31-33).

Insulin-Like Growth Factor-I (IGF-I)

Most of the growth-promoting actions of pituitary GH appear to be mediated by hepatic somatomedin-C, insulin-like growth factor I (IGF-I) (34). IGF-I has been implicated in a negative feedback inhibition of GH secretion at the level of both the pituitary (35-39) and hypothalamus (40-41). The inhibition of rat GH gene expression by IGF-I appears to occur at the level of GH gene transcription (42). A similar negative feedback loop may also exist in humans. Ceda et al. (21) showed that a partially purified somatomedin-C preparation inhibited the release of GH by human pituitary cell cultures. They also demonstrated that human pituitary cells contain specific binding sites for IGF-I. We have extended these studies by characterizing the suppression of human GH secretion and GH mRNA levels in human somatotropinoma cells treated with a purified recombinant human IGF-I analog, Thr-59-IGF-I (10).

IGF-I (13 nM) inhibited GH secretion by somatotropinoma cells incubated in serum-free medium to 65% of that in cultures of untreated cells (P < 0.01). The 50% stimulation of GH secretion induced by GHRH (1 nM) was blocked by simultaneous exposure of the cells to IGF-I (13 nM). GH secretion in the presence of GHRH and IGF-I was not different from that in untreated cells. (10).

To further characterize the effects of IGF-I on GHRH-induced GH secretion, cells from 3 different tumors were treated with GHRH (10 nM) with or without IGF-I (6.5 nM). During 48 hours, GHRH stimulated the accumulation of GH in the medium, and IGF-I blocked this stimulation in

Table 1. Summary of the current
known regulators of human
GH gene expression in
acromegalic cell cultures.

STIMULATORY	SECRETION	mRNA LEVELS
GHRH	▲	▲
VIP	▲	
TRH	▲	
CRF	▲	
INHIBITORY		
SRIF	▼	
IGF-I	▼	▼
DOPAMINE	▼	

each tumor. In each tumor culture, the effects of IGF-I were prevented by addition of alpha-IR3, a specific antibody to the IGF-I receptor (43).

Effects Of IGF-I On mRNA Levels

Relative levels of GH mRNA sequences were measured in adenoma cells by dot blot hybridization with nick-translated GH cDNA. Figure 3 shows the effect of varying IGF-I doses on GH mRNA levels. Maximal inhibition of GH mRNA (40% of basal value) was seen after treatment with 6.5 nM IGF-I ($P < 0.01$). Alpha-IR3 alone (0.1 g/ml) did not alter the levels of GH, but did reverse the suppression of GH mRNA caused by IGF-I (6.5 nM). GHRH (10 nM) stimulated GH mRNA levels by about 35% ($P < 0.05$), and this increase was abolished by simultaneous exposure of the cells to IGF-I (6.5 nM) (10). These data demonstrate, for the first time, the regulation of human GH mRNA in phenotypic human somatotroph cells.

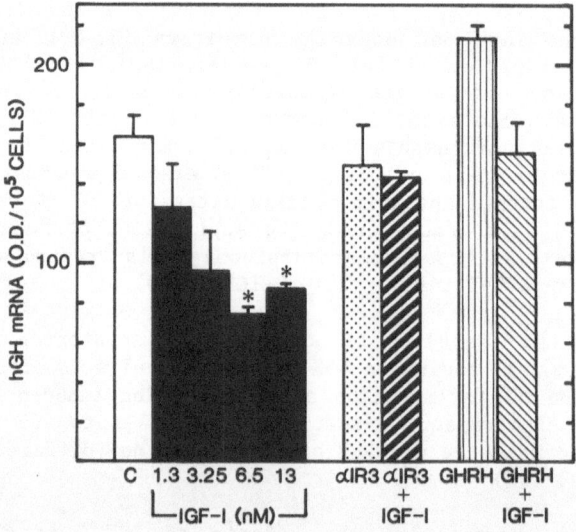

Fig. 3. Regulation of GH mRNA in cultured somatotroph adenoma cells. (From reference 10, with permission.)

REFERENCES

1. Tashjian AH. Colonal strains of hormone-producing cells. In: Jakoby WB, Pasten I, eds. Methods in enzymology. New York: Academic Press, 1979.
2. Melmed S, Odenheimer D, Carlson H, Hershman J. Establishment of functional human pituitary tumor cell cultures. In Vitro 1982; 18:35.
3. Thompson KW, Vincent MM, Jensen FC, Price RT, Schapiro E. Production of hormones by human anterior pituitary cells in serial culture. Proc Soc 1959; 102:403.
4. Reusser F, Smith CG, Smith CL. Investigations on somatrotropin production of human anterior pituitary cells in tissue culture. Proc Soc Exp Biol Med 1962; 109:375.
5. Brauman J, Brauman H, Pasteels JL. Immunoassay of growth hormone in cultures of human hypophysis by the method of complement fixation. Nature 1964; 202:1116.
6. Kohler PO, Bridson WE, Rayford PL, Kohler SE. Hormone production by human pituitary adenomas in culture. Metabolism 1969; 18:782.
7. Batzdorf U, Gold V, Matthews N, Brown J. Human growth hormone in cultures of human pituitary tumors. J Neurosurg 1971; 34:741.
8. Tallo D, Malarkey WB. Adrenergic and dopaminergic modulation of growth hormone and prolactin secretion in normal and tumor-bearing human pituitaries in monolayer culture. J Clin Endocrinol Metab 1981; 53:1278.
9. Ishibashi M, Yamaji T. Direct effects of catecholamines, thyrotropin-releasing hormone, and somatostatin on growth hormone and prolactin secretion from adenomatous and nonadenomatous human pituitary cells in culture. J Clin Invest 1984; 73:66.
10. Yamashita S, Weiss M, Melmed S. Insulin-like growth factor I regulates growth hormone secretion and messenger ribonucleic acid levels in human pituitary tumor cells. J Clin Endocrinol Metab 1986; 63(3):730-5.
11. Robins DM, Paek I, Seeburg PH, Axel R. Regulated expression of human growth hormone genes in mouse cells. Cell 1982; 29:623.
12. Melmed S, Ezrin C, Kovacs K, Goodman RS, Frohman LA. Acromegaly due to secretion of growth hormone by an ectopic pancreatic islet cell tumor. N Engl J Med 1985; 312:9.
13. Pixley S, Geiger M, Melmed S. Growth hormone mRNA regulation: in situ hybridization using biotynylated growth hormone cDNA. Clin Res 1986; 34:25A.
14. Martial JA, Hallewell RA, Baxter JD, Goodman HM. Human growth hormone: cDNA cloning and expression in bacteria. Science 1979; 205:602.
15. Melmed S, Braunstein GD, Chang JR, Becker DP. Pituitary tumors secreting growth hormone and prolactin. Ann Intern Med 1986; 105(2): 238-53.
16. Thorner MD, Perryman RL, Cronin MJ, et al. Acromegaly with somatotroph hyperplasia; successful treatment by resection of a pancreatic tumor secreting GRF. J Clin Invest 1982; 70:965.
17. Guillemin RR, Brazeau P, Bohlen P, Esch F, Ling N, Wehrenberg WB. GRF from a human pancreatic tumor that caused acromegaly. Science 1982; 218:585.
18. Webb CB, Thominet JL, Frohman LA. Ectopic growth hormone releasing factor stimulates growth hormone release from human somatotroph adenomas in vitro. J Clin Endocrinol Metab 1983; 56:417.
19. Lamberts SWJ, Verleun T, Oosterom R. The interrelationship between the effects of somatostatin and human pancreatic growth hormone-releasing factor on growth hormone release by cultured pituitary tumor cells from patients with acromegaly. J Clin Endocrinol Metab 1984; 58:250.

20. Ishibashi M, Yamaji T. Effects of hypophysiotropic factors on growth hormone and prolactin secretion from somatotroph adenomas in culture. J Clin Endocrinol Metab 1985; 60:985.

21. Ceda GP, Hoffman AR, Silverberg GD, Wilson DM, Rosenfeld RG. Regulation of growth hormone release from cultured human pituitary adenomas by somatomedins and insulin. J Clin Endocrinol Metab 1985; 60:1204.

22. Said SI, Porter JC. Vasoactive intestinal polypeptide; release into hypophyseal portal blood. Life Sci 1979; 24:227.

23. Matsushita N, Kato Y, Katakami H, Shimatsu A, Yanaihara N, Imura H. Stimulation of growth hormone release by vasoactive intestinal polypeptide from human pituitary adenomas in vitro. J Clin Endocrinol Metab 1981; 53:1297.

24. Chihara K, Iwasaki J, Minamitani N, et al. Effect of vasoactive intestinal polypeptide on growth hormone secretion in perifused acromegalic pituitary adenoma tissues. J Clin Endocrinol Metab 1982; 54:773.

25. Adams EF, Brajkovich IE, Mashiter K. Hormone secretion by dispersed cell cultures of human pituitary adenomas: effects of theophylline, thyrotropin-releasing hormone, somatostatin, and 2-bromo-a-ergocryptine. J Clin Endocrinol Metab 1979; 49:120.

26. Marcovitz S, Goodyer CG, Guyda H, Gardiner RJ, Hardy J. Comparative study of human feta, normal adult, and somatotropic adenoma pituitary function in tissue culture. J Clin Endocrinol Metab 1982; 54:6.

27. Ishibashi M, Hara T, Tagusagawa Y, et al. Effects of ovine corticotrophin-releasing factor and hydrocortisone on growth hormone secretion by pituitary adenoma cells of acromegaly in culture. Acta Endocrinol (Copenh) 1984; 106:443.

28. Spada A, Sartorio A, Bassetti M, Pezzo G, Giannattasio G. In vitro effect of dopamine on growth hormone (GH) release from human GH secreting pituitary adenomas. J Clin Endocrinol Metab 1982; 55:734.

29. Ishibashi M, Yamaji T. Effect of thyrotropin-releasing hormone and bromoergocriptine on growth hormone and prolactin secretion in perfused pituitary adenoma tissues of acromegaly. J Clin Endocrinol Metab 1978; 47:1251.

30. Peillon F, Cesselin F, Bression D, et al. In vitro effect of dopamine and L-dopa on prolactin and growth hormone release from human pituitary adenomas. J Clin Endocrinol Metab 1979; 49:737.

31. Reubi JC, Landolt AM. High density of somatostatin receptors in pituitary tumors from acromegalic patients. J Clin Endocrinol Metab 1984; 59:1148.

32. Moyse E, Dafniet ML, Epelbaum J, et al. Somatostatin receptors in human growth hormone and prolactin-secreting pituitary adenomas. J Clin Endocrinol Metab 1985; 61:98.

33. Ikuyama S, Nawata H, Kato K, Karashima T, Ibayashi H, Nakagaki H. Specific somatostatin receptors on human pituitary adenoma cell membranes. J Clin Endocrinol Metab 1985; 61:666.

34. Froesch ER, Schmidt CH, Schwander J, Zapf J. Actions of insulin-like growth factors. Annu Rev Physiol 1985; 47:443.

35. Berelowitz M, Szabo M, Frohman LA, Firestone S, Chu L, Hintz RL. Somatomedin-C mediates growth hormone negative feedback by effects on both the hypothalamus and the pituitary. Science 1982; 212:1279.

36. Brazeau P, Guillemin R, Ling N, Van Wyk JJ, Humbel R. Inhibition by somatomedins of growth hormone secretion stimulated by hypothalamic growth hormone releasing factor (somatocrinin, GRF) on the synthetic peptide hpGRF. Computs Rende Acad Sci (Paris) 1982; 295:651.

37. Goodyer CC, De Stephan L, Guyda HJ, Posner BI. Effects of insulin-like growth factor on adult male rat pituitary function in tissue culture. Endocrinology 1984; 115:1568.

38. Yamashita S, Melmed S. Insulin-like growth factor I action on rat anterior pituitary cells: suppression of growth hormone secretion and messenger ribonucleic acid levels. Endocrinology 1986; 118:176.

39. Melmed S, Yamashita S. Insulin-like growth factor I action on hypothyroid rat anterior pituitary cells: suppression of T3-induced GH secretion and mRNA levels. Endocrinology 1986; 118:1483.
40. Abe H, Molitch ME, Van Wyk JJ, Underwood LE. Human growth hormone and somatomedin-C suppress the spontaneous release of growth hormone in unanesthetized rats. Endocrinology 1983; 113:1319.
41. Tannenbaum GS, Guyda HJ, Posner BI. Insulin-like growth factors: a role in growth hormone negative feedback and body weight regulation via brain. Science 1983; 220:77.
42. Yamashita S, Melmed S. Insulin-like growth factor I regulation of growth hormone gene transcription. Clin Res 1986; 34:435A.
43. Kul FC, Jacobs S, Su YF, Svoboda ME, Van Wyk JJ, Cuatrecasas P. Monoclonal antibodies to receptors for insulin and somatomedin C. J Biol Chem 1983; 258:6561.

3

DETECTION OF THE MULTIPLE FORMS OF HUMAN GROWTH HORMONE

U. J. Lewis, R. N. P. Singh, L. J. Lewis, and N. Abadi

The Whittier Institute for Diabetes and Endocrinology
9894 Genesee Avenue
La Jolla, CA

It was not until the introduction of gel electrophoresis that the heterogeneity of preparations of growth hormone was uncovered. Prior to that time, moving boundary electrophoresis in the Tiselius apparatus was the most discriminating method for resolution of protein mixtures (1). A comparison of the resolving power of the Tiselius method with that of gel electrophoresis for separating components of bovine growth hormone can be found in an early paper by Lewis (2). The moving boundary technique only suggested heterogeneity by the nonsymmetry of the protein peak whereas by the polyacrylamide gel disc electrophoresis method of Ornstein and Davis (3,4), three well-separated components were detected. Before the use of polyacrylamide, starch gel was used as the supporting medium. Starch gel was difficult to work with but excellent resolution of components of human GH could be demonstrated as shown by Wallace and Ferguson (5). With the introduction of disc electrophoresis with its simple polyacrylamide gel formation technique, the reports dealing with the heterogeneity of preparations of pituitary proteins multiplied enormously. The technique owes its resolving power to separations on the basis of both charge and molecular size. The method is also versatile with regard to the ability to choose a wide range of pH values for the electrophoresis (6).

Separation of proteins according to size was enhanced with the introduction of the use of sodium dodecyl sulfate during the gel electrophoresis. The detergent imparted a similar negative charge to proteins in a mixture so that migration rate was influenced principally by molecular sieving by the gel (7). Another major advance in the analysis of protein mixtures was isoelectric focusing (8). With this technique, a pH gradient is established in polyacrylamide gel during electrophoresis by use of ampholytes of varying pK values. When a mixture of proteins is placed in such a gradient, each component will seek its isoelectric point. The resolving power of this technique is evidenced by the resulting electrophoretic pattern which often presents an imposing array of bands. For example, if a protein readily deamidates, isoelectric focusing can distinguish the charge difference between a deamidated asparagine and a deamidated glutamine. Neighboring amino acids can also influence the ionization of a charged amino acid. This technique of separating charge isomers can be combined with electrophoresis in sodium dodecyl sulfate to give a two-dimensional analysis which at this time is probably the most discriminating method for examining mixtures of proteins.

We utilized all the techniques referred to above for detection and isolation of the multiple forms of growth hormone (GH). Often, the most difficult part of the work was identifying a particular electrophoretic band as a growth hormone. This was accomplished by cutting the band from the gel and eluting the material for analysis by radioimmunoassay. We now realize that minor forms of the hormone were overlooked in the past simply because they could not be visualized by standard staining techniques. With the introduction of immunoblotting on nitrocellulose paper, the task of identifying a component in an electrophoretic pattern has been greatly simplified (9). In addition, the development of specific antisera to the various GHs has permitted rapid visualization of multiple forms of the peptide in a whole pituitary extract, or in fractions of that extract generated by column chromatography. This battery of techniques will allow us to address important questions regarding the production of various forms of GH by the pituitary gland.

PHYSICOCHEMICAL PROPERTIES

A summary of the various forms of GH identified so far is given in Table 1.

The major 22K-dalton form (GH_{22K}) accounts for approximately 60% of the growth hormone in the pituitary gland. The amino acid sequence was determined by direct sequencing studies (10) and confirmed by elucidation of the structure of the gene (11). The hormone has an acidic isoelectric

Table 1. Multiple forms of GH detected in
pituitary extracts.

Form	Description	% in Pituitary
GH_{22K}	Major form	60
Acidic GH	Blocked NH_2 terminus	5-10
Desamido and/or phosphorylated GH	More acidic than "acidic GH"	10-15
GH_{20K}	Alternative mRNA processing	15
Disulfide dimer	Interchain S-S	5
Stable dimer	S-S or another linkage	5
Alkaline (slow) forms	Sulfone and sulfoxide of methionine	--
GH_{24K}	Glycosylated ?	1-5
GH_{27K}	Intron D variant	1-5
GH_{1-43}	Insulin potentiator	--
5-10K fragment	Diabetogenic peptide	--

point, pH 4.9, and contains two disulfide bridges. There is no consensus sequence for asparagine-linked glycosylation.

The GH_{22K} exists as an interchain disulfide dimer. The linkage of the two chains is thought to be an antiparallel arrangement since no unusual disulfide peptides were found by peptide mapping of tryptic digests (12). The disulfide dimer of human placental lactogen was shown (13) to have this same structure, with the disulfide bridge being at the COOH-terminal disulfide. The precise isoelectric point of the GH dimer is not currently known. However, during chromatography on DEAE-cellulose, the dimer elutes after the desamido forms indicating a more acidic peptide.

The 20K dalton variant (GH_{20K}) results from an alternative splicing procedure for the mRNA of GH_{22K} (14). During the removal of the nucleotide sequence corresponding to intron B, an additional 45 nucleotides are also eliminated so that after splicing, the mRNA is translated into an GH with 15 fewer residues (15). The GH_{20K} has a more alkaline isoelectric point than GH_{22K}, approximately pH 5.8. The variant migrates behind GH_{22K} in disc electrophoresis (pH 7.8 or 10) and elutes from DEAE-cellulose ahead of the major form (16). A disulfide dimer of GH_{20K} has not been isolated but we have observed an immunoreactive 40K component in pituitary fractions during SDS electrophoresis which may in fact be such a dimer. A consensus sequence for glycosylation was not introduced into the GH_{20K} structure during the alternative splicing.

A slightly more acidic form of GH is noted in disc electrophoresis patterns (17) of the hormone. Baumann et al. (18) have also noted the form in serum. Our studies indicated a blocked amino terminus which would explain the change in charge; however, the blocking group has not yet been identified. This form is easily detected by isoelectric focusing since it clearly migrates between the major GH_{22K} and what is thought to be the first deamidated form of the major GH_{22K}.

A common form of GH_{22K} that is seen in even highly purified preparations of the hormone is an acidic modification that migrates well ahead of the major form during disc electrophoresis at an alkaline pH (19). The form is also readily seen by isoelectric focusing. Since concentration of the form increases when GH_{22K} is permitted to stand in an alkaline solution, and because it comigrates with GH_{22K} at pH 4 where ionization of the -COOH group would be suppressed, the form is thought to be a deamidated modification. Although it is generally agreed that the desamido form is produced by alkali, it is not certain whether the acidic form seen in extracts of fresh pituitary glands (20) is a deamidated form of the peptide. Liberti et al. (21) demonstrated phosphorylated ovine GH in their preparations of the hormone and Oetting et al. (22) showed that prolactin is readily phosphorylated in the rat pituitary gland. Using isoelectric focusing, at least 6 acidic components have been seen in purified preparations of GH. These were considered to be minor desamido forms of the hormone but, in addition, one or more forms may be phosphorylated peptides.

Two slower migrating alkaline forms of GH have been detected in many preparations of GH by disc electrophoresis (17). We now think that these are artifacts produced by oxidation of methionines at positions 14 and 125 to either the sulfone or sulfoxide form. However, the methionine at position 170 is not involved in this degradation as determined by migration behavior of the methionine containing tryptic peptides during HPLC. The electrophoretic behavior of the alkaline forms reverts to that of GH_{22K} when treated with a reducing agent. In isoelectric focusing patterns these artifacts are seen as slightly more alkaline components (23).

Immunoblotting of 2-dimensional patterns (isoelectric focusing/SDS electrophoresis) of various pituitary fractions indicate the presence of a 27K-dalton form of GH (unpublished observations). This variant does not bind to concanavalin A or lentil lectin indicating that it is not a glycosylated form of GH. A recent report by Hampson and Rottman (24) suggests a possible structure for this 27K form. These investigators found in bovine pituitary glands a m-RNA for bovine growth hormone in which intron D had not been removed during splicing and, in addition, only the first 50 nucleotides of exon 5 were present. When translated, therefore, a GH with a chain length 42 amino acids longer than the major form GH would be produced. The molecular weight would be near 27K-daltons. A similar alternative mRNA splicing may also occur in human pituitary glands and would explain the 27K variant we have detected.

Immunoblotting experiments also indicate that extracts of human pituitary glands contain a 24K dalton form. We know that it is not a two-chain proteolytic product (25) because it remains intact when treated with reducing agent. Since the GH-V variant (26) contains a consensus sequence for asparagine linked glycosylation, we are examining the possibility that the 24K dalton form is glycosylated GH-V. In support of this hypothesis, Sinha and Lewis (27) recently reported evidence for the presence of an immunoreactive glycosylated GH in pituitary extracts.

BIOLOGIC PROPERTIES

An important question regarding the multiple forms of GH is whether the various peptides have specific roles in growth hormone physiology. The final answer must await the development of specific RIAs which are sensitive and selective for each of the hormonal forms. Such assays will be extremely useful in the measurement of the various peptides in numerous metabolic disorders. To date, this approach has been hindered by lack of discriminating antisera (production of such antisera has not been possible by direct immunization). In the meantime, immunoblotting techniques can be used to give preliminary analyses of sera as demonstrated by Markoff et al. (28) and Sinha et al. (29) for the GH_{20K} while Baumann et al. (30) were the first to detect GH_{20K} in serum by a combined electrophoresis-RIA techniques. Examination of both in vivo and in vitro biologic actions of the multiple forms will, of course, aid in determining physiologic significance. Preliminary studies indicate that certain forms act as GH but with greatly attenuated actions. This does suggest a need for such hormones with restricted activity. Only two of the forms, GH_{20K} and the disulfide dimer of GH_{22K}, have been isolated in quantities sufficient for biologic studies.

The disulfide dimer of GH clearly shows an altered biologic profile. Growth promoting activity in the hypophysectomized rat is extremely low but yet the dimer retained lactogenic activity as measured by the pigeon crop sac assay (12). Interestingly, receptor binding of the dimer to liver membrane receptors is greatly reduced. The suppression of one function with retention of another certainly suggests a role in the regulation of hormone action.

The GH_{20K} variant retains the growth promoting activity of GH_{22K} in rats whereas the insulin-like activity on rat adipose tissue is essentially absent, having been reduced to 3-20% of the GH_{22K}. Frigeri et al. (31), using a single-point test analysis, reported that the ability to stimulate oxidation of glucose to CO_2 in vitro in rat adipose tissue was absent from GH_{20K}. These experiments were recently repeated (unpublished observations) using a 9-point dose response curve and it was concluded that an accurate comparison of the potencies of GH_{22K} and GH_{20K} cannot be made because the dose response curves for CO_2 production are not parallel for the two hormones. At best, the GH_{20K} was only 10% as active as GH_{22K}. Using essentially the same assay, Goodman et al. (32) noted a loss of 80-90% of this in vitro insulin-like activity by GH_{20K}. Kostyo et al. (33) reported that about 80% of this property was absent from the variant. Smal et al. (34) tested the in vitro insulin-like activity of GH_{20K} by measuring lipogenesis in rat adipocytes. When compared to GH_{22K}, GH_{20K} was only 3% as active. This correlated well with the loss of receptor binding for GH_{20K} in adipose tissue. However, Schwartz and Foster (35) were unable to detect a difference between GH_{22K} and GH_{20K} in glucose oxidation in 3T3 adipocytes. This suggests a difference in the glucose oxidation pathways for normal rat adipose tissue and the 3T3 cells.

The in vivo insulin-like activity of GH_{20K} has also been investigated. In rats the experiments were done in fasted hypophysectomized animals. Changes in serum NEFA and glucose concentrations were measured one hour after administering the hormone. In contrast to Frigeri et al. (31) who found no effect of GH_{20K} on these values, we found that the insulin-like activity was reduced but not absent (unpublished observations). The GH_{20K} was about 30% as effective as GH_{22K} on lowering NEFA values and about 40% as active in decreasing blood glucose. In the hypophysectomized rat, therefore, GH_{20K} appears to have more insulin-like activity in vivo than when tested in vitro on adipose tissue. Also, it can be concluded that deletion of the 15 amino acid sequence from GH_{20K} has more effect on metabolism of fatty acids than on glucose. Similarly, Culler et al. (manuscript in preparation) found that in the hypopituitary child, a dose of 2 mg of GH_{20K} failed to lower serum NEFA whereas the same dose of GH_{22K} significantly decreased NEFA values. Neither hormone lowered blood glucose suggesting that GH itself has less effect on glucose production than it does on lipid metabolism.

There are conflicting reports regarding the diabetogenic action of GH_{20K}. Lewis et al. (36) found that at a dosage of 0.25 mg/kg in the dog, the variant did not produce glucose intolerance when given 10 hours before a glucose tolerance test. At the same dosage, however, GH_{22K} produced a small abnormality in the clearance of blood glucose. This was an enormous dose of GH, being equivalent to giving 17.5 mg to a 70-kg individual, and illustrates that in this assay, GH affects blood glucose values only at nonphysiologic doses. Kostyo et al. (33) found that when ob/ob mice were given 75 µg of either GH_{20K} or GH_{22K} over a period of 3 days, the two hormones were equipotent in producing glucose intolerance. This is the equivalent of giving about 50 mg of GH to a 70-kg individual and raises the question of biologic relevance of this observation. Recently, Agajanian et al. (37) have reported that the two forms of GH have diabetogenic activity at physiologic doses. The hormones were administered intravenously to dogs for 12 days at a rate of 20 µg/kg/day. The GH_{22K} produced only a small effect on blood glucose while GH_{20K} caused no detectable changes. However, both hormones induced a marked insulin resistance, indicating a definite diabetogenic activity for the substances. Based on these lines of evidence, the concept of fragmentation of GH to produce a more active diabetogenic form of hormone cannot be eliminated. Although we reported low diabetogenic activity for GH in our dog assay, the activity could be enhanced by proteolytic cleavage (38). A 5-10K peptide has been detected in pituitary fractions (39) but as yet its structure is not known. The low molecular weight peptide was at least 50 times more active than GH_{22K} in producing glucose intolerance in the dog. Our conclusion is that GH_2 is only a mild hyperglycemic agent, but upon proteolytic alteration, a much more potent agent is produced. The possibility exists, therefore, that when given to an animal, GH is cleaved either in the circulation or at the target organ to produce a diabetogenic fragment more active than GH itself. Evidence for another diabetogenic substance also comes from the report by Hart et al. (40) who showed that a preparation of bovine GH with the greatest growth promoting activity was not the most diabetogenic fraction isolated from the pituitary. Another pituitary fraction rich in low molecular weight substances showed the greatest diabetogenic activity.

At this time there is no clear explanation for the multiple forms of GH. The assumption has been that since the newly recognized forms of GH are found in the pituitary gland only in small quantities, they must be of minor importance. What must be kept in mind, however, is that the major form of GH amounts to 5-10% of the dry weight of the pituitary gland, which is an enormous quantity compared to the other pituitary hormones. For example, prolactin is found in only about one hundredth of that amount. Thus, these minor forms then may also function physiologically even though they are stored in much smaller quantities.

REFERENCES

1. Tiselius A. A new apparatus for electrophoretic analysis of colloidal mixtures. Trans Faraday Soc 1937; 33:524.
2. Lewis UJ. Enzymatic transformations of growth hormone and prolactin. J Biol Chem 1962; 237:3141.
3. Ornstein L. Disc electrophoresis. I. Background and theory. Ann NY Acad Sci 1964; 121:321.
4. Davis BJ. Disc electrophoresis. II. Method and application to human serum proteins. Ann NY Acad Sci 1964; 121:404.
5. Wallace ALC, Ferguson KA. Preparation of human growth hormone. J Endocrinol 1961; 23:285.
6. Rodbard D, Chrambach A. Estimation of molecular radius, free mobility and valance using polyacrylamide gel electrophoresis. Anal Biochem 1969; 40:95.
7. Weber K, Osborn M. The reliability of molecular weight determinations by dodecyl sulfate-polyacrylamide electrophoresis. J Biol Chem 1969; 244:4406.
8. Vesterberg O. Physicochemical properties of the carrier ampholytes and some biochemical applications. Ann NY Acad Sci 1973; 209:23.
9. Sinha YN, Gilligan TA, Lee DW. Detection of a high molecular weight variant of prolactin in human plasma by a combination of electrophoretic and immunological techniques. J Clin Endocrinol Metab 1984; 58:752.
10. Li CH, Dixon JS. Human pituitary growth hormone. XXXII. The primary structure of the hormone: revision. Arch Biochem Biophys 1971; 146:233.
11. Goodman HM, DeNoto F, Fiddes JC, et al. Structure and evolution of growth hormone related genes. In: Scott WA, Werner R, Joseph DR, Schultz J, eds. Miami winter symposium. New York: Academic Press, 1980.
12. Lewis UJ, Peterson SM, Bonewald LF, Seavey BK, VanderLaan WP. An interchain disulfide dimer of human growth hormone. J Biol Chem 1977; 252:3697.
13. Schneider AB, Kowalski K, Russell J, Sherwood LM. Identification of the interchain disulfide bonds of dimeric human placental lactogen. J Biol Chem 1979; 254:3782.
14. DeNoto FM, Moore DD, Goodman HM. Human growth hormone DNA sequence and mRNA structure: possible alternative splicing. Nucleic Acids Res 1981; 9:3719.
15. Lewis UJ, Bonewald LF, Lewis LJ. The 20,000-dalton variant of human growth hormone: location of the amino acid deletion. Biochem Biophys Res Commun 1980; 92:511.
16. Lewis UJ, Dunn JT, Bonewald LF, Seavey BK, VanderLaan WP. A nat-

urally occurring structural variant of human growth hormone. J Biol Chem 1978; 253:2679.

17. Lewis UJ, Singh RNP, Bonewald LF, Lewis LJ, VanderLaan WP. Human growth hormone: additional members of the complex. Endocrinology 1979; 104:1256.

18. Baumann G, Stolar MW, Amburn K. Molecular forms of circulating growth hormone during spontaneous secretory episodes and in the basal state. J Clin Endocrinol Metab 1985; 60:1216.

19. Lewis UJ, Singh RNP, Bonewald LF, Seavey BK. Altered proteolytic cleavage of human growth hormone as a result of deamidation. J Biol Chem 1981; 256:11645.

20. Talamantes F, Lopez J, Lewis UJ, Wilson CB. Multiple forms of growth hormone: detection in medium from cultured pituitary adenoma explants. Acta Endocrinol (Copenh) 1981; 98:8.

21. Liberti JP, Antoni BA, Chlebowski JF. Naturally-occurring pituitary growth hormone is phosphorylated. Biochem Biophys Res Commun 1985; 128:713.

22. Oetting WS, Tuazon PT, Traugh JA, Walker AM. Phosphorylation of prolactin. J Biol Chem 1986; 261:1649.

23. Lewis UJ, Singh RNP, Peterson SM, VanderLaan WP. Human growth hormone: a family of proteins. In: Pecile A, Muller EE, eds. Growth hormone and related peptides. International Congress Series No. 381. Amsterdam: Excerpta Medica, 1981.

24. Hampson RK, Rottman FM. A potential variant of bovine growth hormone resulting from non-splicing of an intron. Fed Proc 1986; 45:1703.

25. Singh RNP, Seavey BK, Rice VP, Lindsey TT, Lewis UJ. Modified forms of human growth hormone with increased biological activities. Endocrinology 1974; 94:883.

26. Seeburg PH. The human growth hormone gene family: nucleotide sequences show recent divergence and predict a new polypeptide hormone. DNA 1982; 1:239.

27. Sinha YN, Lewis UJ. Detection of glycosylated growth hormone in the human pituitary gland. Endocrinology 1986; 118(suppl):260.

28. Markoff E, Lee DW, Culler FL, Jones KL, Lewis UJ. Release of the 22,000- and 20,000-dalton variants of growth hormone in vivo and in vitro by human anterior pituitary cells. J Clin Endocrinol 1986; 62:664.

29. Sinha YN, Gilligan TA, Lee DW, Baxi SC, VanderLaan WP. Demonstration of 20K growth hormone in human plasma by gel electrophoretic-immuno-staining-autoradiographic assay (GEISAA). Horm Metab Res 1986; 18:402.

30. Baumann G, MacCart JG, Ambrun K. The molecular nature of circulating growth hormone in normal and acromegalic man: evidence for a principal and minor monomeric form. J Clin Endocrinol Metab 1983; 56:946.

31. Frigeri LG, Peterson SM, Lewis UJ. The 20,000 dalton structural variant of human growth hormone: lack of some early insulin-like effects. Biochem Biophys Res Commun 1979; 91:778.

32. Goodman HM, Grichting G, Coiro V. Growth hormone action on adipocytes. In: Raiti S, Tolman RA, eds. Human growth hormone. New York: Plenum Publishing Corporation, 1986.

33. Kostyo JL, Cameron CM, Olson KC, Jones AJS, Pai R-C. Biosynthetic 20-kilodalton methionyl-human growth hormone has diabetogenic and insulin-like activities. Proc Nat Acad Sci USA 1986; 82:4250.

34. Smal J, Closset J, Hennen G, de Meyts P. Receptor binding and insulin-like effects of 22K human growth hormone and its 20K variant in the rat adipocytes. Endocrinology 1986; 118(suppl):122.

35. Schwartz J, Foster CM. Pituitary and recombinant deoxyribonucleic acid-derived human growth hormones alter glucose metabolism in 3T3 adipocytes. J Clin Endocrinol Metab 1986; 62:791.

36. Lewis UJ, Singh RNP, Tutwiler GF. Hyperglycemic activity of the

20,000 dalton variant of human growth hormone. Endocr Res Commun 1981; 8:155.

37. Agajanian T, Ader M, Bergman RN. Both recombinant DNA-derived 22K and 20K-human growth hormone (hGH) possess diabetogenic activity during chronic low dose infusion in dogs. Endocrinology 1986; 118(suppl):218.

38. Lewis UJ, Singh RNP, VanderLaan WP, Tutwiler GF. Enhancement of the hyperglycemic activity of human growth hormone by enzymic modification. Endocrinology 1977; 101:1587.

39. Singh RNP, Lewis LJ, O'Brien R, Lewis UJ, Tutwiler GF. Characterization of the pituitary hyperglycemic factor as a low molecular weight peptide. Endocrinology 1982; 110(suppl):102.

40. Hart IC, Blake LA, Chadwick ME, Payne GA, Simmonds AD. The heterogeneity of bovine growth hormone. Extraction from the pituitary of components with different biological and immunological properties. Biochem J 1984; 218:573.

4

MOLECULAR HETEROGENEITY OF CIRCULATING GROWTH HORMONE IN ACROMEGALY

Gerhard Baumann

Center for Endocrinology, Metabolism and Nutrition
Northwestern University Medical School
Chicago, Illinois 60611

INTRODUCTION

Growth hormone (GH) is known to consist of several molecular species. In the case of human GH, two general types of heterogeneity can be distinguished, one relating to molecules of similar size but different charge (charge isomerism), the other to molecules of substantially different molecular size (size isomerism). In pituitary extracts, an entire family of GH-related proteins has been described (1,2). This kindred contains both size and charge isomers. The physiological role of the various GH forms is not clear; some of the forms in pituitary extracts could represent extraction and storage artifacts resulting from aggregation, proteolysis, oxidation, or deamidation. Thus, it becomes important to determine which forms are secreted and circulate in vivo. Table 1 lists some of the possible origins/mechanisms of GH heterogeneity. Some have been proven to exist while others are still speculative.

The following will briefly discuss these various possibilities. Two GH genes have been shown to be located in the GH/CS gene cluster on chromosome 17 (3). The GH-N gene codes for the 22kD protein, generally

Table 1. Possible sources of GH heterogeneity.

1) Genetic: 2 - (5) GH-like genes
2) mRNA processing: 22K and 20K GH
3) Precursors: pre-GH
4) Posttranslational processing: - proteolysis
- glycosylation (?)
- acylation
- phosphorylation (?)
- deamidation
5) Polymerization, aggregation: - "simple"
- disulfide interchange
6) Protein-protein interaction: carrier proteins
7) Metabolic conversions → active daughters (?)
8) Metabolic conversions → inactive daughters

known as pituitary GH, while the other—denoted GH-V gene—codes for a similar protein with 13 amino acid substitutions. It is presently not known with certainty whether this GH-V gene is expressed, however. The other three GH-like genes in the gene cluster code for human chorionic somatomammotropin (CS) (3). Alternative mRNA processing at two different splicing sites leads to two proteins derived from the GH-N gene, i.e., the 22kD GH and the 20kD GH variant (4,5). A pre-GH is synthesized at the ribosome, but since the signal (pre-) sequence is cotranslationally cleaved, this precursor is ephemeral and need not be considered as a secreted product. No other GH precursor is either predicted from the genetic code nor has been identified in pituitary tissue.

Proteolytically modified two-chain forms of GH are present in pituitary extracts (6-8); they exhibit the interesting property of enhanced bioactivity with respect to the parent polypeptide (7-9). An N_α-acylated GH has been described in pituitary (10), as have two deamidated GH-forms (11). Aggregates of GH are universally present in pituitary extracts (12); one disulfide dimer has been characterized in detail (13). Very recently, a carrier protein for GH has been discovered in human plasma (14). While metabolic conversion to active daughter products may include the above-mentioned proteolytically cleaved GH forms, the physiological importance of bioactive GH metabolites has not been established. On the other hand, metabolic degradation to inactive daughter products likely occurs, although this has not been investigated in detail. Depending on the assay used, any of the possibilities listed in Table 1 may appear as GH heterogeneity. The difficulty lies in sorting out artifacts from physiologically occurring heterogeneity, and in assigning biological roles to the various components of GH. Several critical questions in this regard exist: "Which of the GH forms found in pituitary extracts are secreted?" "What GH forms circulate in vivo, both as a result of secretion and postsecretory modification?" "Is circulating GH in disease states, such as acromegaly, qualitatively different from the normal state?" This treatise will deal with these three questions.

SECRETED VS. STORED GH

The first step in elucidating the physiologically relevant GH forms is to examine secreted forms. Earlier work (15,16) had identified "little," "big" and "big-big" GH in the media of cultured pituitary tissue, but is was not clear whether this represented active secretion or passive leakage of GH from degenerating cells. These studies also did not allow discrimination between the various monomeric GH forms. Accordingly, a study was undertaken where these issues were addressed by showing de novo biosynthesis, response to secretagogues, and by including high resolution techniques for analysis of secreted as well as intracellularly stored GH in minimally manipulated pituitary organ cultures (17). A major impetus for these studies was the hypothesis that single-chain GH may be a storage form that had to be cleaved, coincident with or immediately preceding secretion, to the more bioactive two-chain forms to express its ultimate bioactivity, analogous to other proteolytic activation pathways (18).

These pituitary cultures, derived from a variety of normal and diseased pituitaries, including acromegaly, showed a predominant secretory product, GH_{22K}, with evidence for GH_{20K} ($\approx$ 5%) and (possibly) an acidic form (< 5%), in addition to big forms (17). No evidence of cleaved forms in detectable amounts was obtained, either extracellularly or intracellularly. This was in marked contradistinction to pituitary extracts, where variable amounts of cleaved forms are universally found (7,8,17), presumably as a result of proteolysis during extraction and storage (19). The molecular characteristics of secreted GH forms were the same in acromegalic pituitaries as in other (including normal) pituitaries. Thus, in vitro, the human pituitary secretes GH_{22K}, GH_{20K} and one or more acidic forms (N_α-acylated or deamidated GH), as well as corresponding oligomers.

CIRCULATING VS. SECRETED VS. STORED GH

Presumably information gained in vitro should be applicable to the in vivo state. However, several other factors, listed in Table 2, come into play in vivo. Some of the degradation products may retain partial immunoreactivity and thereby contribute to heterogeneity of immunoreactive GH. The same may be true for protein-bound GH.

Extensive studies of the nature of circulating GH, obtained by extraction and concentration of GH from plasma, followed by electrophoretic characterization, have yielded the same GH species as those recognized in vitro, although in different proportions (20-23). Thus, among the monomeric GH forms, GH_{22K} is predominant (75%). However, GH_{20K} is proportionally more prevalent in vivo (16%) than in vitro (5%), presumably because of its slower metabolic clearance (24). There is also evidence of acidic GH (8%) in slightly higher proportions than in vitro ($\leq 5\%$). The structure of this acidic GH has not been determined, but it corresponds most likely to N_α-acylated GH or one of the deamidated GH forms. Its consistent presence under all experimental conditions suggests that it is a native form rather than a form generated in the laboratory. No evidence for cleaved two-chain GH forms in the circulation, either derived from pituitary stores or from peripheral metabolism (25,26), has been obtained to date.

In addition to the secreted forms, at least three immunoreactive fragments of molecular weight (mw) 16kD, 30kD, and 12kD have been identified in blood (22). They are particularly evident in the basal state, when little GH is secreted, and presumably derive from GH metabolism in peripheral tissues. Their physiological role, if any, is presently unknown.

The so-called "big" and "big-big" (or "pre-big") GH forms, originally described in 1972 (27,28), were recently shown to represent, at least in part, an oligomeric series ranging from dimeric to pentameric GH (29). The building blocks for these oligomers are the same three monomeric GH forms already mentioned above (i.e., GH_{22K}, GH_{20K} and acidic GH). GH_{20K} is particularly enriched in big (dimeric) plasma GH (29), as is the case in the pituitary dimer fraction (4,30). The plasma oligomers are most likely derived from direct pituitary secretion, as suggested by in vitro data (15-17) and by monoclonal immunochemical evidence (31). In normal plasma, 30 minutes after a GRH stimulus, about 55% of GH consists of monomeric forms, 27% of dimeric forms, and 18% of oligomeric forms (21). Two thirds of the oligomers are non-covalently linked, one third is disulfide-linked, and a small fraction is not dissociable by strong denaturants and sulfhydryl reduction (21,29). The proportion of "big" and

Table 2. Factors affecting circulating GH forms.

- secreted GH forms
- metabolic clearance of individual GH forms
- protein binding/aggregation
- intravascular degradation
- recirculating tissue degradation products
- artifacts (spurious immunoreactivity)

"big-big" GH is substantially higher in plasma (21,27,28,31-34) than in either pituitary extracts (13,27,28,32,34) or pituitary culture media (15-17,35). The reason for this is twofold: (a) oligomers are cleared more slowly from the circulation than monomers (36,37), and (b) part of "big" and "big-big" GH represents GH complexed with a plasma protein (14).

We recently discovered a binding protein for GH in human plasma (14). This protein exhibits high specificity, high affinity and limited binding capacity for GH_{22K} and, to a lesser extent, GH_{20K}. As a result, GH circulates partially as a complex with the binding protein; we estimate that under physiological conditions about half of plasma GH exists in complexed form (38). The 80,000 mw complex, which dissociates upon fractionation, forms part of big-big GH (about one third under standard gel filtration conditions), and also a small part of big GH. The physiological role of the binding protein is not yet clear. Recent evidence indicates that it restricts the distribution of GH in the body and slows its degradation and clearance (39). The binding protein is present in apparently normal amounts in acromegaly (14).

Thus, in the blood stream, three monomeric GH forms and corresponding dimers, trimers, tetramers and pentamers can be identified. In addition, three or more immunoreactive GH fragments circulate. A substantial part of GH is complexed with one or more specific carrier protein(s).

IS THE GH-V GENE EXPRESSED?

The GH-V gene, alluded to above, codes for a protein that has not been identified as a normal pituitary component. The question then arises whether this gene is expressed under normal or pathological circumstances. Clearly the GH-V gene product is neither necessary nor sufficient for normal growth, as patients who lack the GH-N gene but possess the GH-V gene do not grow normally (40), whereas subjects who possess the GH-N gene but lack the GH-V gene exhibit completely normal growth (41). Therefore, it is possible that the GH-V gene is not functional. However, it has been suggested that it may function under pathological conditions such as acromegaly (42). To test this hypothesis, we searched for the GH-V gene product in both normal and acromegalic plasmas.

Some information about the property of this putative GH form can be derived from its predicted structure, as dictated by the genetic code, and from an artificially expressed GH-V gene product (43,44). Some key properties are listed in Table 3; they were used to direct the search for the protein.

Table 3. Properties of the GH-V gene product.

- basic protein: predicted pI = 8.5-9
- potential glycosylation site: $Asn^{140} Gln^{141} Ser^{142}$
- potential proteolysis site: $Arg^{18} Arg^{19}$
- propensity to aggregate
- immunoreactivity: 10%*
- receptor binding activity: 50-100%*
- RRA to RIA ratio: 5-10*

---

*In reference to GH-N

GH-V differs from GH-N in 13 amino acid positions. These substitutions confer a more basic nature, a potential site for tryptic cleavage and a potential site for N-linked glycosylation. Depending on whether posttranslational processing takes place at these sites, the protein may be shorter or more acidic than predicted from the primary structure. A tendency to aggregate and diminished immunoreactivity with antibodies directed against GH-N also result from the substitutions.

With all these limitations in mind, we have searched for the GH-V gene product by immunoextracting large plasma samples, by using wide (pH 3-10) pH gradients in isoelectric focusing, and by examining oligomeric plasma fractions from both normal and acromegalic subjects. In no instance did we find GH forms other than the known forms described above. We thus failed to find evidence for the expression of the GH-V gene in postnatal life. We estimate that we should have detected an expression level of 5% relative to that of the GH-N gene. One condition not examined by us is pregnancy because of technical considerations related to the vast excess of CS in pregnancy plasma. It is conceivable that the GH-V gene, which is wedged between two of the CS genes (3), might be expressed as part of the enormous activation of those genes in the placenta. However, this possibility still needs confirmation.

IS GH IN ACROMEGALY DIFFERENT FROM NORMAL GH?

Speculation has occasionally centered on whether GH in acromegaly is qualitatively abnormal. The principal reason for such speculation is the poor correlation between GH levels and clinical manifestation of GH excess. Examination of the relative proportions of normal monomeric GH forms circulating in acromegaly reveals no significant difference from that in normal subjects (23) (Table 4). In addition, no structurally abnormal molecular forms have been identified in acromegaly. Furthermore, circulating monomeric GH forms seem to be the same in acromegalics with high or low average GH levels.

The composition of oligomeric GH forms is also not different in acromegaly, as the same three monomeric building blocks are identifiable (29). However, Gorden et al. (45) have described that "little" GH constitutes a higher proportion of total plasma GH in acromegaly than in normals. This phenomenon has not been adequately explained to date. In view of the newly recognized binding protein, one possibility is that the saturable nature of the GH-binding protein accounts for this finding. Complexed GH elutes in the region of big-big and big GH on gel filtration (14), while free monomeric GH elutes in the region of little GH. In the presence of high GH levels, such as those encountered in acromegaly, a greater proportion of GH is in the free form because of partial saturation of the binding protein. This could explain the shift toward little GH reported by Gorden et al. (45).

Table 4. Proportions (as percent) of plasma monomeric GH forms (mean ± SEM) in normal subjects and acromegalic patients.

	GH_{22K}	GH_{20K}	Acidic GH
Normals (n = 22) (various secretory stimuli)	77.0±1.1	15.8±1.0	8.1±0.9
Acromegaly (n = 8)	72.6±1.8	16.9±1.7	10.5±2.4

To test this hypothesis, I have calculated the theoretical percentage of complexed GH, based on the saturation curve for the binding protein (14), for the plasma samples included in Gorden's paper, taking into account the endogenous GH level in each plasma. I then correlated the calculated (predicted) percentage of protein-bound GH with the percentage of big and big-big (pre-big) GH reported by Gorden for each sample. The results are shown in Figure 1.

Predicted values for complexed GH correlated highly with measured pre-big and big GH in both normals and acromegalics. Thus, saturation of the binding protein may be responsible for the phenomenon of disproportionately high levels of little GH in acromegaly. It should also be pointed out that under the conditions of fractionation used by Gorden (45) and by us (14), only about one third of big-big and big GH is accounted for by complexed GH (Fig. 1). The remainder is composed of GH oligomers (29) which elute in the same region of the column.

SUMMARY

At least three monomeric GH forms (GH_{22K}, GH_{20K}, and acidic GH) and four corresponding oligomers circulate in normal and acromegalic man. Part of GH is complexed with a specific high-affinity binding protein in plasma. There is no inherent qualitative abnormality in the GH circulating in acromegaly as compared to normal individuals. No evidence has pointed to the expression of the GH-V gene in either normal pituitary or somatotroph tumors. The high proportion of "little" GH in acromegalic plasma is not due to a different GH structure but rather to saturation of the binding protein at high plasma GH levels.

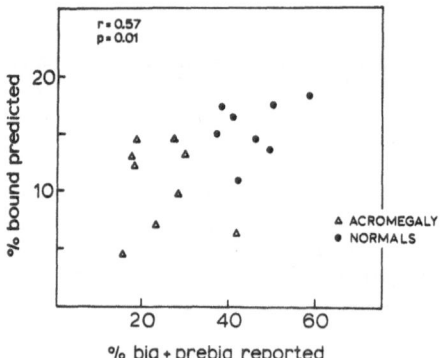

Fig. 1. Correlation of the calculated (predicted) percentage of protein-bound GH, based on the saturation curve for the GH-binding protein (14), and the percentage of pre-big and big plasma GH reported by Gorden et al. (45). Samples from acromegalic patients and normal subjects appear as parts of the same overall data population.

REFERENCES

1. Lewis UJ, Singh RNP, Tutweiler GF, et al. Human growth hormone: a complex of proteins. Recent Prog Horm Res 1980; 36:477.
2. Skyler JS, Baumann G, Chrambach A. A catalogue of isohormones of human growth hormone based on quantitative polyacrylamide gel electrophoresis. Acta Endocrinol (Copenh) 1977; 211(suppl):1.
3. Barsh GS, Seeburg PH, Gelinas RE. The human growth hormone gene family: structure and evolution of the chromosomal locus. Nucleic Acids Res 1983; 11:3939.
4. Lewis UJ, Dunn JT, Bonewald LF, et al. A naturally occurring structural variant of human growth hormone. J Biol Chem 1978; 253:2679.
5. DeNoto FM, Moore DD, Goodman HM. Human growth hormone DNA sequence and mRNA structure: possible alternative splicing. DNA 1981; 9:3719.
6. Chrambach A, Yadley RA, Ben-David M, et al. Isohormones of human growth hormone. I. Characterization by electrophoresis and isoelectric focusing in polyacrylamide gel. Endocrinology 1973; 93:848.
7. Yadley RA, Chrambach A. Isohormones of human growth hormone. II. Plasmin-catalyzed transformation and increase in prolactin biological activity. Endocrinology 1973; 93:858.
8. Singh RNP, Seavey BI, Rice VP, et al. Modified forms of human growth hormone with increased biological activities. Endocrinology 1974; 94:883.
9. Baumann G, Nissley SP. Somatomedin generation in response to activated and non-activated isohormones of human growth hormone. J Clin Endocrinol Metab 1979; 48:246.
10. Lewis UJ, Singh RNP, Bonewald LF, et al. Human growth hormone: additional members of the complex. Endocrinology 1979; 104:1256.
11. Lewis UJ, Singh RNP, Bonewald LF, et al. Altered proteolytic cleavage of human growth hormone as a result of deamidation. J Biol Chem 1981; 256:11645.
12. Ferguson K. In: Raiti S, ed. Advances in human growth hormone research. Washington, DC: US Government Printing Office, 1973; DHEW publication no. (NIH)74-612:526.
13. Lewis UJ, Peterson SM, Bonewald LF, et al. An interchain disulfide dimer of human growth hormone. J Biol Chem 1977; 252:3697.
14. Baumann G, Stolar MW, Amburn K, et al. A specific growth hormone-binding protein in human plasma: initial characterization. J Clin Endocrinol Metab 1986; 62:134.
15. Guyda HJ. Heterogeneity of human growth hormone and prolactin secreted in vitro: immunoassay and radioreceptor assay correlations. J Clin Endocrinol Metab 1975; 41:953.
16. Skyler JS, Rogol AD, Lovenberg W, et al. Characterization of growth hormone and prolactin produced by human pituitary in culture. Endocrinology 1977; 100:283.
17. Baumann G, MacCart JG. Growth hormone production by human pituitary glands in organ culture: evidence for predominant secretion of the single-chain 22,000 molecular weight form (isohormone B). J Clin Endocrinol Metab 1982; 55:611.
18. Lewis UJ, Pence SJ, Singh RNP, et al. Enhancement of the growth promoting activity of human growth hormone. Biochem Biophys Res Commun 1975; 67:617.
19. Ellis S, Nuenke JM, Grindeland RE. Identity between the growth hormone degrading activity of the pituitary gland and plasmin. Endocrinology 1968; 83:1029.
20. Baumann G, MacCart JG, Amburn K. The molecular nature of circulating growth hormone in normal and acromegalic man: evidence for a principal and minor monomeric forms. J Clin Endocrinol Metab 1983; 56:946.
21. Stolar MW, Baumann G, Vance ML, et al. Circulating growth hormone

forms after stimulation of pituitary secretion with growth hormone releasing factor in man. J Clin Endocrinol Metab 1984; 59:235.

22. Baumann G, Stolar MW, Amburn K. Molecular forms of circulating growth hormone during spontaneous secretory episodes and in the basal state. J Clin Endocrinol Metab 1985; 60:1216.

23. Baumann G, Stolar MW. Molecular forms of human growth hormone secreted in vivo: non-specificity of secretory stimuli. J Clin Endocrinol Metab 1986; 62:789.

24. Baumann G, Stolar MW, Buchanan TA. Slow metabolic clearance rate of the 20,000 dalton variant of human growth hormone: implications for biological activity. Endocrinology 1985; 117:1309.

25. Baumann G. Failure of endogenous plasmin to convert human growth hormone to its "activated" isohormones. J Clin Endocrinol Metab 1976; 43:222.

26. Baumann G, Hodgen G. Lack of in vivo transformation of human growth hormone to its "activated" isohormones in peripheral tissues of the rhesus monkey. J Clin Endocrinol Metab 1976; 43:1009.

27. Goodman AD, Tanenbaum R, Rabinowitz D. Existence of two forms of immunoreactive growth hormone in human plasma. J Clin Endocrinol Metab 1972; 35:868.

28. Gorden P, Hendricks C, Roth J. Evidence for "big" and "little" components of human plasma and pituitary growth hormone. J Clin Endocrinol Metab 1973; 36:178.

29. Stolar MW, Amburn K, Baumann G. Plasma "big" and "big-big" growth hormone (GH) in man: an oligomeric series composed of structurally diverse GH monomers. J Clin Endocrinol Metab 1984; 59:212.

30. Chapman GE, Rogers KM, Brittain T, et al. The 20,000 molecular weight variant of human growth hormone: preparation and some physical and chemical properties. J Biol Chem 1981; 256:2395.

31. Stolar MW, Baumann G. Big growth hormone forms in human plasma: immunochemical evidence for their pituitary origin. Metabolism 1986; 35:75.

32. Yalow RS. Heterogeneity of peptide hormones. Recent Prog Horm Res 1974; 30:597.

33. Diamond RD, Wartofsky L, Rosen SW. Heterogeneity of circulating growth hormone in acromegaly. J Clin Endocrinol Metab 1974; 39:1133.

34. Wright DR, Goodman AD, Trimble KD. Studies on "big" growth hormone from human plasma and pituitary. J Clin Invest 1974; 54:1064.

35. Talamantes F, Lopez J, Lewis UJ, et al. Multiple forms of growth hormone: detection in medium from cultured pituitary adenoma explants. Acta Endocrinol (Copenh) 1981; 98:8.

36. Hendricks CM, Eastman RC, Takeda S, et al. Plasma clearance of intravenously administered pituitary human growth hormone: gel filtration studies of heterogeneous components. J Clin Endocrinol Metab 1985; 60:864.

37. Baumann G, Stolar MW, Buchanan TA. The metabolic clearance, distribution and degradation of dimeric and monomeric growth hormone: implications for the patterns of circulating growth hormone forms. Endocrinology 1986; 119(4):1497-501.

38. Baumann G, Amburn K. Human growth hormone circulates in large part as a complex associated with (a) plasma protein(s) [Abstract]. Clin Res 1986; 34:681A.

39. Baumann G, Amburn K, Buchanan TA. Growth hormone binding protein in human plasma: effect on metabolic clearance, distribution and degradation of growth hormone [Abstract 11]. The Endocrine Society 68th Annual Meeting, 1986.

40. Phillips JA, Parks JS, Hjelle BL, et al. Genetic analysis of familial isolated growth hormone deficiency type I. J Clin Invest 1982; 70:489.

41. Wurzel J, Parks JS, Herd JE, et al. A gene deletion is responsible for absence of human chorionic somatomammotropin. DNA 1982; 1:251.

42. Parks JS. Organization and function of the growth hormone gene cluster. In: Raiti S, Tolman RA, eds. Human growth hormone. New York: Plenum, 1986:199.

43. Pavlakis GN, Hizuka N, Gorden P, et al. Expression of two human growth hormone genes in monkey cells infected by simian virus 40 recombinants. Proc Natl Acad Sci USA 1981; 78:7398.

44. Hizuka N, Hendricks CM, Pavlakis GN, et al. Properties of human growth hormone polypeptides purified from pituitary extracts and synthesized in monkey kidney cells and bacteria. J Clin Endocrinol Metab 1982; 55:585.

45. Gorden P, Lesniak MA, Eastman R, et al. Evidence for higher proportions of "little" growth hormone with increased radioreceptor activity in acromegalic plasma. J Clin Endocrinol Metab 1976; 43:364.

5

SOMATOMEDIN GENE EXPRESSION

Andrew R. Hoffman, Susan N. Perkins, Ines Zangger,
James Eberwine, Jack D. Barchas, Phillip James,
Ron G. Rosenfeld, and Raymond L. Hintz

Departments of Medicine, Pediatrics, and Psychiatry
Stanford University Medical Center, Stanford, CA

INTRODUCTION

The Somatomedin Hypothesis

Three independent and seemingly unrelated lines of inquiry led to the discovery and characterization of the family of growth-promoting polypeptides now known as somatomedins (SM) or insulin-like growth factors (IGF):

I. While it had long been appreciated that growth hormone (GH) stimulated the growth and development of bone and cartilage, the precise details of hormone action proved difficult to elucidate. In an elegant series of experiments, Salmon and Daughaday (1) studied the regulation of cartilage metabolism by measuring the in vitro incorporation of [35-S]-sulfate into chondroitin sulfate. They found that cartilage derived from hypophysectomized rats incorporated less [35-S]-sulfate than did cartilage from intact rats. When the rats were treated with GH, [35-S]-sulfate uptake returned to normal, but simply adding GH in vitro to the cartilage derived from the hypophysectomized rats had no effect on sulfation. If the cartilage was incubated in the presence of normal rat serum, however, the rate of [35-S]-sulfate incorporation was restored; serum from hypophysectomized rats did not alter [35-S]-sulfate uptake. Since this sulfation factor could be induced in hypophysectomized rats by GH treatment, it was suggested that the growth-promoting effects of the pituitary hormone were mediated by this nondialyzable serum hormone (the somatomedin hypothesis).

II. In the course of pursuing studies of insulin action, Froesch and his colleagues (2) discovered that the great majority of the insulin-like action of serum on rat adipose tissue was not suppressed in the presence of anti-insulin antibodies, and they suggested that serum contained other insulin-like factors. This nonsuppressible insulin-like activity, (NSILA), was subsequently shown to consist of at least three components: a high molecular weight, acid-ethanol precipitable form, and two ~7000 dalton soluble species.

III. Finally, Temin and colleagues began to characterize serum growth factors that were necessary for cells in culture to multiply. They employed a bioassay that measured the incorporation of [3-H]-thymidine into DNA in chick embryo fibroblasts to purify multiplication stimulating activity (MSA) from bovine serum and Buffalo rat liver cell line (BRL)-3A conditioned medium (3).

During careful characterization of sulfation factor, NSILA and MSA, it became apparent that the properties of sulfation activity, insulin-like activity, and stimulation of cell multiplication co-purified. The generic term "somatomedin" was chosen to designate this group of serum factors. In 1978, the two major somatomedins, now called IGF-I and IGF-II, were purified and sequenced by Rinderknecht and Humbel (4,5). Schoenle and co-workers provided dramatic confirmation of the somatomedin hypothesis when they demonstrated that a subcutaneous infusion of purified IGF-I stimulated growth and [3-H]-thymidine incorporation into costal cartilage in hypophysectomized rats (6).

Peptide Structure of Insulin-Like Growth Factors I and II

The human IGF-I and IGF-II are single chain polypeptides of 70 and 67 amino acids, respectively, with three intrachain disulfide bridges. IGF-I is identical to SM-C, while MSA is highly homologous to IGF-II, and is now considered to be the rat IGF-II. These SMs belong to a family of peptide hormones that includes insulin, relaxin, and, possibly, the beta-subunit of nerve growth factor. Because of their homology to proinsulin, the regions of the IGF molecules are denoted by a nomenclature similar to that for the insulin precursor. While there is a 38-48% homology between the IGFs and proinsulin for the A and B regions, the IGFs differ from insulin in that they each retain a short C-peptide region and possess a carboxy-terminal D domain not found in insulin. The IGFs are even more homologous to each other, sharing 45 amino acids in common. Computer-derived models of the three-dimensional configurations of the IGFs and insulin demonstrate a high degree of homology (7), consistent with the ability of the IGFs and insulin to interact with each other's receptors (see reference 8 for review).

SOMATOMEDIN GENE STRUCTURE

IGF-I Gene

In 1983, Jansen and colleagues cloned a human IGF-I cDNA from a liver cDNA library using an oligonucleotide probe from amino acids 58-62 (9). The IGF-I gene was subsequently identified (10), and localized to chromosome 12 (11,12) where it spans 45 kb of genomic DNA. The peptide sequence deduced from the cDNA suggested that the IGF-I precursor peptide contained another region ("E domain") at its carboxyl terminus, which presumably is clipped from the mature IGF-I during intracellular peptide processing. There is a single copy of the IGF-I gene, yet two different IGF-I cDNAs have been characterized from human liver by Rotwein and his co-workers (13,14). These cDNAs have identical 5' ends and regions coding for the mature peptide, but different 3' extensions. These findings suggest the existence of alternate processing of the heteronuclear RNA. The IGF-I gene contains 5 potential exons and 4 introns. The first intron, 4.8 kb in length, is located in the region that codes for the pre- or prepro-portion of the IGF-I precursor peptide, and intron 2 (> 21 kb) interrupts the section of the gene encoding the B region. The middle of that portion of the gene that codes for the E region is interrupted by an intron segment which can be processed in one of two ways. Removal of a 17 kb intron results in a predicted precursor protein of 153 amino acids, whereas the splicing of a 1.5 kb intron suggests the synthesis of a 195-amino acid polypeptide. Such alternative splicing is not unprecedented; the calcitonin gene has also been shown to undergo alternative splicing, producing two peptides, calcitonin and calcitonin gene-related peptide (CGRP) of potentially varying bioactivities. The differential processing of the IGF-I heteronuclear RNA allows for the possibility of tissue specific processing, and permits another level of control in the regulation of IGF-I synthesis. Moreover, the E domain peptides may have important biological activities of their own. Thus, in an analogous fashion to the pro-opiomelanocortin molecule which is processed into ACTH, beta-endorphin and MSHs, proIGF-I may also serve as the precursor to a family of peptide hormones.

IGF-II Gene

The cDNAs for rat MSA (15,16) and human (17) IGF-II were cloned in 1984, as were the genes encoding for each of these peptides. The single human IGF-II gene spans at least 15 kb of DNA and is located on the short arm of chromosome II (11, pp 14-15), directly contiguous with the insulin gene (18). The two genes are aligned with the same polarity, separated by 12.6 kb of intergenic DNA, in the following configuration: 5'-insulin-IGF-II-3'. These genes are also located near the ras I proto-oncogene.

The cDNA sequence predicts a preproIGF-II of 180 amino acids, including a 24 amino-acid leader (pre-) sequence, the 67 amino-acid mature IGF-II, and an 89 amino-acid E region. Like the IGF-I gene, an intron interrupts the portions of the gene corresponding to the B domain. A single intron is located within the E region and, thus, only one IGF-II precursor peptide is predicted; another intron is located 6 bp 5' to the start of the IGF-II gene.

There is minimal homology between the IGF-II E peptide and the IGF-I E domains, but the IGF-II E region is highly conserved (79%) between the human and the rat. This conservation suggests that this carboxyl terminal fragment may in fact have a biological function. Recently, Hylka and co-workers confirmed the presence of an immunoreactive E peptide in medium from BRL-3A cells and showed that a synthetic IGF-II E-region peptide stimulated the incorporation of [3H]-thymidine in NIL8 hamster cells (19). In addition to the 7.5 kDa, 67 amino acid IGF-II and the E peptide, a 10 kDa variant human IGF-II has also been found (20). This peptide may represent an allelic variant of the IGF-II gene, a translation product of an mRNA-derived from alternate splicing of IGF-II mRNA, or an incompletely processed product of proIGF-II (perhaps containing portions of the E domain).

By comparing the structures of the genes for insulin, IGF-I and IGF-II, it is now clear that these three peptides were all derived from a common ancestral peptide. The insulin gene has one intron 17 bp 5' to the start signal, and a second intron interrupting the portion of the gene corresponding to the C peptide. It is likely that the insulin and the IGF genes arose from duplication of the ancestral gene. The two IGF genes likely diverged later, with each gene subsequently acquiring the dissimilar exon(s) which code for the E domains independently.

SITES OF IGF SYNTHESIS

Source of IGF Peptides

Sulfation factor was initially purified from blood; however, the site(s) of its synthesis was uncertain. Since the liver was known to respond to GH in vitro, and because infusions of radiolabeled GH accumulated in the liver, the somatomedin hypothesis suggested a hepatic source. McConaghey and Sledge (21) showed that the perfused rat liver produced a sulfation factor, and that bovine GH increased the release of this factor by more than sixfold. This finding has since been replicated many times, and investigators have also carefully delineated the production of IGF-II from cultures of fetal and adult rat livers (22,23). These studies indicate that the liver is able to synthesize and secrete both IGFs.

However, other organs have also been shown to synthesize somatomedin peptides. McConaghey and Dehnel reported the presence of a GH-stimulating sulfation factor in kidney in 1972 (24), and, subsequently, D'Ercole and colleagues (25) demonstrated that fetal mouse explants of liver, limb bud, heart, brain, kidney and lung made SM-C. Several laboratories have investigated the synthesis of SMs in cultures of human (26) and rat fibroblasts (27), in myoblasts (28), in ovaries (29) and in pituitary and in brain (30).

SM levels within various tissues have been shown to be regulated by both GH and a variety of other factors. In fetal rat hepatocytes, epidermal growth factor (EGF) stimulates rat IGF-II synthesis, while GH is relatively ineffective (31); in liver cells derived from adult rats, however, GH treatment was a potent inducer of rat IGF-I production (23). D'Ercole and co-workers (32) demonstrated that when ovine GH was administered to hypophysectomized rats, SM-C levels increased in kidney, liver, lung, heart and testes, but not in brain. In cultured embryonic rat fibroblasts, placental lactogen (PL), but not GH, stimulated rat IGF-II production, but during maturation, there was a shift in the hormonal regulation of fibroblast IGFs. While fibroblast rat IGF-II production was not altered by GH or PL in cells derived from adult animals, both somatotropic hormones stimulated IGF-I synthesis in such cells (27). Triiodothyronine increased the production of IGFs in cultures of fetal murine hypothalamic cells (33). The complexity of studying hormonal control of IGF production in vitro, however, was carefully illustrated by Clemmons (34) who emphasized the importance of cell density and serum growth factors in the expression of SM peptides. Both platelet-derived growth factor (PDGF) and fibroblast growth factor (FGF) were potent stimuli for SM-C production by human fibroblasts in serum-free medium. Quiescent cells in serum-free medium did not increase SM synthesis when incubated with hydrocortisone, thyroxine, insulin or EGF. When PDGF was added, however, both hydrocortisone and thyroxine became effective stimulants of SM production.

Tissue Distribution of IGF-I and IGF-II mRNAs

The measurement of immunoreactive IGFs in various tissue extracts is complicated by the fact that IGFs circulate bound to specific carrier proteins at remarkably high concentrations (on the order of 1 µg/ml); even if organs are extensively perfused and washed, there is still a possibility that some of the relatively low concentration of measured "tissue IGF" actually reflects contamination by circulating IGF-binding protein complexes. The techniques of molecular biology now offer an alternative approach to the determination of IGF gene expression by allowing the detection of specific mRNA levels in different tissues. Complementary DNA and RNA probes provide a more sensitive and potentially far more specific assay for the presence of a given peptide than is possible with RIAs or traditional bioassays. When used in conjunction with these latter assays, moreover, mRNA assays may also reveal differences in regulation of gene activation and peptide secretion.

Several laboratories have begun to characterize the distribution and regulation of IGF-I and IGF-II mRNAs. Using cDNAs for the 3' ends of IGF-IA and IGF-IB (see Figure 1), Rotwein (13) found four major mRNA species (ranging in size from 1.1 to 6.3 kb) in human liver. Bell et al. (17) described three major bands in adult human liver (0.9, 5.3 and 7.7 kb), and noted that IGF-I mRNA is distributed in a wide variety of tissues. We have subcloned selected portions of IGF-I and IGF-II cDNA probes (isolated from a library made from adult human liver [9]) into the Riboprobe vectors pSP64 and 65. These vectors contain a promoter site for SP6 RNA polymerase, which synthesizes RNA complementary to DNA. This system allowed us to prepare single-stranded [32-P]-cRNA probes of high specific activity and of greater sensitivity than cDNA probes. For the IGF-I studies, a plasmid containing a portion of the 3'-nontranslated region of the IGF-IA cDNA was constructed. The region chosen has essentially no homology with IGF-II, and we have shown that this IGF-I [32-P]-cRNA probe is specific, as it does not bind to the cDNA coding for the IGF-II peptide. Using this probe, we have found IGF-I mRNA in nearly every organ in the adult rat, including liver, salivary gland, fat, placenta, skeletal muscle, diaphragm, heart, lung, thymus, pancreas, duodenum, adrenal, testis, pituitary and brain. Each tissue showed multiple hybridization bands (ranging from 0.9 to 6 kb), with the duodenum and pancreas demonstrating numerous other, smaller mRNA species.

The expression of the IGF-II gene also displays tissue-specific processing in a similarly complex fashion. Bell and his colleagues (18) described several IGF-II mRNA species in adult human liver (6.0, 5.3, 4.9 kb); they noted that IGF-II mRNA is present in numerous organs, while the insulin gene, which is located adjacent to the IGF-II gene, is expressed only in the pancreas; hence, the regulators of the IGF-II gene do

INSULIN–LIKE GROWTH FACTOR – I

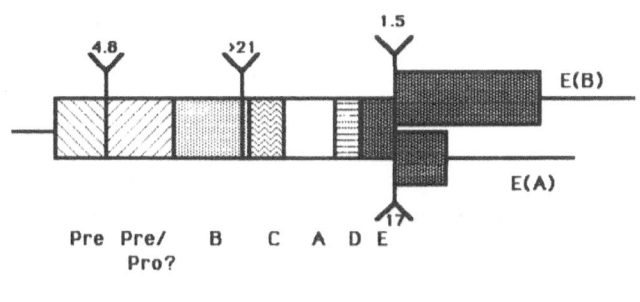

INSULIN–LIKE GROWTH FACTOR – II

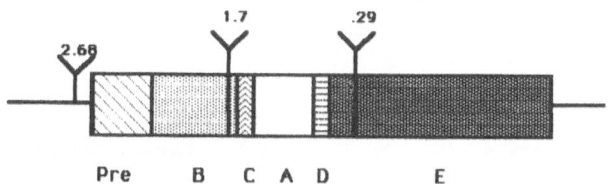

Fig. 1. Exon-intron structure of insulin-like growth factor genes. The IGF-1 gene can be spliced into two different mRNAs, designated by the two different E regions, A and B. The numbers above the forks represent kilobases of DNA within that intron. The letters below the exons denote the regions of the translated protein. Adapted from Rotwein et al. (14).

not activate transcription of insulin. Placenta and human fetal tissue also express IGF-II mRNA (bands of 6.0, 4.9-4.8, and 2.0-1.9 have been described) (35,36). Soares and co-workers (37) have found rat IGF-II mRNA in a variety of neonatal and adult rat tissues. Tissue-specific processing is also evident in the rat, with up to four major mRNA species identified (3.4, 1.75, 1.6, and 1.1 kb in length). Our laboratories have recently begun to screen rat tissues for rat IGF-II gene expression using a 240-base cRNA constructed from the E-peptide domain of the human liver cDNA. We have found that the IGF-II mRNA is expressed in numerous rat organs, and that a variety of mRNAs (most ranging in size from 1.4 to 4.5 kb in length) are exhibited in the various tissues.

The presence of multiple species of IGF mRNAs has increased the potential complexity of the regulation of the IGF genes. The various IGF mRNA transcripts might arise from stepwise splicing and deletion of one or more of the genomic introns. It is not yet known which of the mRNA species are actually translated, or whether the several mRNA species can be differentially regulated within a single tissue.

NONENDOCRINE ROLES FOR THE SOMATOMEDINS

IGFs as Autocrine Factors

The fact that the IGF mRNAs and peptides are synthesized in a wide array of tissues has raised the possibility that somatomedins may act as autocrine or paracrine factors as well as traditional hormones. Thus, changes in the endogenously-produced intracellular levels of IGFs may regulate local cell or organ growth. We are currently investigating 18,54SF cells, a line which both synthesizes and secretes immunoreactive rat IGF-II, and possesses Type II IGF membrane receptors (38). We have detected a single 4.5 kb IGF-II mRNA in these cells; however, unlike most rat tissues examined, no IGF-I mRNA can be detected. Thus, IGF-II may qualify as an autocrine factor in the 18,54SF cell line; after endogenous synthesis and secretion, IGF-II could interact with its specific cell surface receptor and act as a growth factor for its cell of origin.

IGF and Cancer

Proto-oncogenes are normal cellular genes that are potentially oncogenic if their normal structure or regulation is disrupted. Perturbations in the homeostatic regulation of autocrine factors could theoretically result in unimpeded and unregulated cell growth and neoplasia. Wilms' tumor is a malignancy which arises in embryonal kidney cells. In both the hereditary and sporadic forms, deletions in the short arm of chromosome II (11, pp 13-14), an area near the IGF-II gene, have been described. Two groups (35,36) recently reported that there is an increased concentration of IGF-II mRNA present in Wilms' tumors. The three major IGF-II mRNA transcripts seen in the tumor are the same size as those found by these investigators in other tissues. No gene rearrangement or amplification of the IGF-II gene was found, and it was suggested that IGF-II might act in an autocrine fashion to initiate or enhance tumor growth. Finally, a recent study of the human MCF-7 breast cancer cell line suggests that endogenously synthesized IGF-I may act as an "estrogen-induced second messenger," stimulating the growth of breast cancer (39).

CONCLUSION

In the 30 years since the elucidation of sulfation factor and the formulation of the somatomedin hypothesis, our understanding of the physiology of IGF action has expanded to include autocrine and paracrine functions in addition to the classical role of an endocrine factor. The challenge for the near future will be to: (1) elucidate the biology of the various mRNA transcripts and learn which ones are translated in which cells; (2) characterize IGF peptide precursors and study the physiology of potential E-domain fragments; (3) understand the hormonal regulation of IGF synthesis throughout the body; and, (4) define paracrine and autocrine activity in relation to cell growth and oncogenesis.

ACKNOWLEDGMENTS

Supported in part by grants from the Juvenile Diabetes Foundation and the NIH (AM 36054). Dr. Perkins is the recipient of a National Research Service Award (AM 007768), and Dr. Rosenfeld is a recipient of a Research Career Development Award for the NIH.

REFERENCES

1. Salmon WD, Daughaday WH. A hormonally controlled serum factor which stimulates sulfate incorporation by cartilage in vitro. J Lab Clin Med 1957; 49:825.
2. Froesch ER, Burgi H, Ramseier EB, Bally P, Labhart A. Antibody-suppressible and nonsuppressible insulin-like activities in human serum and their significance. An insulin assay with adipose tissue of increased precision and specificity. J Clin Invest 1963; 42:1816.
3. Dlak N, Temin HM. A partially purified polypeptide fraction from rat liver cell conditioned medium with multiplication-stimulating activity for embryo fibroblasts. J Cell Physiol 1973; 81:153.
4. Rinderknecht E, Humbel RE. The amino acid sequence of human insulin-like growth factor I and its structural homology with pro-insulin. J Biol Chem 1978; 253:2769.
5. Rinderknecht E, Humbel RE. Primary structure of human insulin-like growth factor II. FEBS Lett 1978; 89:283.
6. Schoenle E, Zapf J, Humbel RE, Froesch ER. Insulin-like growth factor I stimulates growth in hypophysectomized rats. Nature 1982; 296:252.
7. Honegger A, Blundell T. A computer graphics study of insulin-like growth factors and their receptor interactions. In: Spencer EM, ed. Insulin-like growth factors/somatomedins. Berlin: Walter de Gruyter & Co., 1983.
8. Rosenfeld RG, Hintz RL. Somatomedin receptors: structure, function, and regulation. In: Conn PM, ed. The receptors, vol III. Orlando: Academic Press, Inc., 1986.
9. Jansen M, van Schaik FMA, Ricker AT, et al. Sequence of cDNA encoding human insulin-like growth factor I precursor. Nature 1983; 306:609.
10. Ullrich A, Berman CH, Dull TJ, Gray A, Lee JM. Isolation of the human insulin-like growth factor I gene using a single synthetic DNA probe. EMBO J 1984; 3:361.
11. Brissenden JE, Ullrich A, Francke U. Human chromosomal mapping of genes for insulin-like growth factors I and II and epidermal growth factor. Nature 1984; 310:781.
12. Tricoli JV, Rall LB, Scott J, Bell GI, Shows TB. Localization of insulin-like growth factor genes to human chromosomes 11 and 12. Nature 1984; 310:784.
13. Rotwein P. Two insulin-like growth factor I messenger RNAs are expressed in human liver. Proc Natl Acad Sci USA 1986; 83:77.
14. Rotwein P, Pollock KM, Didier DK, Krivi GG. Organization and sequence of the human insulin-like growth factor I gene. J Biol Chem

1986; 261:4828.

15. Dull TJ, Gray A, Hayflick JS, Ullrich A. Insulin-like growth factor II precursor gene organization in relation to insulin gene family. Nature 1984; 310:777.

16. Whitfield HJ, Bruni CB, Frunzio R, Terrell JE, Nissley SP, Rechler M. Isolation of a cDNA clone encoding rat insulin-like growth factor-II precursor. Nature 1984; 312:277.

17. Bell GI, Merryweather JP, Sanchez-Pescador R, et al. Sequence of a cDNA clone encoding human preproinsulin-like growth factor II. Nature 1984; 310:775.

18. Bell GI, Gerhard DS, Fong NM, Sanchez-Pescador R, Rall LB. Isolation of the human insulin-like growth factor genes: insulin-like growth factor II and insulin genes are contiguous. Proc Natl Acad Sci USA 1985; 82:6450.

19. Hylka VW, Teplow DB, Kent SBH, Straus DS. Identification of a peptide fragment from the carboxyl-terminal extension region (E-domain) of rat pro insulin-like growth factor-II. J Biol Chem 1985; 260:14417.

20. Zumstein PP, Luthi C, Humbel RE. Amino acid sequence of a variant pro-form of insulin-like growth factor II. Proc Natl Acad Sci USA 1985; 82:3169.

21. McConaghey P, Sledge CB. Production of "sulfation factor" by the perfused liver. Nature 1970; 225:1249.

22. Rechler MM, Eisen HJ, Higa OZ, et al. Characterization of a somato-medin (insulin-like growth factor) synthesized by fetal rat organ cultures. J Biol Chem 1979; 254:7942.

23. Scott CD, Martin JL, Baxter RC. Rat hepatocyte insulin-like growth factor I and binding protein: effect of growth hormone in vitro and in vivo. Endocrinology 1985; 116:1102.

24. McConaghey P, Dehnel J. Preliminary studies of "sulfation factor" by rat kidney. J Endocrinol 1972; 52:587.

25. D'Ercole AJ, Applewhite GT, Underwood LE. Evidence that somatomedin is synthesized by multiple tissues in the fetus. Dev Biol 1980; 75:315.

26. Atkinson PA, Weidman ED, Bhaumick B, Bala RM. Release of somato-medin-like activity by cultured WI-38 human fibroblasts. Endocrinology 1980; 106:2006.

27. Adams SO, Nissley SP, Handwerger S, Rechler MM. Developmental patterns of insulin-like growth factor I and II synthesis and regulation in rat fibroblasts. Nature 1983; 302:150.

28. Hill DJ, Crace CJ, Nissley SP, Morrell D, Holder AT, Milner RDG. Fetal rat myoblasts release both rat somatomedin-C (SM-C)/insulin-like growth factor I (IGF I) and multiplication-stimulating activity in vitro: partial characterization and biological activity of myoblast-derived SM-C/IGF I. Endocrinology 1985; 117:2061.

29. Hammone JM, Lino J, Baranao S, et al. Production of insulin-like growth factors by ovarian granulosa cells. Endocrinology 1985; 117:2553.

30. Binoux M, Hossenlopp P, Lassare C, Hardouin N. Production of in-sulin-like growth factors and their carrier by rat pituitary gland and brain explants in culture. FEBS Lett 1981; 124:178.

31. Richman RA, Benedict MR, Florini JR, Toly BA. Hormonal regulation of somatomedin secretion by fetal rat hepatocytes in primary culture. Endocrinology 1985; 116:180.

32. D'Ercole AJ, Stiles AD, Underwood LE. Tissue concentrations of somatomedin-C: further evidence for multiple sites of synthesis and paracrine or autocrine mechanisms of action. Proc Natl Acad Sci USA 1984; 81:935.

33. Binoux M, Faivre-Bauman A, Lassarre C, Barret A, Tixier-Vidal A. Triiodothyronine stimulates the production of insulin-like growth factor (IGF) by fetal hypothalamus cells cultured in serum-free

medium. Brain Res 1985; 21:319.

34. Clemmons DR. Multiple hormones stimulate the production of somato-medin by cultured human fibroblasts. Endocrinology 1984; 58:850.

35. Reeve AE, Eccles MR, Wilkins RJ, Bell GI, Millow LJ. Expression of insulin-like growth factor-II transcripts in Wilms' tumour. Nature 1985; 317:258.

36. Scott J, Cowell J, Robertson ME, et al. Insulin-like growth factor-II gene expression in Wilms' tumour and embryonic tissues. Nature 1985; 317:260.

37. Soares MB, Ishii DN, Efstratiadis A. Developmental and tissue-specific expression of a family of transcripts related to rat insulin-like growth factor II mRNA. Nucleic Acids Res 1985; 13:1119.

38. Lee PDK, Hodges D, Hintz RL, Wyche JH, Rosenfeld RG. Identification of receptors for insulin-like growth factor II in two insulin-like growth factor II producing cell lines. Biochem Biophys Res Commun 1986; 134:595-600.

39. Dickson RB, McManaway ME, Lippman ME. Estrogen-induced factors of breast cancer cells partially replace estrogen to promote tumor growth. Science 1986; 232:1540.

6

SOMATOMEDIN ACTION AND TISSUE GROWTH FACTOR RECEPTORS

Ron G. Rosenfeld, Gian Paolo Ceda, Darrell M. Wilson, and
Andrew R. Hoffman

Department of Pediatrics and Medicine, Stanford University
School of Medicine, and Instituto di Clinica Medica
Generale, Parma, Italy

RECEPTORS FOR THE SOMATOMEDINS

The somatomedins (SMs) are a family of peptide hormones which are growth hormone (GH)-dependent, possess insulin-like activity in extra-skeletal tissue, and promote the incorporation of (35-S)-sulfate into proteoglycans of cartilage. Although their precise role in the control of cellular growth and replication is still unclear, a growing body of evidence supports the hypothesis that the SMs are the major mediators of the anabolic actions of GH: (1) plasma levels of SM are decreased in GH deficiency and rise following treatment with exogenous GH (1); (2) plasma levels of SM are, generally, elevated in acromegaly (2); (3) under in vitro conditions, SM stimulates DNA synthesis in many cell lines (3); and, (4) continuous subcutaneous administration of the SM peptide IGF-I stimulates tibial epiphyseal widening and increased body weight in hypophysectomized rats (4).

In 1978, Rinderknecht and Humbel (5,6) purified and sequenced two SM peptides, which they named insulin-like growth factors (IGF) I and II (IGF-I is identical to the basic peptide, SM-C). IGF-I and II have a 62% identity in amino acid positions, but perhaps even more impressive is their striking structural homology to proinsulin. All three hormones are single-chain polypeptides with three intrachain disulfide bridges, and with significant sequence homology in the B- and A-chain region of the active insulin molecule. The sequences of cDNAs encoding for human preproIGF-I and -II have been elucidated, and the respective 130 and 180 amino acid precursors predicted (7,8). IGF-II has been mapped to the short arm of chromosome 11, tightly linked to both the insulin gene and the c-Ha-ras1 proto-oncogene. IGF-I maps to chromosome 12, which is evolutionarily related to chromosome 11 and carries the gene for the c-Ki-ras2 proto-oncogene (9,10). These striking homologies suggest evolutionary conservation of a common critical peptide skeleton, and raise important questions concerning the precise role of each peptide and how cells specifically mediate each hormone's biological activities.

Initial studies suggested that the biological effects of the SMs were, in fact, mediated through the insulin receptor, since SM-C competed with (125-I)-insulin for binding sites on adipocytes, liver membranes and chondrocytes (11). However, in addition to their relatively weak insulin-like metabolic effects, the IGFs display potent mitogenic activities, and insulin, in turn, can generally mimic IGF's growth-promoting action only at significantly higher concentrations. Accordingly, it was hypothesized that the insulin-like effects of IGF, presumably mediated through the insulin receptor, were secondary phenomena, and that the mitogenic action of IGF must be mediated through a distinct cell receptor (12).

In 1974, Megyesi et al. (13), using liver membranes, and Marshall et al. (14), using human placental membranes, demonstrated separate insulin and IGF receptors, with markedly different affinities. Subsequent studies confirmed the presence of specific IGF-I and -II receptors on a wide variety of tissues, including chondrocytes, adipocytes, fibroblasts, hepatocytes, lymphocytes and erythrocytes, to name a few (15). Despite these observations, it has been exceedingly difficult to fully delineate the structural and functional interrelationship of the insulin and IGF receptors because of: (1) overlapping affinities of insulin and the IGFs for each other's receptors, (2) use of incompletely purified IGF preparations in both binding and biological studies, and (3) possible heterogeneity in binding properties of these receptors in different tissues and species.

Partial clarification of the interrelationship between the insulin and IGF receptors has emerged from efforts to purify and structurally characterize each receptor. These plasma membrane glycoproteins can be readily solubilized in nonionic detergents, and significant purification can be achieved by employing affinity chromatography with lectins or peptide hormones covalently linked to Sepharose. By means of affinity cross-linking and photoaffinity labeling, followed by SDS-polyacrylamide gel electrophoresis, several laboratories have reported a heterotetrameric structure for the insulin receptor, of the form $(\beta-S-S-\alpha)-S-S-(\alpha-S-S-\beta)$, with a Mr of approximately 350,000 (16). Upon complete reduction of the class I and II disulfide bonds, the insulin receptor resolves into α and β subunits of Mr 130,000 and 95,000 respectively. When affinity cross-linking techniques were applied to investigation of IGF receptors, a striking homology was observed to the insulin receptor (17-19). (125-I)-IGF-I was found to bind with high affinity to a heterotetrameric receptor with the same molecular weight and physical properties as the insulin receptor. The subunit stoichiometry was $(\alpha\beta)_2$, mirroring that of the insulin receptor, and upon reduction of the disulfide bonds, the subunits were found to have similar molecular masses to their counterparts in the insulin receptor. Nevertheless, competitive binding studies confirmed that this receptor (termed type 1 by Massague and Czech [17]) was relatively specific for IGF-I, with inhibition of affinity labeling by IGF-I > IGF-II > insulin. Both subunits of the receptor are glycosylated, and are exposed on the external surface of the cell. The α-subunit contains the binding site for insulin or IGF-I; the β-subunit contains a transmembrane domain, an ATP binding site and a probable tyrosine autophosphorylation site. These findings are consistent with the observation that insulin and IGF-I can induce the phosphorylation of a tyrosine residue on the β-subunit of their own receptors as well as on exogenous protein substrates (20,21). Cloned cDNAs encoding for the entire 1370-1382 amino acid sequence of the human insulin receptor precursor have been identified and found to have significant sequence homology to the EGF receptor and to the src family of tyrosine-specific protein kinases (22,23). Nevertheless, the role(s) of phosphorylation in the biological actions of both insulin and IGF-I is still not established.

Studies performed with IGF-II have indicated the existence of a structurally and immunologically distinct receptor (type 2) (17,18). Following cross-linking and SDS-PAGE, this receptor migrates with an apparent Mr of 220,000 in the unreduced state and 250,000 following reduction, suggesting that it is a single-chain polypeptide with internal disulfide bridges. Binding of (125-I)-IGF-II to this receptor is preferentially displaced by IGF-II > IGF-I, but, unlike the type 1 receptor, the type 2 receptor has no affinity for insulin. Rather, insulin appears to activate the appearance of type 2 receptors on the cell surface (24). Although phosphorylation of the type 2 receptor in intact cells has been observed, and can be stimulated by the addition of IGF-II, this action could be mediated through the IGF-I receptor (25). At this time, there is still no definitive evidence for the type 2 receptor having intrinsic tyrosine kinase activity.

Studies employing biosynthetic or cell surface labeling have indicated that, in addition to the two major subunits ($Mr = 135,000$ and $95,000$) of the type 1 receptors, there exist two higher molecular weight bands of $Mr = 210,000$ and $190,000$ (26,27). Pulse-chase studies demonstrate that the $Mr = 190,000$ band is the earliest labeled component, followed by the appearance of the $Mr = 210,000$ band and the α- and β-subunits. Treatment of cells with monensin, which interferes with the biosynthesis of transmembrane and secretory proteins, blocks the appearance of the mature α- and β-subunits. Thus, the $Mr = 190,000$ component represents the high mannose precursor form of the insulin receptor, which normally undergoes carbohydrate processing to produce fully glycosylated $Mr = 210,000$ band, and then undergoes proteolytic cleavage to generate the α- and β-subunits. Jacobs et al. (27) have demonstrated similar maturational processing of the insulin and IGF-I receptors, although the putative precursors could be specifically immunoprecipitated by anti-insulin or anti-IGF-I receptor antibodies, indicating that the precursors for each receptor are distinct polypeptides.

Studies of the IGF-II receptor have indicated that the apparent molecular mass of the receptor in the absence of N-glycosylation is $232,000$, and that glycosylation is required for the acquisition of binding activity (28). The receptor is synthesized initially as a 245,000 Dalton precursor having 4-6 high-mannose oligosaccharide side chains. Mannose removal and terminal sialylation converts this precursor to the 250,000 Dalton functional receptor. Interestingly, recent immunohistochemical studies from our laboratory, employing polyclonal and monoclonal antibodies to the type 2 receptor, have demonstrated high receptor concentrations in the Golgi complex, a major site of terminal glycosylation and proteolytic processing (29).

The discovery of naturally occurring antireceptor antibodies has greatly aided investigation of insulin and IGF receptors, and has permitted researchers to attempt addressing the critical question of which receptor(s) mediates each metabolic and mitogenic action of insulin, IGF-I and IGF-II. Incubation of rat adipocytes and human fibroblasts with Fab fragments derived from such an antibody, resulted in a thirtyfold rightward shift of the dose-response for both insulin and multiplication-stimulating activity (MSA)-stimulated glucose oxidation, but no alteration in insulin- or MSA-stimulated DNA synthesis (12). It was concluded on this basis that the insulin receptor mediates the metabolic effects of both insulin and IGF, while the IGF receptor(s) mediates the mitogenic actions. However, the generality of these conclusions has been questioned in light of the observation that the authors did not investigate the effect of their antireceptor antibody on the type 1 IGF receptor, or on IGF-I action. Rosenfeld et al. (30) have demonstrated that serum from a patient with insulin-resistant diabetes simultaneously inhibits both insulin and IGF-I binding, a finding which has been confirmed for the majority of naturally occurring antireceptor antibodies (31). Studies by Conover et al. (32) have indicated that insulin stimulation of (3-H)-thymidine incorporation in human fibroblasts is, in fact, biphasic, with responses at insulin concentrations of 10-100 ng/ml apparently mediated through the insulin receptor, while responses at 1-100 μg/ml are mediated through the IGF-I receptor. Beguinot et al. (33) have suggested that IGF-I and -II stimulate glucose and amino acid uptake in L6 cells via interaction with their own receptors. Verspohl et al. (34) reached similar conclusions concerning IGF stimulation of glycogen synthesis in HEP-62 cells, while Yu and Czech (35) have concluded that the type 1 IGF receptor mediates the rapid effects of MSA on xylose and amino acid uptake in rat soleus muscle. Finally, in some cell lines, such as Reuber H-35 cells, insulin is capable of acting as a potent mitogen through its own receptor (36).

Due to limitations in the supply and specificity of antisera from insulin-resistant patients, recent efforts have turned to the development of monoclonal and polyclonal antibodies produced by immunization of animals with receptor preparations in various stages of purity (29,37-39). These antibodies are powerful probes of insulin and IGF receptor structure and function. Thus, a monoclonal antibody specific for the type 1 IGF receptor blocks IGF-I-stimulated DNA synthesis in human fibroblasts (40). Recent studies from our laboratory indicate that this antibody also inhibits IGF-II-stimulated DNA synthesis in these cells, and blocks the second phase of insulin-stimulated thymidine incorporation (41). Similar results have been recently reported by Flier et al. (42) and Van Wyk et al. (40), although some controversy persists over the role of the insulin receptor in the stimulation of DNA synthesis. Studies in H-35 hepatoma cells, employing a polyclonal antibody directed at the type 2 IGF receptor, have demonstrated that under conditions where IGF-II binding is inhibited 70-90%, no alteration in IGF-II stimulation of DNA synthesis is observed (43). These data suggest that the type 2 receptor may play little or no role in transmembrane signaling. Rather, it has been suggested that recycling of the type 2 receptor may be an essential role in the cellular degradation of IGF-II, and that this function is stimulated by insulin (24,44).

These data, however, leave unanswered the question as to what the biological roles of IGF-II and its receptor are. Several studies have suggested a specific role for IGF-II in fetal growth, since plasma levels are relatively high in the fetus and newborn, and since rat embryo fibroblasts synthesize large amounts of MSA (45,46). A second potential role for IGF-II is the regulation of cellular growth in the central nervous system and/or the pituitary. Specific receptors for both IGF-I and IGF-II have been identified throughout the rat and human CNS (47,48), as well as in the pituitary (49-51). Bassas et al. (52) have demonstrated that IGF receptors develop in chick embryo brain before insulin receptors, and may play a pivotal role in embryonic brain differentiation and growth. IGF-II, but not IGF-I, immunoreactivity has been identified throughout the human brain (53) as well as the cerebrospinal fluid (54). Recently, Recio-Pinto et al. (55) have reported that neurite outgrowth from chick embryo peripheral ganglion cells is stimulated by IGF-II at concentrations as low as 10 $_p$M, supporting a specific neuritogenic role for IGF-II.

SOMATOMEDIN RECEPTORS IN THE PITUITARY

Specific receptors for the insulin-like growth factors have been identified and characterized in three different pituitary models: (1) normal rat anterior pituitary cells (49,50), (2) human pituitary adenomas (51), and (3) cloned rat pituitary tumor cells (56). In each of these systems, specific high-affinity receptors for IGF-I and -II have been identified, suggesting a potential role for these peptides in the regulation of pituitary growth and function.

58

Normal Rat Pituitary Cells

Initial studies in primary cultures of rat anterior pituitary cells documented the presence of specific somatomedin receptors (49). Specific binding per 100,000 pituitary cells averaged 9.45% for 125-I-IGF-II, 0.83% for 125-I-IGF-I, and only 0.1% for 125-I-insulin. Similar results were reported by Goodyer et al. (50), employing membrane preparations from rat anterior pituitary. Specific binding of IGF-II was 3-5 times higher than that observed for IGF-I, with relatively low insulin binding.

Human Pituitary Adenomas

Specific receptors for insulin, IGF-I and IGF-II were identified in membrane preparations derived from four GH-secreting adenomas (51). Specific binding ranged from 3.3-9.4% per 100 μg protein for 125-I-insulin, from 2.5-9.7% for 125-I-IGF-I, and from 3.3-12.5% for 125-I-IGF-II. Displacement characteristics of each of these receptors was typical for classical insulin, IGF-I and IGF-II receptors.

Cloned Rat Pituitary Tumor Cells

Specific receptors for insulin, IGF-I, and IGF-II were identified on three separate cloned strains of rat pituitary tumor cells: GH_3, GH_1 and GC (56). Similar binding patterns for each peptide were identified in all three cell lines. Competitive binding experiments were consistent with the presence of three discrete high-affinity receptors. Affinity cross-linking studies confirmed the existence of both type 1 and type 2 receptors in these cells.

Significance of Pituitary Receptors for Insulin and IGF

Since hypothalamic-pituitary-end organ axes are frequently regulated by long-loop feedback homeostatic mechanism, it has been suggested that the IGFs might inhibit GH release from the pituitary in a manner similar to glucocorticoid inhibition of ACTH secretion. Studies by Berelowitz et al. (57) demonstrated that IGF-I inhibited both basal and (partially purified) growth hormone releasing factor (GRF)-stimulated GH release from cultured anterior pituitary cells. Additionally, IGF appeared to stimulate the release of somatostatin from hypothalamic tissue, suggesting the presence of an additional level of feedback control. Brazeau et al. (58) reported that both IGF-I and -II, at nanomolar concentrations, inhibit basal and stimulated GH ·secretion from cultured rat adenohypophyseal cells. Melmed and co-workers (59,60) have demonstrated that GH release from rat somatotropinoma cells could be inhibited by both insulin and IGF-I, and Ceda et al. (51) have demonstrated similar inhibition in short-term cultures of human pituitary adenomas. As demonstrated by Abe et al. (61) and Tannenbaum et al. (62), intracerebroventricular administration of IGF-I inhibits the release of GH from the anterior pituitary.

These studies have delineated a hormonal feedback function for the somatomedins, and possibly insulin, in the regulation of GH synthesis and secretion. While it is reasonable to assume that this feedback is mediated through specific insulin and/or IGF receptors, the specific receptor(s) involved has still not been definitively identified. Furthermore, although recent studies suggest that feedback may be regulated at the level of GH mRNA transcription, other sites of feedback control may exist. Thus, the precise role(s) of the IGFs and their receptors in the regulation of pituitary growth and function remains to be elucidated.

ACKNOWLEGMENTS

Supported in part by grants from the Juvenile Diabetes Foundation and by NIH grants AM-28229 and AM-36054. Dr. Rosenfeld is a recipient of a Research Career Development Award (AM-01275) from the NIH.

REFERENCES

1. Rosenfeld RG, Kemp SF, Hintz RL. Constancy of somatomedin response to growth hormone treatment of hypopituitary dwarfism, and lack of correlation with growth rate. J Clin Endocrinol Metab 1981; 53:611.

2. Clemmons DR, Van Wyk JJ, Ridgway EC, Kliman B, Kjellberg RN, Underwood LE. Evaluation of acromegaly by radioimmunoassay of somatomedin-C. N Engl J Med 1979; 301:1138.

3. Conover C, Dollar LA, Hintz RL, Rosenfeld RG. Insulin-like growth factor I/somatomedin-C (IGF-I/SM-C) and glucocorticoids synergistically regulate mitosis in competent human fibroblasts. J Cell Physiol 1983; 116:191.

4. Schoenle E, Zapf J, Humbel RE, Froesch ER. Insulin-like growth factor I stimulates growth in hypophysectomized rats. Nature 1982; 296:252.

5. Rinderknecht E, Humbel RE. The amino acid sequence of human insulin-like growth factor I and its structural homology with proinsulin. J Biol Chem 1978; 252:2769.

6. Rinderknecht E, Humbel RE. Primary structure of human insulin-like growth factor II. FEBS Lett 1978; 89:283.

7. Jansen M, Van Schaik FMA, Ricker AT, et al. Sequence of cDNA encoding human insulin-like growth factor I precursor. Nature 1983; 306:609.

8. Bell GI, Merryweather JP, Sanchez-Pescador R, et al. Sequence of a cDNA clone encoding human preproinsulin-like growth factor II. Nature 1984; 310:775.

9. Brissenden JE, Ullrich A, Francke U. Human chromosomal mapping genes for insulin-like growth factors I and II and epidermal growth factor. Nature 1984; 310:781.

10. Tricoli JV, Rall LB, Scott J, Shows TB. Localization of insulin-like growth factor genes to human chromosomes 11 and 12. Nature 1984; 310:784.

11. Hintz RL, Clemmons DR, Underwood LE, Van Wyk JJ. Competitive binding of somatomedin to the insulin receptors of adipocytes, chondrocytes, and liver membranes. Proc Natl Acad Sci USA 1972; 69:2351.

12. King GL, Kahn CR, Rechler MM, Nissley SP. Direct demonstration of separate receptors for growth and metabolic activities of insulin and multiplication-stimulating activity (an insulin-like growth factor) using antibodies to the insulin receptor. J Clin Invest 1980; 66:130.

13. Megyesi K, Kahn CR, Roth J, et al. Insulin and non-suppressible insulin-like activity (NSILA-s): evidence for separate plasma membrane receptor sites. Biochem Biophys Res Commun 1974; 57:307.

14. Marshall RN, Underwood LE, Viona SJ, Foushee DB, Van Wyk JJ. Characterization of the insulin and somatomedin-C receptors in human placental cell membranes. J Clin Endocrinol Metab 1974; 39:283.

15. Rosenfeld RG, Hintz RL. Somatomedin receptors: structure, function, and regulation. In: Conn PM, ed. The receptors; vol III. New York: Academic Press, Inc., 1986.

16. Pilch PF, Czech MP. The subunit structure of the high-affinity insulin receptor. Evidence of disulfide-linked receptor complex in fat cells and liver plasma membranes. J Biol Chem 1980; 255:1722.

17. Massague J, Czech MP. The subunit structure of two distinct receptors for insulin-like growth factors I and II. J Biol Chem 1982;

257:5038.

18. Kasuga M, Van Obberghen E, Nissley SP, Rechler MM. Demonstration of two subtypes of insulin-like growth factor receptors by affinity cross-linking. J Biol Chem 1981; 256:5305.

19. Chernausek SD, Jacobs S, Van Wyk JJ. Structural similarities between human receptors for somatomedin C and insulin: analysis by affinity labeling. Biochemistry 1981; 20:7345.

20. Kasuga M, Karlsson FA, Kahn CR. Insulin stimulates the phosphorylation of the 95,000-Dalton subunit of its own receptor. Science 1982; 215:185.

21. Jacobs S, Kull KC Jr, Earp HS, Svoboda ME, Van Wyk JJ, Cuatrecasas P. Somatomedin-C stimulates the phosphorylation of the B-subunit of its own receptor. J Biol Chem 1983; 258:9581.

22. Ullrich A, Bell JR, Chen EY, et al. Human insulin receptor and its relationship to the tyrosine kinase family of oncogenes. Nature 1985; 313:756.

23. Ebina Y, Ellis L, Jarnagin K, et al. The human insulin receptor cDNA: the structural basis for hormone-activated transmembrane signalling. Cell 1985; 40:747.

24. Wardzala LJ, Simpson IA, Rechler MM, Cushman SW. Potential mechanism of the stimulatory action of insulin on insulin-like growth factor II binding to the isolated rat adipose cell. J Biol Chem 1984; 259:8378.

25. Haskell JF, Nissley SP, Rechler MN, Sasaki N, Greenstein L, Lee L. Evidence for the phosphorylation of the type II insulin-like growth factor receptor in cultured cells. Biochem Biophys Res Commun 1985; 130:793.

26. Hedo JA, Kahn CR, Hayashi M, Yameda KM, Kasuga M. Biosynthesis and glycosylation of the insulin receptor. Evidence for a single polypeptide precursor of the two major subunits. J Biol Chem 1983; 258:10020.

27. Jacobs S, Kull FC Jr, Cuatrecasas P. Monesin blocks the maturation of receptors for insulin and somatomedin-C: identification of receptor precursors. Proc Natl Acad Sci USA 1983; 80:1228.

28. MacDonald RG, Czech MP. Biosynthesis and processing of the type II insulin-like growth factor receptor in H-35 hepatoma cells. J Biol Chem 1985; 260:11357.

29. Rosenfeld RG, Hodges D, Pham H, Lee PDK, Powell DR. Purification of the insulin-like growth factor II (IGF-II) receptor from an IGF-II-producing cell line, and generation of an antibody which both immunoprecipitates and blocks the type 2 IGF receptor. Biochem Biophys Res Commun 1986; 138(1):304-11.

30. Rosenfeld RG, Baldwin D Jr, Dollar LA, Hintz RL, Olefsky JM, Rubenstein A. Simultaneous inhibition of insulin and somatomedin-C binding to cultured IM-9 lymphocytes by naturally occurring anti-receptor antibodies. Diabetes 1981; 30:979.

31. Kasuga M, Sasaki N, Kahn CR, Nissley SP, Rechler MM. Antireceptor antibodies as probes of insulin like growth factor receptor structure. J Clin Invest 1983; 72:1459-69.

32. Conover CA, Hintz RL, Rosenfeld RG. Comparative effects of somatomedin C and insulin on the metabolism and growth of cultured human fibroblasts. J Cell Physiol 1985; 122:133.

33. Beguinot F, Kahn CR, Moses AC, Smith RJ. Distinct biologically active receptors for insulin, insulin-like growth factor I, and insulin-like growth factor II in cultured skeletal muscle cells. J Biol Chem 1985; 260:15892.

34. Versophl EJ, Roth RA, Vigneri R, Goldfine ID. Dual regulation of glycogen metabolism by insulin and insulin-like growth factors in human hepatoma cells (HEP-G2). Analysis with an anti-receptor monoclonal antibody. J Clin Invest 1984; 74:1436.

35. Yu K-T, Czech MP. The type I insulin-like growth factor receptor

mediates the rapid effects of multiplication stimulating activity on membrane transport systems in rat soleus muscle. J Biol Chem 1984; 259:3090.

36. Koontz JW. The role of the insulin receptor in mediating the insulin-stimulated growth response in Reuber H-35 cells. Mol Cell Biochem 1984; 58:139.

37. Roth RA, Cassell DJ, Wong KY, Madduz BA, Goldfine ID. Monoclonal antibodies to the human insulin receptor block insulin binding and inhibit insulin action. Proc Natl Acad Sci USA 1982; 79:7312.

38. Kull FC Jr, Jacobs S, Su Y-F, Svoboda ME, Van Wyk JJ, Cuatrecasas P. Monoclonal antibodies to receptors for insulin and somatomedin-C. J Biol Chem 1983; 258:6561.

39. Oka Y, Rozek LM, Czech MP. Direct demonstration of rapid insulin-like growth factor II receptor internalization and recycling in rat adipocytes. J Biol Chem 1985; 260:9435.

40. Van Wyk JJ, Graves DC, Casella SJ, Jacobs S. Evidence from monoclonal antibody studies that insulin stimulates deoxyribonucleic acid synthesis through the type I somatomedin receptor. J Clin Endocrinol Metab 1985; 61:639.

41. Conover CA, Misra P, Hintz RL, Rosenfeld RG. Effect of an anti-insulin-like growth factor I receptor antibody on insulin-like growth factor II and insulin stimulation of DNA synthesis in human fibroblasts. Biochem Biophys Res Commun 1986; 139(2):501-8.

42. Flier JS, Usher P, Moses AC. Monoclonal antibody to the type I insulin-like growth factor (IGF-I) receptor blocks IGF-I receptor-mediated DNA synthesis: clarification of the mitogenic mechanisms of IGF-I and insulin. Proc Natl Acad Sci USA 1986; 83:664.

43. Motolla C, Czech MP. The type II insulin-like growth factor receptor does not mediate increased DNA synthesis in H-35 cells. J Biol Chem 1984; 259:12705.

44. Oka Y, Mottola C, Oppenheimer CL, Czech MP. Insulin activates the appearance of insulin-like growth factor II receptors on the adipocyte cell surface. Proc Natl Acad Sci USA 1984; 81:4028.

45. Moses AC, Nissley SP, Short PA, et al. Increased levels of multiplication-stimulating activity, an insulin-like growth factor, in fetal serum. Proc Natl Acad Sci USA 1980; 77:3649.

46. Adams SO, Nissley SP, Greenstein LA, Yang YW-H, Rechler MM. Synthesis of multiplication-stimulating activity (rat insulin-like growth factor II) by rat embryo fibroblasts. Endocrinology 1983; 112:979.

47. Sara VR, Hall K, Von Holtz H, Humbel R, Sjogren B, Wettenberg L. Evidence for the presence of specific receptors for insulin-like growth factors I (IGF-I) and 2 (IGF-2) and insulin throughout the adult human brain. Neurosci Lett 1982; 34:39.

48. Sara VR, Hall K, Misaki M, Fryklund L, Christensen N, Wettenberg L. Ontogenesis of somatomedin and insulin receptors in the human fetus. J Clin Invest 1983; 71:1084.

49. Rosenfeld RG, Ceda G, Wilson DM, Dollar LA, Hoffman AR. Characterization of high affinity receptors for insulin-like growth factors I and II on rat anterior pituitary cells. Endocrinology 1984; 114:1571.

50. Goodyer CG, De Stephano L, Lai WH, Guyda HJ, Posner BI. Characterization of insulin-like growth factor receptors in rat anterior pituitary, hypothalamus and brain. Endocrinology 1984; 114:1187.

51. Ceda GP, Hoffman AR, Silverberg GD, Wilson DM, Rosenfeld RG. Regulation of growth hormone release from cultured human pituitary adenomas by somatomedins and insulin. J Clin Endocrinol Metab 1985; 60:1204.

52. Bassas L, De Pablo F, Lesniak MA, Roth J. Ontogeny of receptors for insulin-like peptides in chick embryo tissues: early dominance of insulin-like growth factors over insulin in brain. Endocrinology 1985; 117:2321.

53. Haselbacher GK, Schwab ME, Pasi A, Humbel RE. Insulin-like growth factor II (IGF-II) in human brain: regional distribution of IGF-II and of higher molecular mass forms. Proc Natl Acad Sci USA 1985; 82:2153.

54. Backstrom M, Hall K, Sara V. Somatomedin levels in cerebrospinal fluid from adults with pituitary disorders. Acta Endocrinol (Copenh) 1984; 107:171.

55. Recio-Pinto E, Rechler MM, Ishii DN. Effects of insulin, insulin-like growth factor-II, and nerve growth factor on neurite formation and survival in cultured sympathetic and sensory neurons. J Neurosci 1986; 6:1211.

56. Rosenfeld RG, Ceda G, Cutler CW, Dollar LA, Hoffman AR. Insulin and insulin-like growth factor (somatomedin) receptors on cloned rat pituitary tumor cells. Endocrinology 1985; 117:2008.

57. Berelowitz M, Szabo M, Frohman LA, Firestone S, Chu L, Hintz RL. Somatomedin-C mediates growth hormone negative feedback by effects on both the hypothalamus and the pituitary. Science 1981; 212:651.

58. Brazeau P, Guillemin R, King N, Van Wyk J, Humbel R. Inhibition by somatomedins of growth hormone secretion stimulated by hypothalamic growth hormone releasing factor (somatocrinin, GRF) or the synthetic peptide hpGRF. Computs Rende Acad Sci (Paris) 1982; 295:651.

59. Melmed S. Insulin suppresses growth hormone secretion by rat pituitary cells. J Clin Invest 1984; 73:1425.

60. Yamashita S, Melmed S. Insulin-like growth factor I action on rat anterior pituitary cells: suppression of growth hormone secretion and messenger ribonucleic acid levels. Endocrinology 1986; 118:176.

61. Abe H, Molitch ME, Van Wyk J, Underwood LE. Human growth hormone and somatomedin C suppress the spontaneous release of growth hormone in unanesthetized rats. Endocrinology 1983; 113:1319.

62. Tannenbaum GS, Guyda HJ, Posner BI. Insulin-like growth factors: a role in growth hormone negative feedback and body weight regulation via brain. Science 1983; 220:77.

7

THE MECHANISM OF THE GROWTH-PROMOTING ACTION OF GROWTH HORMONE

E. Martin Spencer,* Nicole Schlechter,[2] Sharon Russell,[2] and Charles Nicoll[2]

*Department of Medicine, Children's Hospital and University of California, San Francisco, CA, and [2]Department of Physiology/Anatomy, University of California, Berkeley, CA

INTRODUCTION

The mechanism of the growth-promoting action of growth hormone has been under investigation for many years. Freud et al. in 1939 found that in vivo administration of partially purified growth hormone preparations were able to increase the width of the tibial epiphysis (1). Ellis et al. in 1953 demonstrated that the stimulatory action of growth hormone was associated with an increase in the incorporation of sulfate into glycosaminoglycans (2). Although unable to elicit a direct stimulatory effect of growth hormone on sulfate incorporation into cartilage in vitro, Salmon and Daughaday in their 1957 pioneering discovery showed that there resided in serum a growth hormone-dependent activity, designated "sulfation factor," which possessed this property (3). They observed that the serum of hypophysectomized (hypox) rats contained very little sulfation activity, but serum from hypox rats treated with growth hormone contained increased amounts. Although the name sulfation factor was changed in 1972 to somatomedins, these observations were the birth of the somatomedin hypothesis: The growth-promoting effect of growth hormone is mediated by the somatomedins.

The somatomedin hypothesis was seemingly established by the failure of other researchers to elicit a direct action of growth hormone on cartilage or bone cells, and by the ability of somatomedins to stimulate growth in vivo in the absence of growth hormone (4-6). This led to an in-depth investigation of the biological properties of the somatomedins, their purification, elucidation of their amino acid sequence and genetic structure, and successful cloning.

SOMATOMEDINS

Nomenclature and Growth Hormone Dependence

The two principal human somatomedins were purified and sequenced by Rinderknecht and Humbel (7). Since they were homologous to insulin, and the somatomedin hypothesis had not been established, these peptides were named insulin-like growth factors, which is now used synonymously with somatomedins.

Somatomedin-C/insulin-like growth factor-I (SM-C/IGF-I) is a basic polypeptide with a molecular weight of approximately 7,500. It is somatomedin-C which is primarily responsible for growth hormone-dependent postnatal growth. The normal plasma level is 230 ± 70 (SD) ng/ml in adults; plasma levels are elevated in acromegaly and depressed in growth hormone deficiency (9-12). During human development, plasma levels of SM-C are low at birth, rise throughout childhood, and increase into the acromegalic range at puberty before falling to the normal adult value (10). Although growth hormone is the primary regulator of plasma levels of SM-C, other hormones can stimulate its production, e.g., estrogen, thyroxin, insulin, and platelet-derived growth factor (14).

The other identified somatomedin is a neutral polypeptide of approximately 7,300 molecular weight and is referred to as IGF-II (8). Originally, the neutral somatomedin was called somatomedin-A (SM-A), and thus IGF-II should be equivalent to SM-A. Although approximately 70% of the somatomedins in plasma are IGF-II (10), the purification procedures yield highly variable amounts of IGF-II in the neutral isoelectric region which is frequently contaminated with significant amounts of a deaminated form of SM-C/IGF-I (61; unpublished data; personal communications, Rinderknecht and Hintz et al.). Failure to appreciate these facts led Enberg et al. (15) to isolate from crude SM-A the deaminated form of SM-C/IGF-I instead of IGF-II, and then erroneously to equate SM-A to SM-C. Since the majority of somatomedins in plasma are neutral, the appropriate designation in somatomedin terminology logically should be SM-A/IGF-II which shall be used in this review. SM-A/IGF-II is weakly growth hormone dependent. The plasma level is normal in acromegaly but low in growth hormone deficiency. It may have a role in fetal growth, but thus far no role has been found postnatally (10,16-18).

Genetics

Knowledge of the amino acid sequence led to the identification of the genomic structure of both somatomedins. There is only one copy of each gene in the human genome (19-21,64). Rotwein has identified an alternate prepro form of SM-C generated by alternative splicing at the 5' end of the mRNA (22). This transcript has only been identified in fibroblast-conditioned media (personal communication, Clemmons). An alternate form of SM-A/ IGF-II has also been found, but the mechanism of its generation is unknown (62,63). Insulin and SM-A/IGF-II are adjacent on the 11th chromosome while SM-C/IGF-I is located on the 12th chromosome (23,24). It should be noted that both somatomedins are situated near ras oncogenes.

Insulin-like Activity

The basis of the insulin-like activity of the somatomedins is the 47% structural homology to insulin which confers essentially the same three-dimensional structure (7,8,25). Thus, the somatomedins are part of the insulin gene family. However, the growth factor gene could have been the primordial gene which duplicated and diverged during evolution.

The insulin-like activity can be demonstrated in vitro on isolated fat cells where somatomedins have about 1% of insulin's potency. Recently, free SM-C has been shown to dramatically lower blood sugar when given intravenously to rats and humans (27,28). The potency in both systems was 1/16th that of insulin on a molar basis but surprisingly more active than previously considered. The homology of somatomedins to insulin also explains why, at pharmacologic doses, insulin can act as a mitogen, since it can interact with type 1 somatomedin receptors (29,30).

Mitogenicity

Although bone has been considered the primary target tissue for somatomedins, these peptides are also mitogenic for a large variety of other endodermal, mesodermal and ectodermal cell types. Somatomedins exert their mitogenic effect on postnatal cells primarily, if not exclusively, by interacting with the type 1 somatomedin receptor (29,30). The action of somatomedins has been shown to be cell cycle specific for BALBc/3T3 cells and fibroblasts (31). Somatomedins stimulate DNA synthesis by acting at a restriction site in G1 phase of the cell cycle. The mitogenic effect can only be exerted on cells rendered competent by previous interaction with a competence factor, such as platelet-derived growth factor. The latter has been shown to regulate somatomedin receptors (32). The intracellular events triggered by the somatomedins are unknown.

Carrier Proteins

The somatomedins are unique in that, although polypeptide hormones, they are transported in plasma bound to a large molecular weight carrier protein (33,34). The free level of somatomedins has never been measured, but should be on the order of 1% of the total circulating peptide (bound and free). The carrier protein blocks the biologic activity of somatomedins after binding, but on dissociation they are still active (35-37). Binding prolongs the half-life of somatomedins from less than 1 hour to about 24 hours or more, and is thought to be responsible for the observed steady plasma levels. The principal function of the carrier protein has been thought to be the transport of somatomedins to their target tissues in an inactive form.

There appear to be two classes of plasma proteins that bind somatomedins. A large 150 kd protein carries almost all of the plasma somatomedins and is growth hormone dependent, being increased in acromegaly and decreased in growth hormone deficiency (33,39-42). This protein is composed of an acid stable binding subunit of approximately 40 kd. It has been suggested that the entire 150 kd carrier protein is made up of subunits of about 25 kd (43). The other type of binding protein which is also approximately 40 kd in size is present in human amniotic fluid, fetal, neonatal and adult serum, and is synthesized by BRL tumor cells (44-48). It is not growth hormone dependent, transports very little of the plasma somatomedins and appears to make up the majority of unsaturated somatomedin binding in plasma. A partial sequence is available (47). Antibody studies have indicated that the 40 kd binding proteins from the above-mentioned sources are either the same, or very closely related species, and different from the 150 kd protein or its acid stable subunit (48,49). Exogenously added labeled somatomedins react with the unsaturated 40 kd binding protein. In contrast, there is little exchange with the 150 kd complex, presumably because it has a higher affinity for somatomedins.

New Concepts of Carrier Protein Action

According to the somatomedin hypothesis, somatomedins are produced primarily in the liver and then transported in an inactive form to peripheral target tissues by the carrier protein where they are released and act (50). However, there is now substantial evidence that local tissue production of somatomedins is more important than hepatic production (51,52). Using DNA-RNA hybridization techniques, almost all cells of the body tested have been shown to express the somatomedin gene (53-55). (It remains to be determined in which cells somatomedin gene expression is growth hormone dependent, constitutive or regulated by other factors.) If somatomedins exert their action by autocrine and paracrine mechanisms rather than endocrine, it raises the question of whether the 150 kd carrier protein is actually transporting somatomedins to or from tissues. Its primary action may be to regulate the activity of free somatomedins at the cellular level by blocking their action on binding and then transporting them away for subsequent catabolism. The 40 kd binding protein, on the other hand, could have an entirely different function. It has recently been shown to potentiate the mitogenic activity of SM-C on smooth muscle cells and fibroblasts (58; personal communication, Clemmons).

MECHANISM OF GROWTH HORMONE ACTION

In spite of numerous failures by other investigators to obtain direct effects of growth hormone on cartilage, Isaksson et al. achieved unilateral tibial epiphyseal growth by direct injections of growth hormone (57). Russell and Spencer were able to repeat this work and also demonstrated that as little as 100 ng per day of SM-C for 4 days also stimulated epiphyseal growth (58). Schlechter et al. obtained this same result by continuous infusion of growth hormone and SM-C into the hind limbs of rats for 7 days (59). One interpretation of these results was that growth hormone stimulated epiphyseal growth by stimulating local production of SM-C at the epiphysis. This was suggested by previous studies of Bennington and Spencer who noted that growth hormone stimulated production of SM-C by epiphyseal chondrocytes (52). In their investigations the growth hormone deficient Little (lit/lit) mouse was injected with 50 μg of growth hormone daily for 7 days and a control group with the vehicle. After sacrifice, the epiphyses from both groups were stained for somatomedin production by the PAP (peroxidase-antiperoxidase) immunohistochemical procedure. Control mice showed no staining for SM-C; however, growth hormone-treated mice showed that large numbers of cells in the hypertrophic zone and in articular cartilage were positive for SM-C production.

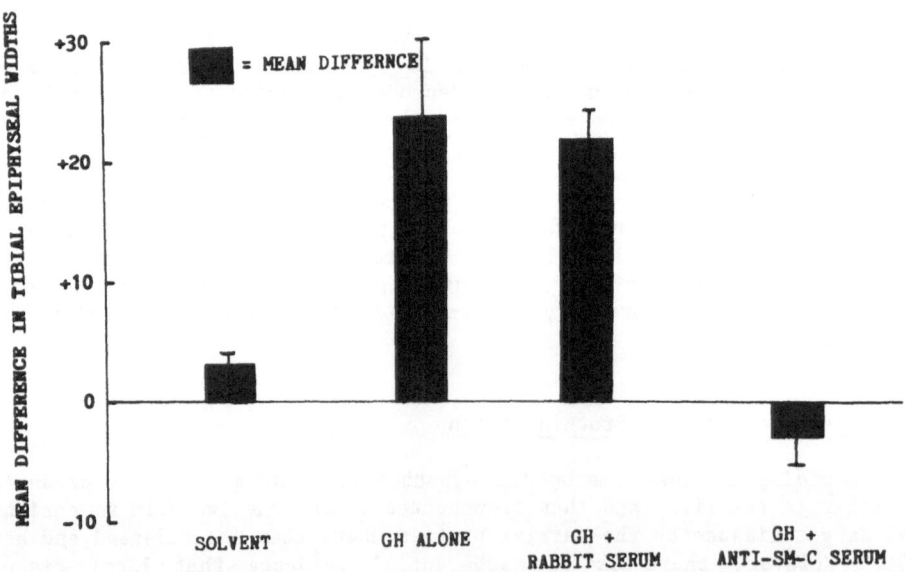

Fig. 1. The effect of somatomedin-C blocking action on the growth-promoting effect of growth hormone at the rat tibial epiphysis.

To establish that the "direct" growth-promoting action of growth hormone employed somatomedin as an intermediary, the right hind limbs of rats were perfused intraarterially for 7 days by Alzet Osmotic Minipumps (60). The substances infused were either saline, growth hormone, growth hormone plus normal rabbit serum or growth hormone plus SM-C antiserum. In all experiments the uninfused left limb was the control. The effect of growth hormone on epiphyseal width was blocked by coinfusion of anti-SM-C antiserum but not normal rabbit serum (Fig. 1). From these results we concluded that the direct growth-promoting action of growth hormone also requires SM-C as an intermediary.

ACKNOWLEDGMENT

This research was supported by N.I.H grant AM 35496.

REFERENCES

1. Freud J, Levie LH, Kroon DB. Observations on growth (chondrotrophic) hormone and localization of its point of attack. J Endocrinol 1939; 1:56-64.

2. Ellis S, Huble J, Simpson ME. Influence of hypophysectomy and growth hormone on cartilage sulfate metabolism. Proc Soc Exp Biol Med 1953; 84:603.

3. Salmon WD Jr, Daughaday WH. A hormonally controlled serum factor which stimulates sulfate incorporation by cartilage in vitro. J Lab Clin Med 1957; 49:825-36.

4. Holder AT, Preece MA, Spencer EM. Effect of bovine growth hormone and a partially pure preparation of somatomedin on various growth parameters in hypopituitary dwarf mice. J Endocrinol 1981; 89: 275-82.

5. Schoenle E, Zapf J, Humbel RE, Froesch ER. Insulin-like growth factor I stimulates growth in hypophysectomized rats. Nature 1982; 206:252-3.

6. Schoenle E, Zapf J, Froesch ER. Long-term in vivo effects of insulin-like growth factors (IGF) I and II on growth indices: direct evidence in favor of the somatomedin hypothesis. In: Spencer EM, ed. Insulin-like growth factors—somatomedins. New York: Walter De Gruyter, 1983:51.

7. Rinderknecht E, Humbel RE. The amino acid sequence of human insulin-like growth factor I and its structural homology with proinsulin. J Biol Chem 1978; 253:2769-76.

8. Gospodarowicz D, Bialecki H, Greenburg G. Purification of the fibroblast growth factor activity from bovine brain. J Biol Chem 1978; 253:3736-43.

9. Furlanetto RW, Underwood LE, Van Wyk JJ, D'Ercole AJ. Estimation of somatomedin-C levels in normals and patients with pituitary disease by radioimmunoassay. J Clin Invest 1977; 60:648-57.

10. Zapf J, Morell B, Walter H, Laron Z, Froesch ER. Serum levels of the insulin-like growth factor (IGF) and its carrier. Acta Endocrinol (Copenh) 1980; 95:507-17.

11. Spencer EM, Uthne E, Mims R. Somatomedin A levels measured by radioreceptor assay in acromegaly: relation to growth hormone levels. In: Giordano G, Van Wyk JJ, Minuto F, eds. Somatmedins and growth. London: Academic Press, 1979:335.

12. Underwood LE, D'Ercole AJ, Van Wyk JJ. Somatomedin-C and the assessment of growth. Pediatr Clin North Am 1980; 27:771.

13. Copeland KC, Johnson DM, Kuehl TJ, Castracane VD. Estrogen stimulates growth hormone and somatomedin-C in castrate and intact female baboons. J Clin Endocrinol Metab 1984; 58:698-703.

14. Clemmons DR, Shaw DS. Variables controlling somatomedin production by cultured human fibroblasts. J Cell Physiol 1983; 115:137-43.

15. Enberg G, Carlquist M, Jornvall H, Hall K. The characterization of somatomedin A isolated by microcomputer controlled chromatography reveals an apparent identity to insulin-like growth factor I. Eur J Biochem 1984; 143:117-24.

16. Moses AC, Nissley SP, Short PA, et al. Increased levels of multiplication-stimulating activity, and insulin-like growth factor, in fetal rat serum. Proc Natl Acad Sci USA 1980; 77:3649-53.

17. Adams SO, Nissley SP, Greenstein LA, Yang YW-H, Rechler M. Synthesis of multiplication-stimulating activity (rat insulin-like growth factor II) by rat embryo fibroblasts. Endocrinology 1983; 112:979-87.

18. Gavin JR III, Trivedi B. IGF-II receptor expression in developing tissues: models in vivo and in vitro. In: Spencer EM, ed. Insulin-like growth factors—somatomedins. New York: Walter De Gruyter, 1983:531.

19. Jansen M, van Schaik FMA, Ricker AT, et al. Sequence of cDNA encoding human insulin-like growth factor I precursor. Nature 1983; 306.

20. Dull TJ, Gray A, Hayflick JS, Ullrich A. Insulin like growth factor II precursor gene organization in relation to insulin gene family. Nature 1984; 310.

21. Bell GI, Merryweather JP, Sanchez-Pescador R, et al. Sequence of a cDNA clone encoding human preproinsulin-like growth factor II. Nature 1984; 310.

22. Rotwein P. Two insulin-like growth factor I messenger RNAs are expressed in human liver. Proc Natl Acad Sci USA 1986; 83:77-81.

23. Tricoli JV, Rall LB, Scott J, Bell GI, Shows TB. Location of insulin-like growth factor genes to human chromosomes 11 and 12. Nature 1984; 310:784.

24a Hoppener JWM, Pagter-Holthuizen P, van Kessel AHMG, et al. The human gene encoding insulin-like growth factor I is located on chromosome 12. Hum Genet 1985; 69:157-60.

24b Pagter-Holthuizen P, Hoppener JWM, Jansen M, van Kessel AHMG, van Ommen GJB, Sussenbach JS. Chromosomal localization and preliminary characterization of the human gene encoding insulin-like growth factor II. Hum Genet 1985; 69:170-3.

25. Blundell TL, et al. Insulin-like growth factor: a model for tertiary structure accounting for immunoreactivity and receptor binding. Proc Natl Acad Sci USA 1978; 75:180.

26. Nissley SP, Short PA, Rechler MM, Podskalny JM, Coon HG. Proliferation of buffalo rat liver cells in serum-free medium does not depend upon multiplication stimulating activity (MSA). Cell 1977; 11:441.

27. Valliant SW, Peters M, Finley S, Fagin K. Insulin-like growth factors I(THR59): hypoglycemic potency and pharmacokinetics in conscious rats [Abstract]. The Endocrine Society 68th Annual Meeting 1986:392.

28. Guler HP, Zenobi P, Zapf J, et al. IGF I and II and recombinant human (RH) IGF I are hypoglycemic in the rat, mini-pig and men. The Endocrine Society 68th Annual Meeting 1986:394.

29. Kasuga M, Van Obberghen E, Nissley SP, Rechler MM. Demonstration of two subtypes of insulin-like growth factor receptors by affinity cross-linking. J Biol Chem 1981; 256:5305-8.

30. Massague J, Czech MP. The subunit structures of two distinct receptors for insulin-like growth factors I and II and their relationship to the insulin receptor. J Biol Chem 1982; 257:5038-45.

31. Stiles CD, Capone GT, Scher CD, Antoniades HN, Van Wyk JJ, Pledger WJ. Dual control of cell growth by somatomedins and platelet derived growth factor. Proc Natl Acad Sci USA 1979; 76:1279-83.

32. Clemmons DR, Van Wyk JJ, Pledger WJ. Sequential addition of platelet factor and plasma to BALB/c 3T3 fibroblast cultures stimulates somatomedin-C binding early in cell cycle. Proc Natl Acad Sci USA 1980; 77:6644.

33. Hintz RL, Liu F. Demonstration of specific plasma protein binding sites for somatomedin. J Clin Endocrinol Metab 1977; 45:988.

34. Zapf J, Waldvogel M, Froesch ER. Binding of nonsuppressible insulin-like activity to human serum: evidence for a carrier protein. Arch Biochem Biophys 1975; 168:638.

35. Meuli C, Zapf J, Froesch ER. NSILA-carrier protein abolishes the action of nonsuppressible insulin-like activity (NSILA-S) on perfused rat heart. Diabetologia 1978; 14:255.

36. Zapf J, Schoenle E, Jagars G, Sand I, Grunwald J, Froesch ER. Inhibition of the action of nonsuppressible insulin-like activity on isolated rat fat cells by binding to its carrier protein. J Clin Invest 1979; 63:1077.

37. Knauer DJ, Smith GL. Inhibition of biological activity of multi-plication-stimulating activity by binding to its carrier protein. Proc Natl Acad Sci USA 1980; 77:7252-6.

38. Copeland KC, Johnson DM, Kuehl TJ, Castracane VD. Estrogen stim-ulates growth hormone and somatomedin-C in castrate and intact female baboons. J Clin Endocrinol Metab 1984; 58:698-703.

39. Furlanetto RW. The somatomedin-C binding protein: evidence for a heterologous subunit structure. J Clin Endocrinol Metab 1980; 51:12.

40. Hintz RL, Liu F, Rosenfeld RG, Kemp SF. Plasma somatomedin-binding proteins in hypopituitarism: changes during growth hormone therapy. J Clin Endocrinol Metab 1981; 53:100.

41. White RM, Nissley SP, Moses AC, Rechler MM, Johnsonbaugh RE. The growth hormone dependence of somatomedin-binding protein in human serum. J Clin Endocrinol Metab 1981; 53:49.

42. D'Ercole AJ, Willson DF, Underwood LE. Changes in the circulating form of serum somatomedin-C during fetal life. J Clin Endocrinol Metab 1980; 51:674.

43. Wilkins JR, D'Ercole AJ. Affinity-labeled plasma somatomedin-C/-insulin-like growth factor I binding proteins. J Clin Invest 1985; 75:1350-8.

44. Cochinov RH, Mariz IK, Hajek AS, Daughaday WH. Characterization of a protein in mid-term human amniotic fluid which reacts in the somato-medin-C radioreceptor assay. J Clin Endocrinol Metab 1977; 44:902.

45. Drop SLS, Kortleve DJ, Guyda HJ. Isolation of a somatomedin-binding protein from preterm amniotic fluid. Development of a radioimmuno-assay. J Clin Endocrinol Metab 1984; 59:899.

46. Drop SLS, Kortleve DJ, Guyda HJ, Posner BI. Immunoassay of a somato-medin-binding protein from human amniotic fluid levels in fetal, neonatal, and adult sera. J Clin Endocrinol Metab 1984; 59:908.

47. Povoa G, Enberg G, Jornvall H, Kerstin H. Isolation and characteri-zation of a somatomedin-binding protein from mid-term human amniotic fluid. Eur J Biochem 1984; 144:199-204.

48. Romanus JA, Terrell JE, Yang YW-H, Nissley SP, Rechler MM. Insulin-like growth factor carrier proteins in neonatal and adult rat serum are immunologically different: demonstration using a new radioim-munoassay for the carrier protein from BRL-3A rat liver cells. Endocrinology 1986; 118:1743-58.

49. Martin JL, Baxter RC. Antibody against acid-stable insulin-like growth factor binding protein detects 150,000 mol wt growth hormone-dependent complex in human plasma. J Clin Endocrinol Metab 1985; 61:799.

50. Spencer EM. The use of cultured rat hepatocytes to study the synthesis of somatomedin and its binding proteins. FEBS Lett 1979; 99:157.

51. D'Ercole AJ, Applewhite GT, Underwood LE. Evidence that somatomedin is synthesized by multiple tissues in the fetus. Dev Biol 1980; 75:315.

52. Bennington J, Spencer EM, Reber K. Immunoperoxidase localization of insulin-like growth factor-I containing tissues. In: Spencer EM, ed. Insulin-like growth factors—somatomedins. New York: Walter De Gruyter, 1983:563-70.

53. Lund PK, Hynes MA, Moats-Staats B, D'Ercole AJ, Jansen M, Van Wyk JJ. Somatomedin/insulin-like growth factor mRNAs in rat fetal, neonatal and adult tissues. The Endocrine Society 68th Annual Meeting 1986;251.

54. Perkins SN, Zangger I, Eberwine JH, et al. Tissue distribution of insulin-like growth factor I and insulin-like growth factor II messenger RNA. The Endocrine Society 68th Annual Meeting 1986;252.

55. Van Wyk JJ, Moats-Staats BM, Jansen M, Lund PK. Rat brain IFG-II mRNAs after hypophysectomy and growth hormone replacement. The Endocrine Society 68th Annual Meeting 1986;253.

56. Clemmons DR, Elgin RG, Han VKM, Casella SJ, D'Ercole AJ, Van Wyk JJ. Cultured fibroblast monolayers secrete a protein that alters the cellular binding of somatomedin-C/insulin-like growth factor I. J Clin Invest 1986; 77:1548-56.

57. Isaksson OGP, Jansson J-O, Gause IAM. Growth hormone stimulates longitudinal growth directly. Science 1982; 216:1237-9.

58. Russell SM, Spencer EM. Local injections of human or rat growth hormone or of purified human somatomedin-C stimulate unilateral tibial epiphyseal growth in hypophysectomized rats. Endocrinology 1985; 116:2583-7.

59. Schlechter NL, Russell SM, Greenberg S, Spencer EM, Nicoll CS. A direct growth effect of growth hormone in rat hindlimb shown by arterial infusion. Am J Physiol 1986; 250:231-5.

60. Schlechter NL, Russell SM, Spencer EM, Nicoll CS. Evidence that the direct growth-promoting effects of growth hormone on cartilage in vivo are mediated by local production of somatomedin. Proc Natl Acad Sci USA 1986; 83(20):7932-4.

61. Spencer EM, Ross M, Smith B. The identity of human insulin-like growth factors I and II with somatomedins C and A: homology with rat IGF I and II. In: Spencer EM, ed. Insulin-like growth factors—somatomedins. New York: Walter De Gruyter, 1983:563-70.

62. Jansen M, van Schaik FMA, van Tol H, van den Brande JL, Sussenbach JS. Nucleotide sequences of cDNAs encoding precursors of human insulin-like growth factor II (IGF-II) and an IGF-II variant. FEBS Lett 1985; 179:243-6.

63. Zapf J, Walter H, Froesch ER. Radioimmunological determination of insulinlike growth factors I and II in normal subjects and in patients with growth disorders and extrapancreatic tumor hypoglycemia. J Clin Invest 1981; 68:1321-30.

64. Whitefield HJ, Bruni CB, Frunzio R, Terrell JE, Nissley SP, Recher MM. Isolation of a cDNA clone encoding rat insulin-like growth factor-II precursor. Nature 1984; 312:277.

II. REGULATION OF GROWTH HORMONE SECRETION

8

SOMATOSTATIN AND THE SYNDROME OF ACROMEGALY

Richard J. Robbins, M.D.

Section of Neuroendocrinology
Yale University School of Medicine
New Haven, CT 06410

THE DISCOVERY OF SOMATOSTATIN

Regulation of pituitary growth hormone (GH) secretion by the hypo-thalamus was first suspected when it was clear that rodents who had lesions of the hypothalamus grew abnormally. That these lesions, which were designed to create "hypothalamic obesity," were resulting in a decrease in pituitary GH secretion was first suggested by Bogdanove and Lipner (1) in 1952. This possibility was directly confirmed by Reichlin (2) who demonstrated that full replacement of thyroid, gonadal, adrenal, and posterior pituitary hormones did not prevent the growth retardation induced by large medial basal hypothalamic lesions. After Franz and co-workers (3) reported that acetone/acetic acid extracts of porcine hypothalamus contained somatotrophic hormone releasing activity, a number of laboratories including those of Guillemin, McCann, Meites, Saffran, Schally, and Reichlin began an intensive search for this GH-releasing factor (GRF). During the search for this factor, Krulich et al. (4) noted that hypothalamic extracts also contained a GH release-inhibiting factor (Fig. 1), an observation later confirmed by Knobil et al. (5). In a similar fashion, Brazeau, Vale, and colleagues in the laboratory of Roger Guillemin, found a GH inhibitory activity inside fractions of ovine hypothalamic extracts (6,7) which were prepared for the search for GRF and which were used to isolate and identify the first hypothalamic releasing factor, TRH. The somatotropin release-inhibiting factor (SRIF) was isolated, sequenced, and found to be a tetradecapeptide which was named "somatostatin" (SS).

The publication of the primary sequence of somatostatin (SS-14) was quickly followed by the availability of synthetic peptide and, within one year, specific and sensitive radioimmunoassays were available. It became rapidly clear that this peptide was not unique to the hypothalamus as it was found in virtually every mammalian tissue (Fig. 2) (8,9) and that it had a long evolutionary history being present in plants (10) and unicel-lular organisms (11).

The GH inhibiting role of SS-14 soon lost its luster as the peptide was demonstrated to play an important role in regulating other pituitary hormones, islet hormones, gastrointestinal secretions, and to meet the criteria as a neurotransmitter in the central and peripheral nervous systems (12).

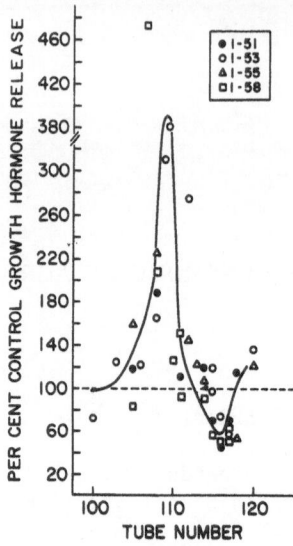

Fig. 1. Growth hormone-releasing
activity in ovine hypothalamic
extracts. Sephadex G-25 fractions
107-110 had GH-releasing activity;
fractions 116-118 had GH release
inhibitory activity. Reprinted
with permission from Krulich et
al., 1968 (4).

The earliest chromatographic separations of immunoreactive somatostatin (IRS) confirmed the bioassay data (13) that there were several
different molecular species of the peptide in the hypothalamus. Multiple
forms were also found in virtually every tissue which had appreciable IRS
content (9). The structure of one of these larger forms was found by
Pradayrol et al. (14) to consist of the tetradecapeptide with an additional 14 amino acids on the N-terminus, now designated somatostatin-28
(SS-28). In 1980 the structure of prosomatostatin was deduced from
anglerfish islet complementary DNA sequences (15,16). The structures of
both rat (17,18) and human (19) preprosomatostatins soon followed. Most
recently, the structure of the mammalian somatostatin gene has been
elucidated using recombinant DNA techniques by Montminy and co-workers
(20). Unlike fish, where at least two separate genes encode different IRS
species, mammals seem to have a single gene for the production of somatostatin. Therefore, SS-14 and SS-28 both arise from the same precursor,
and in some tissues SS-14 may arise from SS-28. The somatostatin gene is
1.2 kilobases in length and consists of one intervening sequence flanked
by two exons, the second of which contains the coding regions for both
SS-14 and SS-28 (20).

TISSUES CONTAINING SOMATOSTATIN CELLS

CENTRAL NERVOUS SYSTEM
    BASAL FOREBRAIN NUCLEII
    CEREBRAL CORTEX
    STRIATUM
    HIPPOCAMPUS
    AMYGDALA
    HYPOTHALAMUS
    MID-BRAIN NUCLEII
    SPINAL CORD

AUTONOMIC GANGLIA
RETINA
THYROID PARAFOLLICULAR CELLS
GASTROINTESTINAL MUCOSA
PANCREATIC ISLETS
POSTERIOR PITUITARY
SALIVARY GLANDS
ADRENAL MEDULLA
PLACENTA

Fig. 2. Tissues in which cell bodies containing
immunoreactive somatostatin have been identified.

Somatostatin alters the secretory activity of target cells, including somatotrophs, in several ways. The most well-established mechanism is via potent inhibition of cyclic AMP accumulation in response to secretagogues known to stimulate adenylate cyclase. The observations that somatostatin binding can be altered by guanine nucleotides and that its effects can be attenuated by pertussis toxin have led to the hypothesis that SS receptors in many cells interact with the inhibitory nucleotide regulatory subunit (N_i) of the adenylate cyclase complex (12).

SS also inhibits hormone secretion via cyclic AMP independent ion channel modulation. In several GH-producing cell lines SS lowers both basal and stimulated free cytosolic calcium levels (21,22). In pancreatic islet cells, Pace et al. (23) have demonstrated that SS can hyperpolarize cells by increasing K^+ conductances. Finally, it has recently been recognized that SS can dephosphorylate proteins which have been phosphorylated by the kinase activity of the EGF receptor (24). In summary, SS can interfere with hormone secretion by blocking the generation of "second messengers" such as cyclic AMP, calcium, and phosphorylation. The ability of a single agent to attack diverse and multiple secretory mechanisms explains the widespread tissue distribution and evolutionary conservation of this remarkable and versatile inhibitor.

SS can inhibit basal GH release as well as GH responses to exercise, sleep, meals, arginine, hypoglycemia, L-dopa, and GRF (12,25,26). The ability to lower GH levels in vivo could occur at multiple sites. Experiments performed in cultured pituitary cells demonstrate that somatotrophs respond directly to SS (7,27). It has further been documented that SS is released into the portal circulation in episodic bursts (28) and that SS withdrawal may be responsible, in part, for GH surges (29). GH inhibition by SS-28 seems to be of greater magnitude than that of SS-14 (30) although the existence of unique SS-28 receptors is still not unequivocally established.

SS receptors and responsiveness are present in several pituitary tumor cell lines. These include ACTH-producing AtT-20 cells (31), GH-producing GH_4C_1 (32) and GH_3 cells (22), and in nonendocrine tumor cells such as fibroma and HeLa cells (33).

Soon after the discovery of SS and its actions on GH secretion, it was administered to human volunteers. SS decreased basal GH levels as well as GH responses to arginine, L-dopa (34), and hypoglycemia (35). SS also blocked the sleep-associated GH surge (36,37) and exercise-induced GH secretion (38). Although direct effects on somatotrophs are a certainty, it is possible that SS may decrease GRF release (39). Effects of SS on GRF receptor levels, or on the action of GH to stimulate somatomedin production, require further investigation. Finally, in addition to its GH inhibiting role it has been suggested that full GH pulses seen in vivo may depend on SS withdrawal as much as on the pulsatile GRF release (29). Autoregulation of SS release by SS has been demonstrated to partially explain declines in SS secretory rates (40).

THE ROLE OF SOMATOSTATIN IN THE ACROMEGALY SYNDROME

Within months of the discovery and synthesis of pure SS-14 the peptide was administered to patients with acromegaly (35). Yen et al. (41) reported that SS also inhibited prolactin and insulin secretion in these patients and that a rebound GH surge occurred after the cessation of the SS infusion (Fig. 3). The hyperglycemia of acromegaly also diminished during SS-14 infusions (42). Several investigators reported that the GH-lowering effects of SS correlated with GH responses to dopamine agonists (43,44) and that individual responses to SS were highly variable. Pieters et al. (45) suggested that this variability was due to the presence of two subgroups of acromegalics (Fig. 4). The first of these consisted of individuals whose elevated GH levels could be returned to normal during an SS-14 infusion, associated with a rebound hypersecretion of GH after the end of the infusion. The second group consisted of acromegalics whose GH levels were resistant to suppression by SS-14. They also noted that LH-RH only caused a paradoxical rise in GH in Group 1 patients. These results confirmed earlier observations by Hanew et al. (46). Neither Pieters et al. (45) nor Lamberts et al. (47) found a good correlation between the GH suppression from SS and the GH suppression by dopaminergic agonists.

One source of variability in GH responses to SS may reside in the number or affinity of SS receptors on the neoplastic somatotrophs. Reubi and Landolt (48) were the first to demonstrate the presence of SS receptors on human somatotrophic tumors. When compared to other types of pituitary tumors, the SS receptors present in somatotrophic tumors had similar affinities (K_d in the 0.1 to 1 nM range) but they were present in much higher numbers (Fig. 5) (49,50). A negative correlation between plasma GH levels and the number of SS receptors may exist (49). This latter possibility could be due to high portal SS levels since GH is known to stimulate hypothalamic SS secretion (51) assuming receptor downregulation at the pituitary level. It is also possible that a subset of GH cells may lose the ability to express a functional SS receptor, thereby leading to excess GH secretion and acromegaly.

The recent development of a long-acting SS analog, SMS 201-995, by Sandoz resulted in a new series of clinical studies in acromegalics (52,53). The results of these studies are summarized in detail in other

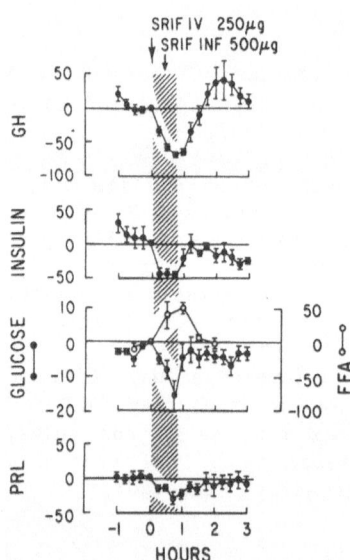

Fig. 3. Mean percent change in GH, prolactin, insulin, glucose, and free fatty acids in acromegalic patients during an infusion of SS-14. Reprinted with permission from Yen et al., 1974 (41).

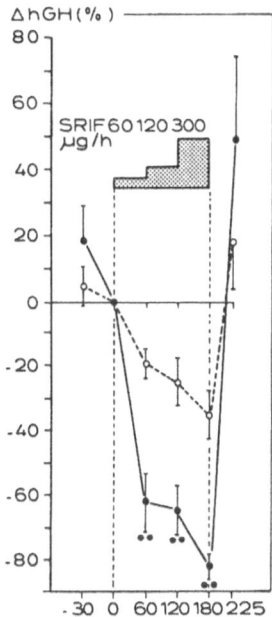

Fig. 4. Mean percent change in GH
levels in acromegalic patients
during an SS-14 infusion. Group 1
patients (closed circles) normalized their GH levels during the
infusion while Group 2 patients
(open circles) did not. Reprinted
with permission from Pieters et
al., 1982 (45).

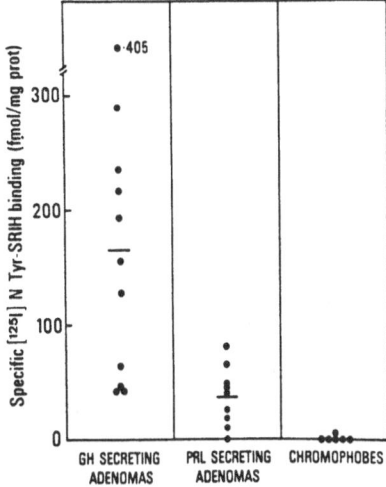

Fig. 5. Density of somatostatin
receptors on membranes of human
pituitary tumors. Horizontal
lines indicate mean values. Reprinted with permission from Moyse
et al., 1985 (49).

chapters in these proceedings. In addition to a direct effect on somato-trophs, SMS 201-995 has been shown to decrease GRF secretion from ectopic GRF-secreting tumors (54,55), although this same action has not been demonstrated in the hypothalamus. In certain patients, bromocriptine may augment the GH-lowering effects of SMS 201-995 (47).

The interesting possibility that a hypothalamic deficiency of SS may be responsible for some cases of acromegaly was raised by Besser et al. (42) soon after SS was shown to lower GH levels in acromegalics. Although peripheral and CSF somatostatin levels are not decreased in acromegaly (56), levels in the hypophyseal-portal circulation have not been measured in vivo.

REFERENCES

1. Bogdanove E, Lipner H. Intestinal absorption of glucose in hypotha-lamic obesity. Proc Soc Exp Biol Med 1952; 81:410.
2. Reichlin S. Growth and the hypothalamus. Endocrinology 1960; 67:760.
3. Franz J, Haselbach C, Libert O. Studies of the effect of hypotha-lamic extracts on somatotrophic pituitary functions. Acta Endocrinol (Copenh) 1962; 41:336.
4. Krulich L, Dhariwal A, McCann S. Stimulatory and inhibitory effects of purified hypothalamic extracts on growth hormone release from rat pituitary in vitro. Endocrinology 1968; 83:783.
5. Knobil E, Meyer V, Schally A. Hypothalamic extracts and the secre-tion of growth hormone in the rhesus monkey. In: Pecile A, Muller E, eds. Growth hormone. Amsterdam: Exerpta Medica Foundation, 1968:226.
6. Vale W, Brazeau P, Grant G, et al. Premieres observations sur le mode d'action de la somatostatine, un facteur hypothalamique qui inhibe la secretion de l'hormone de croissance. C R Acad Sci [III] (Paris) 1972; 275:2913.
7. Brazeau P, Vale W, Burgus R, et al. Hypothalamic polypeptide that inhibits the secretion of immunoreactive pituitary growth hormone. Science 1973; 179:77.
8. Brownstein M, Arimura A, Sato H, Schally A, Kizer J. The regional distribution of somatostatin in the rat brain. Endocrinology 1975; 96:1456.
9. Patel Y, Reichlin S. Somatostatin in hypothalamus, extra-hypotha-lamic brain and peripheral tissues of the rat. Endocrinology 1978; 102:523.
10. LeRoith D, Pickens W, Wilson G, et al. Somatostatin-like material is present in flowering plants. Endocrinology 1985; 117:2093.
11. Berelowitz M, LeRoith D, von Schenk H, et al. Somatostatin-like immunoreactivity and biological activity is present in tetrahymena pyriformis, a ciliated protozoan. Endocrinology 1982; 110:1939.
12. Reichlin S. Somatostatin. N Engl J Med 1983; 309:1495;1556.
13. Burgus R, Brazeau P, Vale W. Isolation and determination of the primary structure of somatostatin of ovine hypothalamic origin. In: Raiti S, ed. Advances in human growth hormone research. US DHEW, Government Printing Office, 1974:144.
14. Pradayrol L, Jornvall H, Mutt V, Ribet A. N-terminally extended somatostatin, the primary structure of somatostatin 28. FEBS Lett 1980; 109:55.
15. Hobart P, Crawford R, Shen L, Pictet R, Rutter W. Cloning and sequence analysis of cDNA encoding two distinct somatostatin precur-sors found in the endocrine pancreas of anglerfish. Nature 1980; 288:137.
16. Goodman R, Jacobs J, Chin W, Lund P, Dee P, Habener J. Nucleotide

sequence of a cloned structural gene coding for a precursor of pancreatic somatostatin. Proc Natl Acad Sci USA 1980; 77:5869.

17. Goodman R, Jacobs J, Dee P, Habener J. Somatostatin-28 encoded in a cloned cDNA obtained from a rat medullary thyroid carcinoma. J Biol Chem 1982; 257:1156.

18. Goodman R, Aron D, Roos B. Rat preprosomatostatin. J Biol Chem 1983; 258:5570.

19. Shen L, Pictet R, Rutter W. Human somatostatin I: sequence of the cDNA. Proc Natl Acad Sci USA 1982; 79:4575.

20. Montminy M, Goodman R, Horovitch S, Habener J. Primary structure of the gene encoding rat preprosomatostatin. Proc Natl Acad Sci USA 1984; 81:3337.

21. Schonbrunn A, Dorflinger L, Koch B. Mechanisms of somatostatin action in pituitary cells. Adv Exp Med Biol 1985; 188:305-24.

22. Schlegel W, Wuarin F, Wollheim C, Zahnd G. Somatostatin lowers the cytosolic free calcium concentration in clonal rat pituitary GH3 cells. Cell Calcium 1984; 5:223.

23. Pace C. Somatostatin: control of stimulus-secretion coupling in pancreatic islet cells. In: Bloom F, ed. Peptides: integrators of cell and tissue function. New York: Raven Press, 1980:163.

24. Hierowski M, Liebow C, duSapin K, Schally A. Stimulation by somato-statin of dephosphorylation of membrane proteins in pancreatic cancer MIA PaCa-2 cell line. FEBS Lett 1985; 179:252.

25. Brazeau P, Epelbaum J, Benoit R. Somatostatin: physiological studies and blood determinations. In: Collu R, Barbeau A, Ducharme J, Rochefort J, eds. Central nervous system effects of hypothalamic hormones and other peptides. New York: Raven Press, 1979:367.

26. Brazeau P, Ling N, Bohlen P, Esch F, Ying S, Guillemin R. Growth hormone releasing factor, somatocrinin releases pituitary growth hormone in vitro. Proc Natl Acad Sci USA 1982; 79:7909.

27. Cuttler L, Welsh J, Szabo M. The effect of age on basal, GRF stimu-lated, and cyclic AMP stimulated GH release from rat pituitary cells in monolayer culture. Endocrinology 1986; 119:152.

28. Kasting N, Martin J, Arnold M. Pulsatile somatostatin release from the median eminence of the unanesthetized rat and its relationship to plasma GH. Endocrinology 1981; 109:1739.

29. Kracier J, Cowan J, Sheppard M, Lussier S, Moor B. Effect of somato-statin withdrawal and GRF on GH release in vitro: amount available for release after disinhibition. Endocrinology 1986; 119:2047.

30. Tannenbaum G, Ling N, Brazeau P. Somatostatin-28 is longer acting and more selective than somatostatin-14 on pituitary and pancreatic hormone release. Endocrinology 1982; 111:101.

31. Morel G, Pelletier G, Heisler S. Internalization and subcellular distribution of radiolabeled somatostatin-28 in mouse anterior pituitary tumor cells. Endocrinology 1986; 119:1972.

32. Presky D, Schonbrunn A. Receptor-bound somatostatin and EGF are processed differently in GH4C1 rat pituitary cells. J Cell Biol 1986; 102:878.

33. Mascardo R, Sherline P. Somatostatin inhibits rapid centrosomal separation and cell proliferation induced by EGF. Endocrinology 1982; 111:1394.

34. Siler T, VandenBerg G, Yen S. Inhibition of growth hormone release in humans by somatostatin. J Clin Endocrinol Metab 1973; 37:632.

35. Hall R, Besser G, Schally A, et al. Actions of growth hormone release inhibitory hormone in healthy men and in acromegaly. Lancet 1973; 2:581.

36. Parker D, Rossman L, Siler T, Rivier J, Yen S, Guillemin R. Inhibi-tion of the sleep-related peak in physiologic human growth hormone release by somatostatin. J Clin Endocrinol Metab 1974; 38:496.

37. Besser G, Mortimer G, McNeilly A, et al. Long term infusion of

growth hormone release inhibiting hormone in acromegaly: effects on pituitary and pancreatic hormones. Br Med J 1974; 4:622.

38. Hansen AP, Orskov H, Seyer-Hansen K, Lundbaek K. Some actions of growth hormone release inhibiting factor. Br Med J 1973; 3:523.

39. Frohman L, Jansson J. Growth hormone releasing hormone. Endocr Rev 1986; 7:223.

40. Richardson S, Twente S. Inhibition of rat hypothalamic somatostatin release by somatostatin: evidence for somatostatin ultrashort feedback loop. Endocrinology 1986; 118:2076.

41. Yen S, Siler T, DeVane G. Effect of somatostatin in patients with acromegaly: suppression of GH, prolactin, insulin, and glucose levels. N Engl J Med 1974; 290:935.

42. Besser G, Mortimer G, Carr D, et al. Growth hormone release inhibiting hormone in acromegaly. Br Med J 1974; 1:352.

43. Dunn J, Donald R, Espiner E. A comparison of the effect of levodopa and somatostatin on the plasma GH, insulin, glucagon, and prolactin in acromegaly. Clin Endocrinol (Oxf) 1976; 5:167.

44. Oppizzi G, Botalla L, Verde G, Cozzi R, Liuzzi A, Chiodini P. Homogeneity in the GH lowering effect of dopamine and somatostatin in acromegaly. J Clin Endocrinol Metab 1980; 51:616.

45. Pieters G, Romeijn J, Smals A, Kloppenborg P. Somatostatin sensitivity and growth hormone responses to releasing hormones and bromocriptine in acromegaly. J Clin Endocrinol Metab 1982; 54:942.

46. Hanew K, Kokubun M, Sasaki A, Mouri T, Yoshinaga K. The spectrum of pituitary growth hormone responses to pharmacologic stimuli in acromegaly. J Clin Endocrinol Metab 1980; 51:292.

47. Lamberts S, Zweens M, Verschoor L, del Pozo E. A comparison among the GH lowering effects in acromegaly of the somatostatin analog SMS 201-995, bromocriptine, and the combination of both. J Clin Endocrinol Metab 1986; 63:16.

48. Reubi J, Landolt A. High density of somatostatin receptors in pituitary tumors from acromegalic patients. J Clin Endocrinol Metab 1984; 59:1148.

49. Moyse E, Le Dafniet M, Epelbaum J, et al. Somatostatin receptors in human growth hormone and prolactin secreting pituitary adenomas. J Clin Endocrinol Metab 1985; 61:98.

50. Ikuyama S, Nawata H, Kato K, Karashima T, Ibayashi H, Nakagaki H. Specific somatostatin receptors on human pituitary adenoma cell membranes. J Clin Endocrinol Metab 1985; 61:666.

51. Robbins R, Leidy J, Landon R. The effects of GH, prolactin, corticotropin, and thyrotropin on the production and secretion of somatostatin by hypothalamic cells in vitro. Endocrinology 1985; 117:538.

52. Plewe G, Beyer J, Krause U, Neufeld M, del Pozo E. Long acting and selective suppression of GH secretion by somatostatin analog SMS 201-995 in acromegaly. Lancet 1984; 2:782.

53. Lamberts S, Oosterom R, Neufeld M, del Pozo E. The somatostatin analog SMS 201-995 induces long acting inhibition of growth hormone secretion without rebound hypersecretion in acromegalic patients. J Clin Endocrinol Metab 1985; 60:1161.

54. von Werder K, Losa M, Stalla G, et al. Long term treatment of a metastasizing GRFoma with SMS 201-995 in a girl with gigantism. Scand J Gastroenterol 1986; 21(suppl 119):238.

55. Barkan A, Shenker Y, Grekin R, Vale W, Lloyd R, Beals T. Acromegaly due to ectopic GRF production: dynamic studies of GH and ectopic GRF secretion. J Clin Endocrinol Metab 1986; 63:1057.

56. Wass J, Penman E, Medbak S, Rees L, Besser G. CSF and plasma somatostatin levels in acromegaly. Clin Endocrinol (Oxf) 1980; 13:235.

9

GROWTH HORMONE SECRETION IN ACROMEGALY

Hiroo Imura, Yuzuru Kato, and Eiji Ishikawa

Department of Medicine, Kyoto University Faculty of
Medicine, Kyoto, and Department of Biochemistry
Miyazaki Medical College, Miyazaki, Japan

INTRODUCTION

Although striking clinical features of acromegaly had been noticed
for a long time, their association with hypersecretion of growth hormone
(GH) was first suggested by Cushing. Since then, many attempts have been
made to demonstrate an increase of GH in plasma from acromegalic patients.
Early studies using the tibia epiphyseal bioassay method revealed the
presence of growth-promoting factors in lyophilized plasma from acromegalic patients (1). It was difficult, however, to quantify plasma GH
levels using this bioassay method. The hemoagglutination inhibition assay
offered greater sensitivity but this procedure was still not satisfactory
for measuring the small amounts of GH present in plasma (2). More recently the sensitive and reliable measurement of plasma GH was made
possible by the introduction of a radioimmunoassay (RIA) for GH (3,4).
Since then, RIAs for GH have been extensively used for studying GH secretion in patients with acromegaly. In this article, we discuss GH secretion in acromegalic patients based on results obtained from studies
conducted in our laboratory as well as findings reported in the literature.

GH SECRETION UNDER PHYSIOLOGICAL CONDITION OR IN RESPONSE TO
PHYSIOLOGICAL STIMULI

Soon after the introduction of the RIA for GH, it became evident that
plasma GH levels fluctuated in response to a variety of stimuli. In
addition, studies on 24-hour profiles of plasma GH levels in normal
subjects revealed a pulsatile GH release pattern which appeared more
frequently during sleep and, particularly, in association with slow-wave
sleep (5). In acromegalic patients, plasma GH levels also show some
fluctuations, suggesting episodic secretion of GH from tumors (Fig. 1).
Although sleep-related GH release is not observed in acromegalic patients
(6), a broad increase, not related with slow-wave sleep, is seen in some
patients with acromegaly (Table 1). We observed also that bromocriptine
treatment lowered plasma GH levels more markedly during the waking state
than during sleep, as shown in Figure 1 (7). Higher GH levels during
sleep were seen even when bromocriptine was given immediately before sleep
(7). The reason for the elevated plasma GH levels during sleep in these
patients on bromocriptine treatment is still unknown.

Table 1. Plasma GH responses to physiological stimuli in acromegalic patients.

	No. of patients	Increase	No change	Decrease
Sleep	13	23%	77%	0%
Exercise	8	25	75	0
Glucose	36	11	89	0
Insulin	33	36	61	3
Arginine	28	29	71	0

Increase means the value more than 150% of the basal level. Decrease means the value less than 50%.

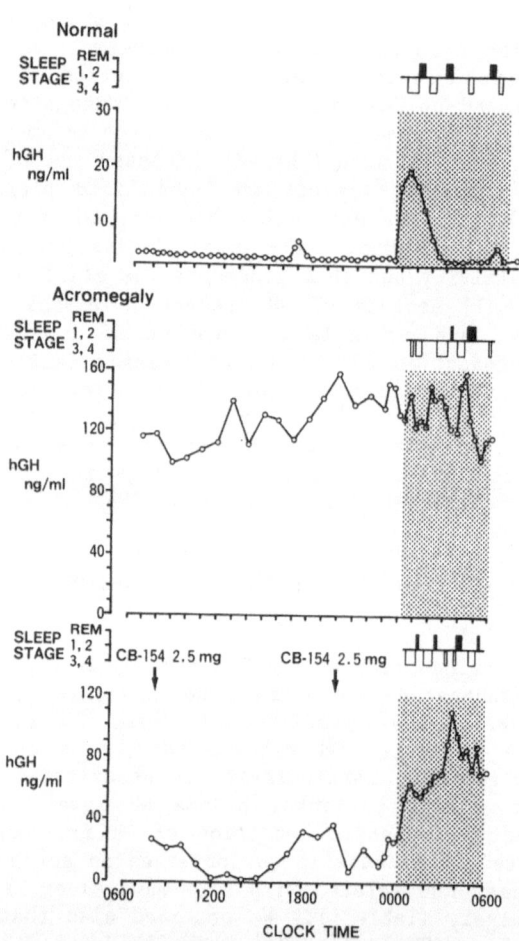

Fig. 1. Twenty-four-hour profile of plasma human GH (hGH) in a normal subject and in a patient with acromegaly before and during bromocriptine (CB-154) treatment.

It is well known that plasma GH levels change in response to "physiological" stimuli in some acromegalic patients. Table 1 shows results from studies in our series of patients. Exercise, which causes a rise in plasma GH in normal subjects, did not significantly increase plasma GH levels in most acromegalic patients, which coincided with previous findings (8). Oral or intravenous glucose administration, which lowers plasma GH in normal subjects, has been shown to cause no significant changes, a paradoxical increase, or even a decrease, in plasma GH in most acromegalic patients (9). Even in suppressed cases, however, plasma GH does not reach normal levels. Therefore, glucose loading test has been used as a useful tool in the diagnosis of acromegaly. In our series, plasma GH levels increased in response to either insulin-induced hypoglycemia or arginine infusion in approximately 30% of the patients studied (Table 1). This is consistent with previous observations (8,10,11). Those who responded to insulin-induced hypoglycemia tended to respond to arginine, although this ·was not not necessarily the case in our patients. These results suggest that GH-producing adenoma in acromegaly is not completely autonomous but is under the control of the hypothalamus to variable extents since insulin and arginine are considered to act through the central nervous system. This is consistent with observations that acromegalic patients respond to hypothalamic hormones as discussed in the following section.

GH SECRETION IN RESPONSE TO HYPOTHALAMIC HORMONES

Plasma GH Response to Nonspecific Hypothalamic Hormones

A paradoxical response of plasma GH to thyrotropin-releasing hormone (TRH) was first reported by Irie and Tsushima (12). In our series, 64% of the patients showed a rise of plasma GH which was greater than 150% of basal levels in response to TRH. The percentage of positive response was 70% in 460 patients reported by a collaborative study in Japan and 78% in patients collected from literature (13). Normalization of the TRH test following treatment seems to suggest the cure, whereas the positive response suggests the presence of residual tumor even if plasma GH falls to below 5 ng/ml (14,15). The absence of TRH responsiveness, however, does not necessarily mean the cure of the disease (13). The significance of TRH responsiveness after therapy, in terms of the relapse of acromegaly, must await further evaluation.

Luteinizing hormone-releasing hormone (LH-RH) also induces a paradoxical rise of plasma GH (16). The frequency of positive test is far less than that of TRH test, being 13% in our series and 28% in collected cases (460 patients) in Japan (Table 2). Corticotropin-releasing factor (CRF) induces less frequent positive response (17,18). Vasoactive intestinal polypeptide (VIP) is now considered to be a prolactin-releasing factor (19). We have observed that VIP stimulates GH release from GH-producing adenoma cells cultured in vitro (20), and further that the intramuscular injection of VIP raises plasma GH at least in some patients (Fig. 2) (21). Peptide with histidine and isoleucine (PHI) share the precursor with VIP and is known to release prolactin from the pituitary. In our observation, PHI also stimulated GH release from cultured adenoma cells obtained from acromegalic patients (22). Thus acromegalic patients respond to nonspecific hypothalamic peptide hormones to variable extents.

The mechanism responsible for paradoxical responses of plasma GH to hypothalamic hormones remains elusive. TRH, LH-RH, VIP and PHI stimulate GH release in cultured adenoma cells (20-23). In addition, we observed that TRH and/or LH-RH increased cyclic AMP content in adenoma cells in vitro, coinciding with plasma GH responses to TRH and/or LH-RH in vivo (24). These results suggest that paradoxical responses of plasma GH are

Table 2. Plasma GH responses to hypothalamic hormones in
patients with acromegaly.

	No. of patients	Increase	No change	Decrease
TRH	36	64%	36%	0%
LH-RH	32	13	87	0
CRF	7	0	100	0
VIP	6	33	67	0
GRF	20	80	20	0

Increase means the value more than 150% of the basal level.
Decrease means the value less than 50%.

related to intrinsic abnormalities of the tumor cells, possibly to altered
receptor mechanisms. Paradoxical responses of plasma GH to TRH and less
frequently to LH-RH are, however, observed in patients with nontumorous
disorders. Moreover, plasma GH responses to TRH are observed in patients
with growth hormone-releasing factor (GRF)-producing tumors (25). This
suggests that increased GRF secretion, which may exist also in acromegaly,
induces pituitary somatotroph dysfunction. Further studies are required
to elucidate the underlying mechanism which induces paradoxical GH responses.

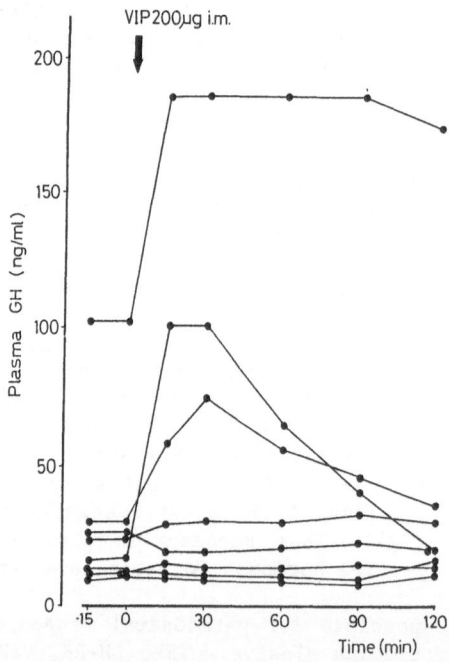

Fig. 2. Effects of a single intramuscular injection of 200 μg vasoactive intestinal polypeptide on plasma
GH levels in 8 acromegalic patients.

GH secretion from the pituitary is known to be under the dual control of hypothalamic hormones, an inhibiting factor, somatostatin, and growth hormone-releasing factor, GRF. It is well known that intravenous infusion of somatostatin causes a decrease in plasma GH to different extents in most acromegalic patients (26). The differential responses of plasma GH to somatostatin are reported to be related to variations in somatostatin receptors on adenoma cell membranes (27). Since the action of somatostatin is of short duration, a rebound rise is observed after the cessation of infusion. More recently, a potent, long-acting analog of somatostatin, SMS 201-995, has been introduced. The suppressive effect of SMS 201-995 is more long-lasting and not followed by a rebound rise of plasma GH (28). Thus, this long-acting analog has now been used successfully for the medical treatment of acromegaly.

GRF was first isolated from human pancreatic tumors and identified to be a 40 amino acid peptide or a 44 amino acid peptide amide. Synthetic peptides (GRF 1-40 and GRF 1-44 amide) are both bioactive and have provided a tool for studying the responsiveness of somatotrophs. A bolus injection of synthetic GRF is known to cause a significant increase in plasma GH in most acromegalic patients (29-31). Our results are shown in Figure 3, indicating that 80% of the patients studied showed a GH increase of more than 150% of the basal level, although the magnitude of the response varied widely. Plasma GH response to GRF significantly decreased following surgery. Although the magnitude of GH responses to GRF decreases with age in normal subjects, no significant relationship was found between age and GH responses in our series and previous studies (32,33). Plasma GH responses were also reported not to be related to basal GH levels nor sex. The reason for variable responses to GRF among different patients may be explained by different sensitivity of adenoma cells to GRF since variable responses to GRF were observed also in vitro (34). However, other factors such as endogenous somatostatin secretion and negative feedback by plasma GH or somatomedin must be considered also. In vitro studies using somatotroph adenoma cells have shown that GRF and somatostatin interact in regulating GH secretion (34). It appears, therefore, that in vivo GH secretion is also affected by both GRF and somatostatin in most acromegalic patients.

Plasma GH Responses to Dopaminergic Agents

Although L-dopa increases plasma GH in normal subjects, it was found to lower plasma GH levels in some patients with acromegaly (35). More potent dopaminergic agonist, bromocriptine, suppresses plasma GH levels in about half of the patients (36) and has been used for the treatment of acromegaly (37). In our series, 29% and 56% of the patients studied responded to L-dopa and bromocriptine, respectively (Table 3). Intravenous infusion of dopamine provides more clear-cut results, since plasma GH lowers below 50% of the basal level, followed by a rebound rise in responders (Fig. 4). The percentage of responders to dopamine (74%) was higher than those to L-dopa or bromocriptine in our series (Table 3). Such response to dopamine disappears following the successful treatment, indicating that the response to dopamine has become a marker of tumor like the response to TRH. The suppressive effect of dopamine given intravenously suggests that the site of action is in the pituitary. This is supported by the observation that dopamine inhibits basal GH release and the response to secretagogues in perifused pituitary adenoma cells in vitro (20,23). It is now generally accepted that dopamine is a major prolactin-inhibiting factor, acting directly on lactotrophs. Therefore, the decrease of plasma GH in response to dopaminergic agonists in acromegaly can be regarded as a type of paradoxical responses to hypothalamic hormones.

Unlike the action of dopamine agonists, the effect of dopamine antagonists on GH secretion in acromegaly is less consistent. In our series, haloperidol increased plasma GH only in 1 out of 7 patients, whereas chlorpromazine did not increase hormone levels (Table 3). Arosi et al. (38) reported that sulpiride, a dopamine antagonist, increased plasma GH while dopamine was infused. Since dopamine does not cross the blood-brain barrier, this observation suggests that sulpiride stimulates GH release from tumor cells in the presence of dopamine.

Interrelationships Between GH Responses to Various Secretagogues

It is of interest to know whether GH-producing adenomas can be divided into subgroups in terms of their responses to various hypothalamic hormones. If adenoma cells have membrane receptors similar to those of lactotrophs, they will respond to TRH and bromocriptine. In fact, Liuzzi et al. (39) reported that TRH and bromocriptine responders were concordant. Such concordance was not significant in our series or in the series of Tolis et al. (13) although there was a similar trend. Lamberts et al. (40) reported that bromocriptine suppressed plasma GH levels more markedly in patients with mixed GH/prolactin tumors than in pure GH tumors. In our series, however, there was no relationship between plasma prolactin levels and GH responses to either TRH or bromocriptine. Chiodini et al. (32) found an inverse correlation between the percentage of GH changes after GRF and after bromocriptine. They suggested that tumoral somatotrophs are sensitive to their specific releasing hormone and that adenoma cells with surface receptors similar to those on lactotrophs have lower sensitivity to GRF. Such a tendency was not significant in our series. Hanew et al.

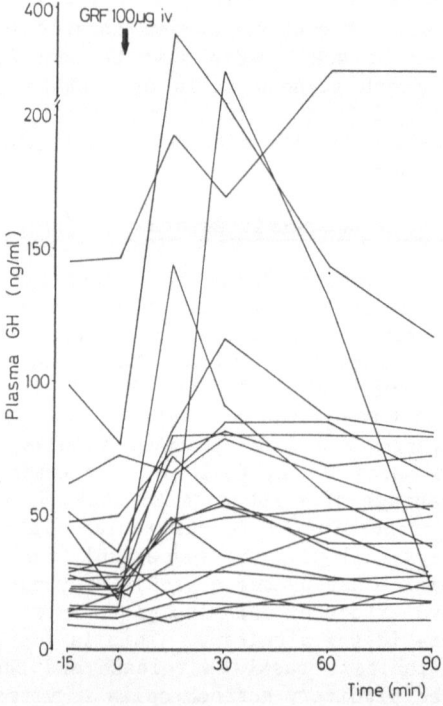

Fig. 3. Effects of an intravenous bolus injection of 100 μg growth hormone-releasing factor on plasma GH levels in 20 acromegalic patients.

Table 3. Plasma GH responses to antagonists or agonists of
putative neurotransmitters in patients with acromegaly.

	Normal	No.	Increase	No change	Decrease
			Acromegaly		
Haloperidol	Inhibit*	7	13%	75%	13%
Chlorpromazine	Inhibit*	12	0	90	10
L-dopa	Stimulate	28	7	64	29
Bromocriptine	Stimulate	34	6	38	56
Phentolamine	Inhibit*	12	0	33	67
Propranolol	Stimulate*	3	33	67	0
Cyproheptadine	Inhibit*	12	8	67	25

*Affect GH responses to a variety of stimuli.
Increase means the value more than 150% of the basal level.
Decrease means the value less than 50%.

(41) observed the presence of two subgroups in acromegaly, one sensitive to somatostatin as well as bromocriptine and TRH, and others less sensitive to these stimuli. Pieters et al. (42) confirmed the presence of two distinct subgroups characterized by different sensitivity to somatostatin. But the responses to TRH or bromocriptine were not parallel to somatostatin sensitivity. Although there are some acromegalic patients who do not respond to a variety of stimuli, it seems difficult to clearly distinguish subgroups in terms of the response to hypothalamic hormones.

GH SECRETION IN RESPONSE TO PUTATIVE NEUROTRANSMITTERS

GRF and somatostatin are released into the pituitary portal vessels from nerve terminals in the median eminence. This release is regulated by

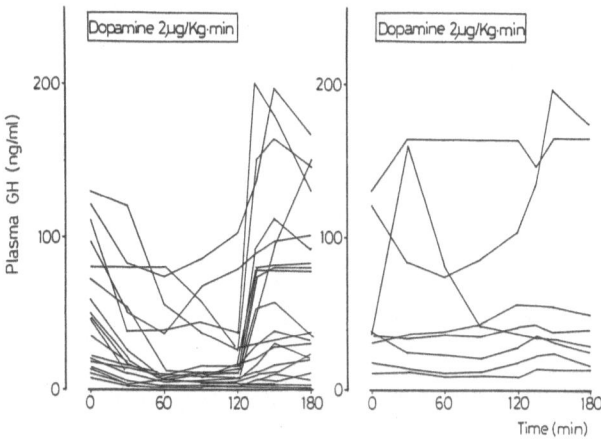

Fig. 4. Plasma GH changes during and after the intravenous infusion of dopamine (2.0 μg/kg body weight/min) in acromegalic patients. In 18 responders (left), plasma GH was lowered during the infusion followed by a rebound rise in hormone levels whereas the change was not significant in 8 nonresponders (right).

other neurons via the action of neurotransmitters. Several neurotransmitters are considered to be involved in the regulation of GH secretion, acting on either GRF or somatostatin neurons. The organization of neural circuits is, however, complex and not completely understood.

Opioid peptides are known to stimulate GH secretion in animals. A potent analog of enkephalin, FK-33-824, is known to stimulate GH secretion in man and this action is blocked by naloxone, a specific opiate antagonist. The administration of FK 33-824 into acromegalic patients failed to evoke GH release in our series of patients as reported by other investigators (43). The administration of naloxone alone lowered plasma GH in 2 of 10 acromegalic patients in our series (44), suggesting that endogenous opioid peptides may be involved in GH secretion in some acromegalic patients.

Noradrenergic and scrotoninergic mechanisms are known to be involved in GH secretion, possibly acting on GRF neurons. Although the central α-adrenoreceptor agonists, clonidine and guanfacine, raise plasma GH in normal subjects, these compounds elevate GH levels in only some acromegalic patients (45). On the other hand, phentolamine, an α-adrenoreceptor antagonist blunts plasma GH responses to secretagogues in normal subjects. This antagonist also lowers plasma GH in some acromegalic patients as shown in Table 3. A β-adrenoreceptor antagonist, propranolol, augments plasma GH responses to various secretagogues in normal subjects but increased plasma GH levels only in one-third of acromegalic patients tested (Table 3). Feely et al. (46) also reported a rise in plasma GH by propranolol in acromegalic subjects. These results suggest that an adrenergic mechanism may be involved in GH secretion in some acromegalic patients. The site of action of these drugs is assumed to be somewhere in the central nervous system but direct action on the pituitary cannot be ruled out at this time.

Serotonin is another monoamine that is involved in the regulation of GH secretion. A serotonin precursor, 5-hydroxytryptophan, stimulates GH secretion while the serotonin antagonists, cyproheptadine and methysergide, inhibit GH secretion in normal subjects. These agents do not significantly affect plasma GH levels in most acromegalic subjects, but we found that cyproheptadine suppressed GH levels in some patients (47). In addition, daily oral administration of cyproheptadine significantly lowered plasma GH levels in two acromegalic patients who did not respond to bromocriptine, as shown in Fig. 5 (47). It may act directly on the pituitary or at higher level centers in the central nervous system. The site of action of cyproheptadine is unknown. The former site seems to be important, since cyproheptadine was reported to inhibit GH release from cultured adenoma cells in vitro (48). Based on these results, it has been suggested that cyproheptadine may have a use in the treatment of acromegaly (Fig. 5). Another serotonin antagonist, metergoline, also inhibits GH secretion in certain patients but this effect has been ascribed to the dopamine agonist properties of this compound.

USE OF HIGHLY SENSITIVE IMMUNOASSAY FOR STUDYING GH SECRETION

The conventional RIA for GH is usually satisfactory for studying GH secretory dynamics in acromegaly. It is also useful in the diagnosis of acromegaly since almost all untreated patients have basal GH levels of greater than 5 ng/ml. However, a few untreated patients, and many treated patients, give values below 5 ng/ml. Such discrepancies are usually due to the limit of sensitivity of the assay. We have developed a sandwich enzyme immunoassay (EIA) using a polyclonal antihuman GH rabbit antibody as the solid phase-bound antibody and its Fab' fragment as the horseradish

Case 1

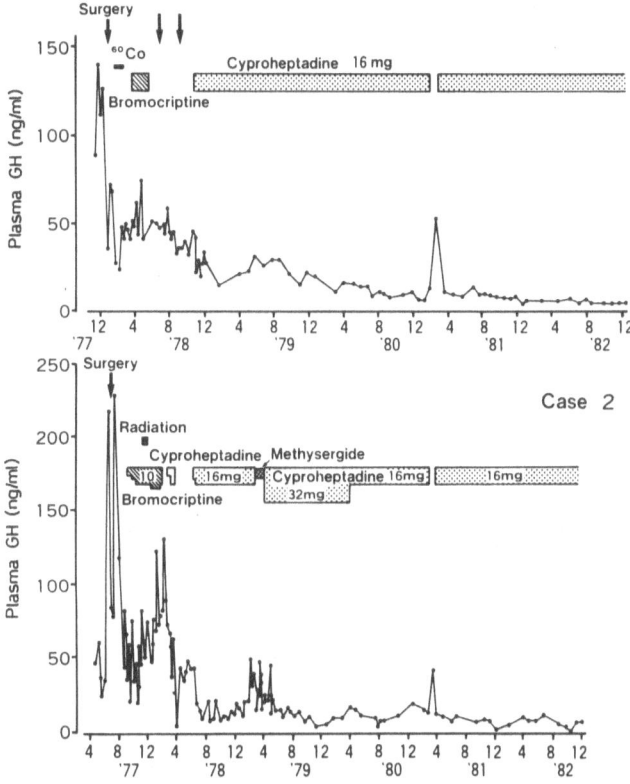

Fig. 5. Effect of daily administration of cyproheptadine (16–32 mg in 4 divided doses) on plasma
GH levels in 2 acromegalic patients in whom
surgery, radiation and bromocriptine only partially lowered plasma GH levels.

peroxidase-labeled second antibody (49). The minimal detectable limit of
this EIA was 60 fg/tube or 3 pg/ml. When blood was collected from normal
adults after an overnight fast and at resting state, plasma GH levels were
widely distributed between 50 pg/ml and 2 ng/ml (Fig. 6). Repeated blood
samplings over a period of 4 hours showed considerable fluctuations in
plasma GH levels (50). The wide distribution in plasma GH levels observed
during a single blood sampling period is likely due to such fluctuations.
Patients with untreated acromegaly gave values greater than 8 ng/ml, while
successfully-treated patients still showed values which were slightly
higher than normal subjects (Fig. 6). Such minor differences can only be
demonstrated using an adequately sensitive EIA.

SUMMARY

GH secretion in acromegaly is not completely autonomous; rather it is
partially regulated by a hypothalamic control mechanism(s). This is
evident from observations that circulating levels of GH respond to
insulin-induced hypoglycemia, arginine, somatostatin and GRF in at least
one-half of the patient population. Acromegalic patients show some
abnormal features in GH secretion, most notably, the lack of diurnal
variation and paradoxical responses to nonspecific hypothalamic hormones.
The latter phenomenon can be explained by an altered receptor mechanism on

tumorous somatotroph cells. However, other factors which contribute to the paradoxical GH responses must be considered. These include the continuous stimulation of somatotrophs possibly by hypothalamic GRF, disconnection from the central control mechanism and abnormalities in the hypothalamic control of GH secretion.

The pathogenesis of the pituitary GH-producing adenoma still remains obscure. It may result from either an intrinsic defect in the somatotrophs, or hypothalamic dysfunction leading to the increased GRF or decreased somatostatin secretion. In addition, if there are abnormalities in the central catecholaminergic mechanisms, GRF secretion may be altered, i.e., increased. The observation that dopaminergic agents lower plasma GH levels suggests a hypothalamic catecholaminergic defect. This can be explained, however, by speculating that tumorous somatotrophs have gained dopamine receptors, thus the hypothalamic effect is masked by direct action of dopamine on the pituitary. The lack of response to the opioid peptide, FK 33-824, may suggest hypothalamic dysfunction but again this may result as a consequence of pituitary GH hypersecretion. The present knowledge of GH secretion in acromegaly does not provide definite evidence to support either a primary pituitary defect or a hypothalamic lesion as the origin of this disorder.

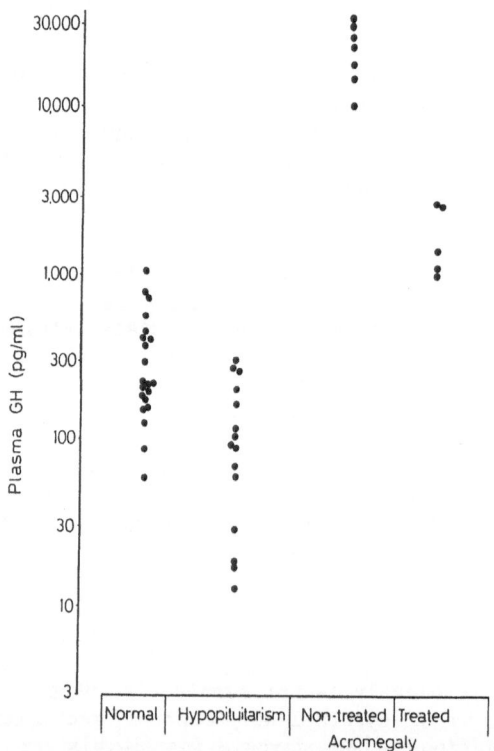

Fig. 6. Plasma GH levels in normal subjects and in patients with pituitary disorders. Growth hormone was measured by the highly sensitive enzyme immunoassay described above.

ACKNOWLEDGMENTS

The preparation of this article and the work presented were supported by grants from the Ministry of Education, Culture and Science, Japan, and the Ministry of Health and Welfare, Japan. We gratefully acknowledge the secretarial assistance of Ms. Y. Mitsuda and Ms. K. Kitamura in the preparation of this manuscript.

REFERENCES

1. Kinsell LW, Michaels GD, Li CH, Larsen WE. Studies in growth. I. Interrelationship between pituitary growth factor and growth-promoting androgens in acromegaly and gigantism. II. Quantitative evaluation of bone and soft tissue growth in acromegaly and gigantism. J Clin Endocrinol 1947; 8:1013.

2. Read CH, Bryan GT. The immunological assay of human growth hormone. Recent Prog Horm Res 1960; 16:187.

3. Utiger RD, Parker ML, Daughaday WH. Studies on human growth hormone. I. A radioimmunoassay for human growth hormone. J Clin Invest 1962; 41:254.

4. Glick SM, Roth J, Yalow RS, Berson SA. Immunoassay of human growth hormone in plasma. Nature 1963; 199:784.

5. Takahashi Y, Kipnis DM, Daughaday WH. Growth hormone secretion during sleep. J Clin Invest 1968; 47:2079.

6. Cryer PE, Daughaday WH. Regulation of growth hormone secretion in acromegaly. J Clin Endocrinol Metab 1969; 29:386.

7. Chihara K, Kato Y, Abe H, Furumoto M, Maeda K, Imura H. Sleep-related growth hormone release following 2-bromo-α-ergocriptine treatment in acromegalic patients. J Clin Endocrinol Metab 1977; 44:78.

8. Lawrence AM, Goldfine ID, Kirstein L. Growth hormone dynamics in acromegaly. J Clin Endocrinol Metab 1970; 31:239.

9. Glick SM, Roth J, Yalow RS, Berson SA. The regulation of growth hormone secretion. Recent Prog Horm Res 1965; 21:241.

10. Hartog M, Gaafar MA, Meisser B, Fraser TR. Immunoassay of serum growth hormone in acromegalic patients. Br Med J 1964; 2:1229.

11. Beck P, Schalch DS, Parker ML, Kipnis DM, Daughaday WH. Correlative studies of growth hormone and insulin plasma concentrations with metabolic abnormalities in acromegaly. J Lab Clin Med 1965; 66:366.

12. Irie M, Tsushima T. Increase in serum GH after TRH injection in patients with acromegaly and gigantism. J Clin Endocrinol Metab 1972; 35:97.

13. Tolis G, Koutsilieris M, Bertrand G. Endocrine diagnosis of growth hormone-secreting pituitary tumors. In: Black PM, et al., eds. Secretory tumors of the pituitary gland. New York: Raven Press, 1984.

14. Faglia G, Paracchi A, Ferrari C, Beck-Peccoz P. Evaluation of the results of transsphenoidal surgery in acromegaly by assessment of the growth hormone response to thyrotropin-releasing hormone. Clin Endocrinol (Oxf) 1978; 8:373.

15. Watanabe M, Kuwayama A, Nakane T, et al. Long-term growth hormone responses to nonspecific hypothalamic hormones in acromegalic patients. Surg Neurol 1985; 24:449.

16. Faglia G, Beck-Peccoz P, Travaglini P, Paracchi A, Spada A, Lewin A. Elevations in plasma growth hormone concentration after luteinizing hormone-releasing hormone (LHRH) in patients with active acromegaly. J Clin Endocrinol Metab 1973; 37:338.

17. Tanaka K, Watanabe T, Yoshida H, Shimizu N. Effect of synthetic ovine corticotropin-releasing factor on growth hormone secretion in patients with acromegaly. Endocrinol Jpn 1984; 31:353.

18. Pieters GFFM, Hermus ARMM, Smals AGH, Kloppenborg PWC. Paradoxical responsiveness of growth hormone to corticotropin-releasing factor in acromegaly. J Clin Endocrinol Metab 1984; 58:560.

19. Kato Y, Matsushita N, Ohta H, Tojo K, Shimatsu A, Imura H. Regulation of prolactin secretion. In: Imura H, ed. The pituitary gland. New York: Raven Press, 1985.

20. Matsushita N, Kato Y, Katakami H, Shimatsu A, Yanaihara N, Imura H. Stimulation of growth hormone release by vasoactive intestinal polypeptide from human pituitary adenoma in vitro. J Clin Endocrinol Metab 1981; 53:1297.

21. Kato Y, Shimatsu A, Matsushita N, Ohta H, Imura H. Role of vasoactive intestinal polypeptide (VIP) in regulating the pituitary function in man. Peptides 1984; 5:389.

22. Kato Y, Shimatsu A, Matsushita N, et al. Regulation of pituitary hormone secretion by VIP and related peptides. In: Labrie F, Proulx L, eds. Endocrinology. Amsterdam: Elsevier Science Publishers, 1984.

23. Ishibashi M, Yamaji T. Direct effects of catecholamines, thyrotropin-releasing hormone and somatostatin on growth hormone and prolactin secretion from adenomatous and nonadenomatous human pituitary cells in culture. J Clin Invest 1984; 73:66.

24. Matsukura S, Kakita T, Hirata Y, et al. Adenylate cyclase of GH and ACTH producing tumors of human: activation by non-specific hormones and other bioactive substances. J Clin Endocrinol Metab 1977; 44:392.

25. Thorner MO, Perryman RL, Cronin MJ, et al. Successful treatment of acromegaly by removal of a pancreatic islet tumor secreting a growth hormone releasing factor. J Clin Invest 1982; 70:965.

26. Hall R, Besser GM, Schally AV, et al. Action of growth-hormone-release inhibitory hormone in healthy men and in acromegaly. Lancet 1973; 2:581.

27. Ikuyama S, Nawata H, Kato K, Ibayashi H, Nakagaki H. Plasma growth hormone responses to somatostatin (SRIH) and SRIH receptors in pituitary adenomas in acromegalic patients. J Clin Endocrinol Metab 1986; 62:729.

28. Lamberts SWJ, Oosterom R, Nenfeld M, del Pozo E. The somatostatin analog SMS 201-995 induces long-acting inhibition of growth hormone secretion without rebound hypersecretion in acromegalic patients. J Clin Endocrinol Metab 1985; 60:1161.

29. von Werder K, Muller OA, Hartl R, Losa M, Stalla GK. Growth hormone releasing factor (hpGRF)-stimulation test in normal controls and acromegalic patients. J Endocrinol Invest 1984; 7:185.

30. Wood SM, Ch'ng JLC, Adams EF, et al. Abnormalities of growth hormone release in response to human pancreatic growth hormone releasing factor (GRF[1-44]) in acromegaly and hypopituitarism. Br Med J 1983; 286:1687.

31. Shibasaki T, Shizume K, Masuda A, et al. Plasma growth hormone response to growth hormone-releasing factor in acromegalic patients. J Clin Endocrinol Metab 1984; 58:215.

32. Chiodini PG, Liuzzi A, Pallabonzana D, Oppizzi G, Verde GG. Changes in growth hormone (GH) secretion induced by human pancreatic GH releasing hormone-44 in acromegaly: a comparison with thyrotropin-releasing hormone and bromocriptine. J Clin Endocrinol Metab 1985; 60:48.

33. Gelato MC, Marrian GR, Vance ML, et al. Effects of growth hormone-releasing factor on growth hormone secretion in acromegaly. J Clin Endocrinol Metab 1985; 60:255.

34. Ishibashi M, Yamaji T. Effects of hypophysiotropic factors on growth hormone and prolactin secretion from somatotroph adenomas in culture. J Clin Endocrinol Metab 1985; 60:985.

35. Liuzzi A, Chiodini PG, Botalla L, Cremascolli G, Silvestrini F.

Inhibitory effect of L-dopa on GH release in acromegalic patients. J Clin Endocrinol Metab 1972; 35:951.

36. Camanni F, Massara F, Belforte L, Molinatti GM. Changes in plasma growth hormone levels in normal and acromegalic subjects following administration of 2-bromo-α-ergocryptine. J Clin Endocrinol Metab 1975; 40:363.

37. Besser GM, Thorner MO, Wass JAH, et al. Bromocriptine treatment of acromegaly. Q J Med 1976; 45:695.

38. Arosi M, Moriondo P, Tranaglini P, et al. Modifications in serum growth hormone concentration induced by sulpiride in acromegalic patients pretreated with dopamine, bromocriptine and metergoline. J Clin Endocrinol Metab 1980; 51:454.

39. Liuzzi A, Chiodini PG, Botalla L, Silvestrini F, Muller EE. Growth hormone (GH)-releasing activity of TRH and GH-lowering effect of dopaminergic drugs in acromegaly: homogeneity in the two responses. J Clin Endocrinol Metab 1974; 39:871.

40. Lamberts SWJ, Klijn JGM, van Vroonhoven CCJ, Stefanko SZ, Liuzzi A. The role of prolactin in the inhibitory action of bromocriptine on growth hormone secretion in acromegaly. Acta Endocrinol (Copenh) 1983; 103:446.

41. Hanew K, Kokubun M, Sasaki A, Mouri T, Yoshinaga K. The spectrum of pituitary growth hormone responses to pharmacological stimuli in acromegaly. J Clin Endocrinol Metab 1980; 51:292.

42. Pieters GFFM, Romeijn JE, Smals AGH, Kloppenborg PWC. Somatostatin sensitivity and growth hormone responses to releasing hormones and bromocriptine in acromegaly. J Clin Endocrinol Metab 1982; 54:942.

43. Demura R, Suda T, Wakabayashi I, et al. Plasma pituitary hormone responses to the synthetic enkephalin analog (FK 33-824) in normal subjects and patients with pituitary diseases. J Clin Endocrinol Metab 1981; 52:263.

44. Kato Y, Katakami H, Imura H. Role of neuropeptides in the control of growth hormone secretion in man and rats. In: Shizume K, Takano K, eds. Growth and growth factors. Tokyo: University of Tokyo Press, 1980.

45. Lamberts SWJ, Klijn JGM, van Vroonhoven LCJ, Stefanko SZ. Different responses of growth hormone secretion to guanfacine, bromocriptine, and thyrotropin-releasing hormone in acromegalic patients with pure growth hormone (GH)-containing and mixed GH/prolactin-containing pituitary adenomas. J Clin Endocrinol Metab 1985; 60:1148.

46. Feely J. Beta-adrenoreceptor-blocking drugs, growth hormone and acromegaly. Postgrad Med J 1980; 56:230.

47. Kato Y, Kabayama Y, Ohta H. Effective long-term treatment with cyproheptadine of patients with acromegaly [Abstract]. 65th Annual Meeting of the Endocrine Society, San Antonio, TX, 1983.

48. Ishibashi M, Fukushima I, Yamaji T. Cyproheptadine-mediated inhibition of growth hormone and prolactin release from pituitary adenoma cells of acromegaly and gigantism in culture. Acta Endocrinol (Copenh) 1985; 109:474.

49. Ishikawa E, Hashida S, Kakogawa K, Ohtaki S. Human growth hormone. In: Bergmeyer HU, ed. Methods of enzymatic analysis. 3rd ed. Weinheim FRG: VCH Verlagsgesellschaft, 1986.

50. Hashida S, Nakagawa K, Ishikawa E, Ohtaki S. Basal level of human growth hormone (hGH) in normal serum. Clin Chim Acta 1985; 151:185.

10

ACTIONS OF GRF IN MAN

Michael O. Thorner, Mary Lee Vance, William S. Evans,
Alan D. Rogol, Jean S. Chitwood, Robert M. Blizzard,
Georgeanna Jones Klingensmith, Jennifer Najjar, Ian Burr,
Seymour Reichlin, Patricia Smith, Charles Brook, Richard
Furlanetto, Kalman Kovacs, Jean Rivier, and Wylie Vale

University of Virginia Medical School, Charlottesville,
VA (MOT, MLV, WSE, ADR, JSC, RMB), The Children's Hospital
and The University of Colorado School of Medicine, Denver,
CO (GJK), Vanderbilt University School of Medicine,
Nashville, TN (JN, IB), Tufts New England Medical Center,
Boston, MA (SR), The Middlesex Hospital, London, England
(PS, CB), Children's Hospital of Philadelphia, Philadel-
phia, PA (RF), Department of Pathology, St. Michael's
Hospital, Toronto, Ontario, Canada (KK), and The Clayton
Foundation Laboratories for Peptide Biology, The Salk
Institute, San Diego, CA (JR, WV)

INTRODUCTION AND HISTORICAL PERSPECTIVE

In 1980 we investigated a 21-year-old woman with Turner's syndrome,
acromegaly, and hyperprolactinemia (1). A head CT scan revealed an
enlarged pituitary gland but no discreet pituitary adenoma was detected.
It was assumed that she had a growth hormone-secreting adenoma and she
subsequently underwent transsphenoidal surgery. After surgery she was not
cured of her acromegaly. The surgical specimen was sent to Dr. Kalman
Kovacs and he astutely diagnosed somatotroph hyperplasia and not a pituitary adenoma. At about this time, a paper by Dr. Frohman and colleagues
appeared describing the partial characterization of a GH-releasing factor
(GRF) from peripheral tumors which also caused acromegaly (2). Based on
this information and the pituitary histology, a search was then made for
an ectopic GRF source which may have resulted in somatotroph hyperplasia.
A CT scan of the abdomen revealed a 5 cm tumor in the tail of the pancreas. The tumor was resected and preserved under ideal conditions for
possible extraction, isolation and characterization of GRF. The bulk of
the tumor was sent to Drs. Wylie Vale and Jean Rivier at the Salk Institute; portions were also sent to several other investigators in the
hope of establishing a cell line which secreted GRF. Within a few weeks
(September 1981) Vale and Rivier had demonstrated that this tumor contained a GRF peptide which had similar chromatographic characteristics to
GRF activity from rat hypothalamic extract. About this time, Dr. F.
Zeitin, who was able to culture cells from our tumor, moved to the Laboratories for Neuroendocrinology at the Salk Institute. She requested
permission to take the tissue, which had been sent by us to Dr. Tashjian,
with her from Boston to Dr. Roger Guillemin at the Laboratories for

Neuroendocrinology. Permission was granted. Additionally, the remaining tissue we had was also sent to Dr. Guillemin. Within a few weeks the amino acid composition of GRF was obtained by Dr. Guillemin and colleagues (3). Dr. Vale then provided Dr. Guillemin with half (approximately 7 grams) of the tumor which we had sent him. In the summer of 1982, the structure of GRF was obtained by Dr. Vale and his group from our tumor and by Dr. Guillemin and his group from a tumor from a patient in France and from our tumor (4,5,6). The Charlottesville tumor contained only GRF (1-40)-OH while the French tumor contained 3 peptides, 60% in the form of GRF(1-40), 20% as GRF(1-44)-NH$_2$ and 20% as GRF(1-37)-OH. Subsequently, 2 groups, those of Gubler and colleagues at the Roche Institute and Mayo and colleagues at the Salk Institute, obtained cDNA probes using messenger RNA from the French and Charlottesville tumors, respectively (7,8). Mayo and colleagues then used this probe to characterize the single copy GRF gene on human chromosome 20 and demonstrated that the gene consisted of 10 kilo bases containing 5 exons (9). The third exon coded for GRF 1-31 which is the biologically-active portion of the molecule since GRF 1-29 contains full biologic potency.

The characterization and sequencing of human GRF and its subsequent synthesis resulted in a new era in the study of GH secretion. The necessary permissions to administer GRF to humans were obtained after toxicologic studies were performed. GRF was first administered by us to man on December 2, 1982. The results of the first study (Fig. 1) demonstrated that GRF-stimulated GH secretion in normal young men after a single intravenous dose of 1 μg/kg (10). However, the amplitude of the GH response was variable among subjects. This has been observed in all subsequent studies performed by us and by all other investigators. We next explored the effect of varying the dose of GRF. Although 1 μg/kg gave the maximum peak response, higher doses led to a prolongation in the stimulation of GH release (11).

We next administered GRF to adults who had been GH-deficient during childhood (12). Of the 12 subjects studied only 4 had a small GH response

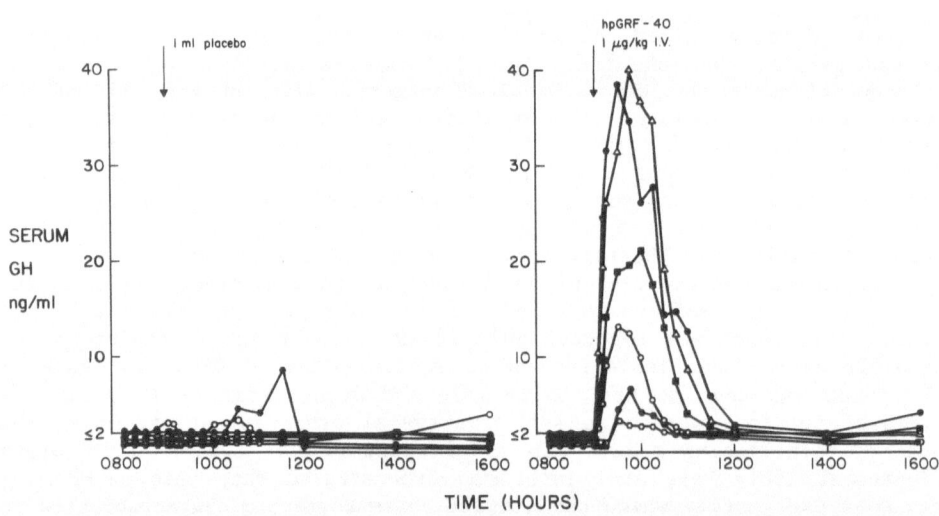

Fig. 1. Serum GH before and after placebo (left panel) and GRF-40 (right panel) in 6 normal men. Each symbol represents an individual patient. Note the variability of response among the subjects. (Reprinted with permission from Thorner et al., 1983.)

to GRF. However, 8 of 10 had an increase in serum somatomedin-C levels 24 hours after GRF administration. Six of these subjects were then given repeated GRF injections (0.3 µg/kg every 3 hours intravenously over 5 days). This resulted in an increase in somatomedin-C levels in all 6 subjects which suggested that GRF was able to stimulate sufficient GH release to raise somatomedin-C levels to normal (13).

A minority of children with short stature are GH-deficient. In GH-deficient children it was important to determine whether these children had a pituitary abnormality or a hypothalamic neurosecretory defect which resulted in the inability to release GH because of lack of stimulation by GRF. We studied 40 children with short stature by administering a single intravenous GRF dose (14). The results (Fig. 2 and 3) demonstrate that children with constitutional delay (CD) of growth and adolescence, and children with intrauterine growth retardation (IUGR) had GH responses to GRF which were similar to those of normal adults. Children with isolated GH deficiency were also studied; a few had no response to GRF, but the majority responded in a similar manner to that of normal adults. Growth hormone-deficient children with an organic lesion (usually a hypothalamic tumor) who had previously been treated (surgery and/or irradiation) had the smallest GH responses to GRF. We believe that this is likely a result of pituitary damage from the prior therapy.

Further studies in normal subjects were also conducted. Continuous intravenous infusions of GRF were administered. There was an acute stimulation of GH release which was not sustained through the 6 and 24 hours of infusions (15,16). At the end of a 6-hour infusion a supramaximal dose of GRF was administered; a smaller GH response occurred as compared with the response to the bolus after a 6-hour placebo infusion. In contrast, when the subjects became hypoglycemic from insulin at the end of a 6-hour GRF infusion, an augmented GH response occurred (17). We interpreted these data to indicate that the pituitary clearly was not depleted of GH by the GRF infusion (if depletion occurred, then hypoglycemia would not have caused an augmented GH response). Additionally, it is likely that insulin-induced hypoglycemia increased GH secretion not only by releasing GRF but also by possibly stimulating the release of another GH-releasing factor, or by suppression of hypothalamic somatostatin secretion. Continuous 24-hour GRF infusions resulted in an augmentation in the pulsatile pattern of GH secretion observed during placebo infusion; a monophasic increase in GH release did not occur.

These observations and the extensive and elegant studies in the rat performed by Tannenbaum and colleagues (18) suggest that pulsatile GH secretion is mediated by pulsatile GRF secretion in concert with intermittent withdrawal of hypothalamic somatostatin secretion. Unfortunately, this question cannot be directly addressed in the rat except by portal blood collection which requires both pituitary extirpation and anesthesia. However, the circumstantial evidence is very supportive of this hypothesis (Fig. 4).

In addition to these infusions in normal subjects, we also measured GRF and GH levels every 20 minutes in a patient with ectopic GRF secretion (16). It is to be noted that in this patient, GRF levels were greater than 5 ng/ml throughout the 24-hour period (Fig. 5). In spite of this, growth hormone secretion was pulsatile which indicated that presumably another factor must be involved in producing pulsatile GH secretion. In our infusion studies, we found that a minimum plasma level of 300 pg/ml of GRF was necessary to stimulate growth hormone secretion. Therefore, this patient's pituitary was exposed to supramaximal levels of GRF at all times.

From the preliminary results of GRF administration to children with short stature, it appeared unlikely that many GH-deficient children suffered from a primary pituitary problem. Therefore, the administration of GRF might be expected not only to increase GH release, but also to increase linear growth. We considered this to be the most important question, i.e., would GRF stimulate growth in GH-deficient children? After the necessary studies in normal subjects were performed, and after obtaining permission from the Food and Drug Administration, we initiated a program to treat GH-deficient children with GRF. Since the majority of healthy children have approximately 8 pulses of GH throughout a 24-hour period, we elected to administer GRF every 3 hours in an attempt to stimulate pituitary GH secretion approximately 8 times over 24 hours. The intravenous administration of GRF was not practical. Based on information of subcutaneous and intranasal GRF dose response studies in normal men, we observed that approximately 30 times the intravenous dose was required via the subcutaneous route (3 µg/kg) to reliably stimulate GH release in nor-

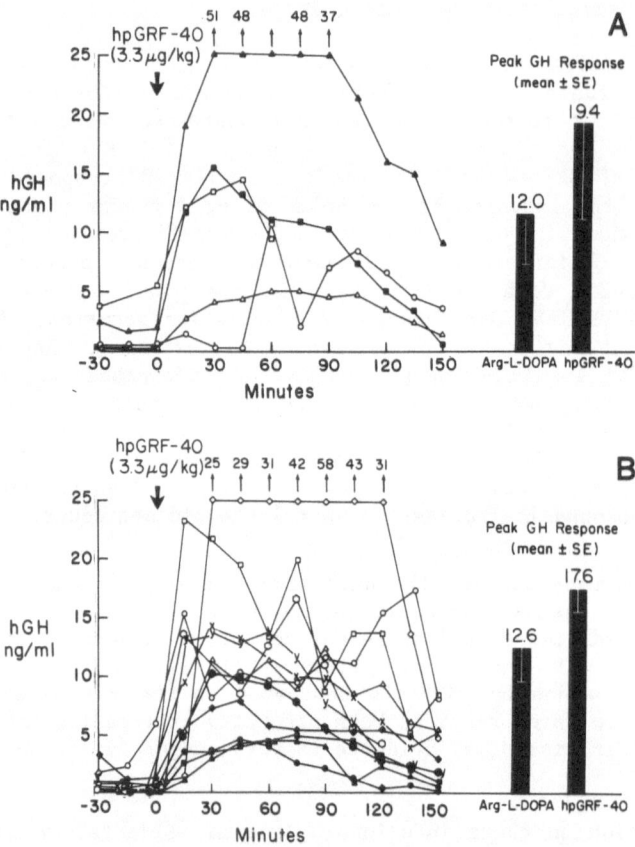

Fig. 2. GH release in response to GRF-40 in children with short stature. Each symbol represents an individual patient. (A) IUGR; (B) CD and/or familial short stature. Bars at the right of each panel are the mean ± SEM of the peak GH responses to the arginine/L-dopa and GRF-40. (Reprinted with permission from Rogol et al., 1984 [14].)

mal adults. We selected the dose of 1-3 μg/kg GRF by the subcutaneous route for therapy which was administered by an automated pump (PULSAMAT, courtesy Ferring, Inc., New Jersey); 12 children were treated for at least 6 months. Our results in the first two children were encouraging (20). The average growth velocity of the 12 children increased from a mean ± SEM of 2.8 ± .41 cm per year to 8.9 ± .75 cm per year. In collaboration with Drs. Patricia Smith and Charles Brook in London, an additional 10 children received subcutaneous GRF every 3 hours by pump overnight only. The growth velocity in these children increased from 3.5 ± .31 to 5.9 ± .45 cm per year and 2 children did not respond. We have also treated 5 children with twice daily subcutaneous GRF injections. All 5 children have had acceleration in growth with this treatment.

These results suggest that GRF is efficacious not only in stimulating GH secretion, but also in increasing growth velocity in GH-deficient children. The optimal dose, route of administration and frequency of administration has yet to be determined.

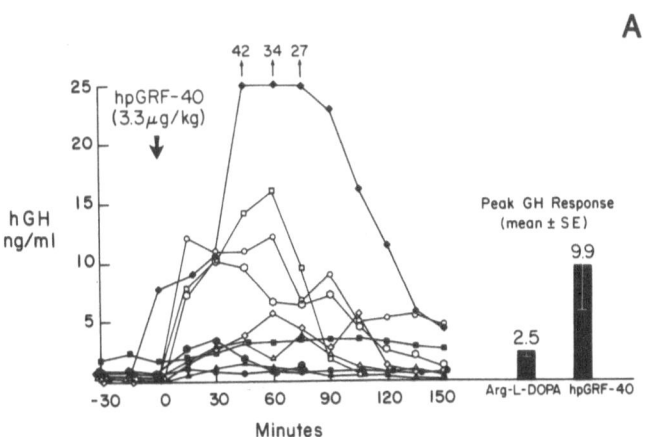

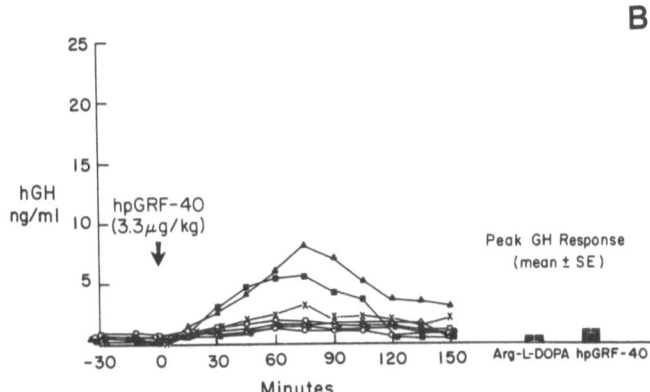

Fig. 3. GH release in response to GRF-40 in children with short stature. Each symbol represents an individual patient. (A) IGHD; (B) organic hypopituitarism. Bars at the right of each panel are the mean ± SEM of the peak GH responses to the arginine/L-dopa and GRF-40. (Reprinted with permission from Rogol et al., 1984 [14].)

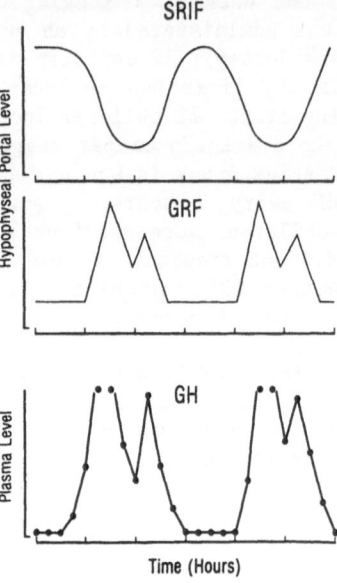

Fig. 4. Schematic representation
of the postulated rhythmic secretion of SRIF and GRF with the net
result on GH secretion. (Reprinted with permission from Tannenbaum
et al., 1984 [18].)

The results of 6 and 24 hours of continuous administration of GRF in
normal subjects over 24 hours suggest that prolonged exposure to GRF can
sustain and augment pulsatile GH secretion. The next step in determining
whether a depot preparation of GRF might have therapeutic potential
involved administration of GRF by continuous infusion to 5 normal men over
two weeks. Each subject received 10 ng/kg/min intravenously. Prior to
the GRF infusion, basal serum somatomedin-C was measured and GH secretion
was monitored by sampling every 20 minutes for 24 hours. Serum somatomedin-C levels were measured at intervals over the 14-day infusion and
over the 14 days following discontinuation. Growth hormone levels were
measured on days 0, 14 and 28 every 20 minutes for 24 hours. There was a

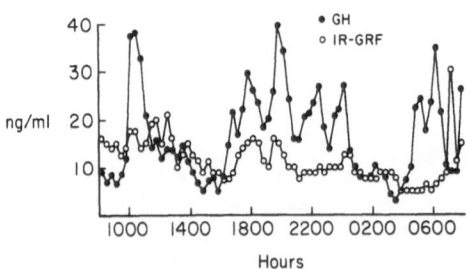

Fig. 5. Serum GH (ng/ml) and
plasma immunoreactive GRF (ng/ml)
levels in a patient with acromegaly and ectopic GRF secretion.
●, GH; o, IR-GRF. (Reprinted with
permission from Vance et al., 1985
[16].)

doubling of the level of somatomedin-C and an increase in the amount of GH secreted over 24 hours on day 14 of the GRF infusion (21). We therefore suggest that a depot preparation of GRF has potential as a useful therapeutic agent in treating children with GH deficiency. We are now extending this study to include GH-deficient children.

CONCLUSIONS

In the 3½ years since the first administration of GRF to man, GRF appears to hold promise as a therapeutic agent. The presence of a growth hormone response to an acute dose of GRF indicates the presence of functioning somatotrophs in the pituitary. However, the absence of such a response does not necessarily indicate the absence of such cells but could reflect either lack of "priming" of the somatotroph by GRF or suppression of the somatotroph by oversecretion of somatostatin. The development of longer-acting and more potent analogs of GRF is urgently needed to make GRF a practical alternative therapy to growth hormone in GH-deficient children.

REFERENCES

1. Thorner MO, Perryman RL, Cronin MJ, et al. Somatotroph hyperplasia: successful treatment of acromegaly by removal of a pancreatic islet tumor secreting a growth hormone releasing factor. J Clin Invest 1982; 70:965.
2. uz Zafar MS, Mellinger RC, Fine G, Szabo M, Frohman LA. Acromegaly associated with a bronchial carcinoid tumor: evidence for ectopic production of growth hormone-releasing activity. J Clin Endocrinol Metab 1979; 48:66.
3. Bohlen P, Thorner M, Cronin M, Shively J, Scheithauer B. Isolation from human neoplastic tissue and partial characterization of a growth hormone releasing factor (GRF) [Abstract 540]. 64th annual meeting of the Endocrine Society Program and Abstracts, 1982.
4. Rivier J, Spiess J, Thorner M, Vale W. Characterization of a growth hormone-releasing factor from a human pancreatic islet tumour. Nature 1982; 300:276.
5. Guillemin R, Brazeau P, Bohlen P, Esch F, Ling N, Wehrenberg W. Growth hormone-releasing factor from a human pancreatic tumor that caused acromegaly. Science 1982; 218:585.
6. Esch FS, Bohlen P, Ling NC, et al. Characterization of a 40 residue peptide from a human pancreatic tumor with growth hormone releasing activity. Biochem Biophys Res Commun 1982; 109:152.
7. Gubler U, Monahan JJ, Lomedico PT, et al. Cloning and sequence analysis of cDNA for the precursor of human growth hormone-releasing factor, somatocrinin. Proc Natl Acad Sci USA 1983; 80:4311.
8. Mayo KE, Vale W, Rivier J, Rosenfeld MG, Evans RM. Expression-cloning and sequence of a cDNA encoding human growth hormone-releasing factor. Nature 1983; 306:86.
9. Mayo KE, Cerelli GM, Lebo RV, Bruce BD, Rosenfeld MG, Evans RM. Gene encoding human growth hormone-releasing factor precursor: structure, sequence, and chromosomal assignment. Proc Natl Acad Sci USA 1985; 82:63.
10. Thorner MO, Rivier J, Spiess J, et al. Human pancreatic growth-hormone-releasing factor selectively stimulates growth-hormone secretion in man. Lancet 1983; 1:24.
11. Vance ML, Borges JLC, Kaiser DL, et al. Human pancreatic tumor growth hormone releasing factor (hpGRF-40): dose response relationships in normal man. J Clin Endocrinol Metab 1984; 58:838.
12. Borges JLC, Blizzard RM, Gelato MC, et al. Effects of human pancre-

atic growth hormone releasing factor on growth hormone and somato-medin C levels in patients with idiopathic growth hormone deficiency. Lancet 1983; ii:119.

13. Borges JLC, Blizzard RM, Evans WS, et al. Stimulation of growth hormone (GH) and somatomedin C in idiopathic GH-deficient subjects by intermittent pulsatile administration of synthetic human pancreatic tumor GH-releasing factor. J Clin Endocrinol Metab 1984; 59:1.

14. Rogol AD, Blizzard RM, Johanson AJ, et al. Growth hormone release in response to human pancreatic tumor growth hormone releasing factor-40 in children with short stature. J Clin Endocrinol Metab 1984; 59:580.

15. Vance ML, Kaiser DL, Evans WS, et al. Evidence for a limited growth hormone (GH)-releasing hormone (GHRH)-releasable quantity of GH: effects of 6-hour infusions of GHRH on GH secretion in normal man. J Clin Endocrinol Metab 1985; 60:370.

16. Vance ML, Kaiser DL, Evans WS, et al. Pulsatile growth hormone secretion in normal man during a continuous 24-hour infusion of human growth hormone releasing factor (1-40): evidence for intermittent somatostatin secretion. J Clin Invest 1985; 75:1584.

17. Vance ML, Kaiser DL, Rivier J, Vale W, Thorner MO. Dual effects of GHRH infusion in normal men: somatotroph desensitization and in-crease in releasable growth hormone. J Clin Endocrinol Metab 1986; 62:591.

18. Tannenbaum GS, Ling N. The interrelationship of growth hormone-releasing factor and somatostatin in generation of the ultradian rhythm of growth hormone secretion. Endocrinology 1984; 115:1952.

19. Evans WS, Vance ML, Kaiser DL, et al. Effects of intravenous, subcutaneous, and intranasal administration of human growth hormone releasing factor-40 on serum growth hormone concentration in normal men. J Clin Endocrinol Metab 1985; 61:846.

20. Thorner MO, Reschke J, Chitwood J, et al. Acceleration of growth in two children treated with human growth hormone releasing factor. N Engl J Med 1985; 312:4.

21. Vance ML, Evans WS, Thorner MO. Growth hormone secretion is aug-mented during 14 days of continuous growth hormone releasing hormone infusion in normal man. American Federation for Clinical Research, 1986.

11

GRF SECRETION IN MAN

M. D. Page, C. Dieguez,* I. Weeks, S. Woodhead, and
M. F. Scanlon

Neuroendocrine Unit, Department of Medicine, University of
Wales College of Medicine, Cardiff, Wales, U.K., and
*Department of Physiology, Santiago de Compostela, Spain

INTRODUCTION

The isolation and characterization of the growth hormone (GH) releasing peptides 1-37 (GRF 37), 1-40 (GRF 40) and 1-44 (GRF 44) have led to the generation of antibodies which have been used for immunocytochemistry techniques and the development of assays based on standard competitive protein binding principles. These procedures are now being used to measure circulating levels of GRF in man in both normal and disease states and to investigate abnormalities associated with the release of this peptide. Recently, GRF 40 and GRF 44, which are immunologically and biochemically identical to GRF of pancreatic origin, have been demonstrated in human hypothalamic extracts (1,2). Immunohistochemical studies in both rats and primates have demonstrated the presence of GRF-positive neurons in the hypothalamus and median eminence (3). Further immunohistochemical studies have also demonstrated the presence of immunoreactive GRF in several pancreatic endocrine tumors (4-6). In a large retrospective study, GRF immunoreactivity was detected in 4/24 pancreatic carcinoids, 1/5 bronchial carcinoids, 2/15 gut carcinoids, 1/2 thymic carcinoids, 2/20 medullary carcinomas of thyroid, 1/12 pheochromocytomas and 5/20 small cell carcinomas of lung (7). In this series, clinical features of acromegaly were present in only 2 of the 4 pancreatic carcinoids and in the single patient with a bronchial carcinoid tumor. These data are concordant with earlier case reports of acromegaly associated with bronchial and foregut carcinoids (8-11). Furthermore, the recent findings reported by Asa et al. suggest a link between the presence of hypothalamic gangliocytomas, all of which were immunopositive for GRF, with pituitary GH-producing adenomas; 4 of these 6 cases had clinical features of acromegaly (12). It appears, therefore, that GRF occurs quite frequently in association with a variety of other endocrine neoplasia. In this chapter we will review the findings of alterations in GRF secretion in disease states and then discuss the results of physiological and pharmacological studies of GH secretion in normal subjects.

ASSESSMENT OF GRF LEVELS

Several standard radioimmunoassays for immunoreactive GRF have been described with sensitivities ranging from less than 1 pmol to 1000 pg/ml

(13-20). In pharmacokinetic studies, it has been estimated that the half-life of GRF in the circulation is approximately 60 min (21). This contrasts with the much shorter half-life of peptides such as TRH and somatostatin which is about 3-4 min. In light of these differences, it is possible that the hypothalamic release of GRF into the hypophyseal portal blood system contributes significantly to the circulating levels of peptide.

We have recently developed an assay which employs a chemiluminescent label bound to an acridinium ester for the measurement of GRF in human plasma. The major advantages of this non-isotopic assay are enhanced sensitivity and increased stability of the luminescent-labeled ligand. Crude, labeled GRF 1-40 was prepared by reacting known amounts of GRF with the acridinium-label complex which binds to the lysine residues in the peptide molecule. The excess label was removed by adding a thousandfold excess of lysine residues and separating the labeled GRF on a Sephadex G25 column. Labeled GRF 1-40 was further purified on HPLC using a micro-Bondapak C18 column with a gradient of 18-54% acetonitrile in 0.1% TFA. Typically, the immunoreactive material eluted in fractions 20-26 (Fig. 1). The antibodies used in this assay showed equimolar cross reactivity with GRF 1-44; however, GRF 1-29 was one hundredfold less sensitive. There was no significant cross reactivity with somatostatin-28, somatostatin-14, VIP, bombesin, glucagon or a variety of other gut peptides and anterior pituitary hormones (Fig. 2). Antibody dilution studies (Fig. 3) showed a standard profile with maximum sensitivity being achieved using an initial dilution of 1:320,000. The absolute sensitivity of the assay was less than 0.5 pg/tube using 100 μl of unextracted plasma. The precision profile analysis, based on triplicate measurements, indicated that the working range of the assay was 2.5 to 25 pg/tube with a coefficient of variation of less than 10% (Fig. 4).

MEASUREMENT OF GRF LEVELS IN NORMAL AND DISEASE STATES

Using standard radioimmunoassay techniques, immunoreactive GRF levels have been estimated in plasma and CSF in normal subjects in a variety of disease states, and during pharmacological and physiological manipulation

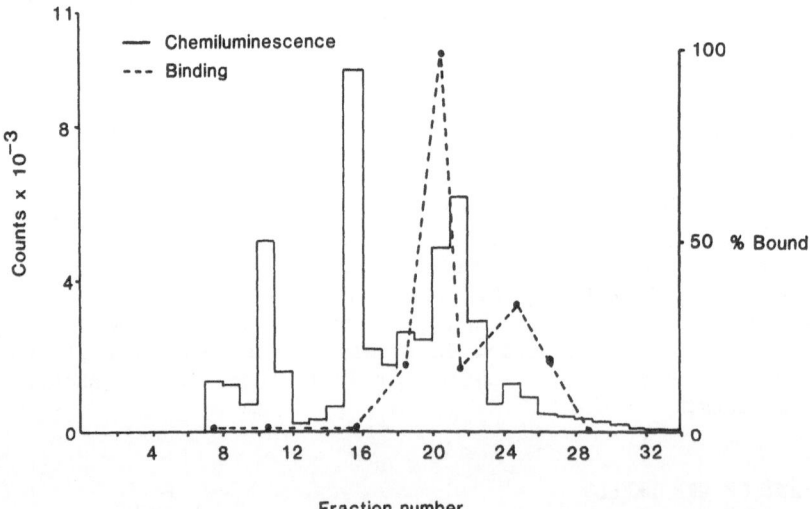

Fig. 1. HPLC profile of total counts and binding activity of labeled GRF.

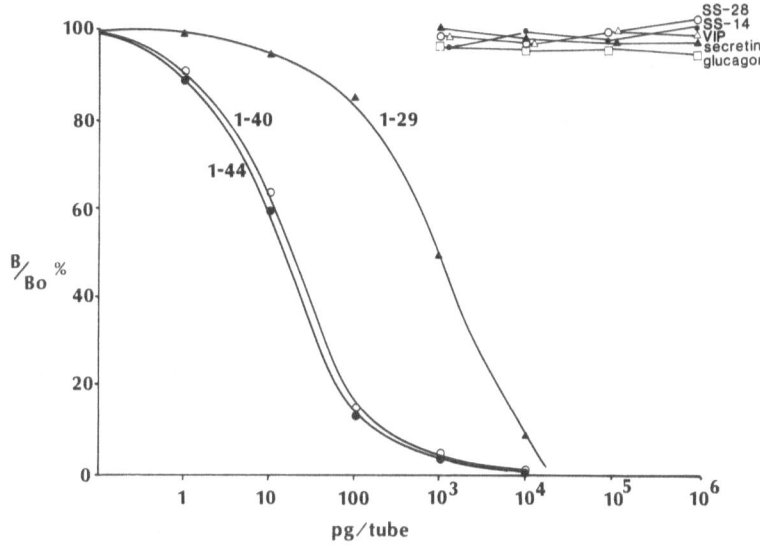

Fig. 2. Cross-reactivity study of different peptides on the binding of labeled GRF against anti-GRF antibodies.

of normal volunteers (Table 1). It has been reported that GRF levels are undetectable in the CSF of patients with hypothalamic disease, whereas levels are not different between normal subjects and patients with acromegaly (16). However, GRF levels are lower than normal in patients with idiopathic growth hormone deficiency (16). Most assays for plasma GRF indicate that circulating levels of peptide in normal individuals are less than 60 pg/ml (19,20). As expected, grossly elevated GRF levels can be detected easily in the relatively few acromegalic patients with ectopic

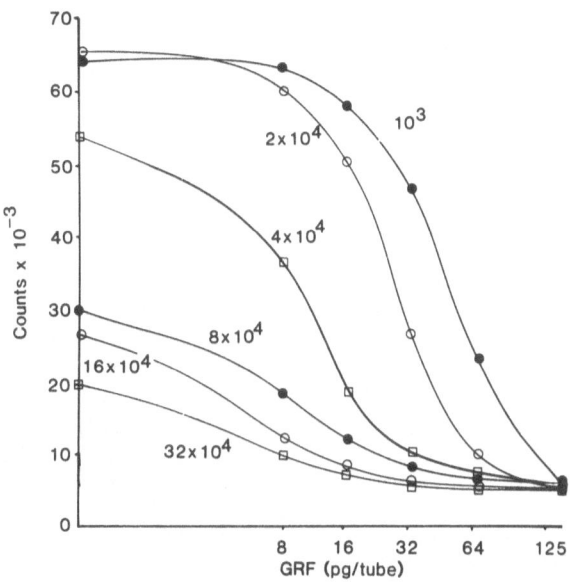

Fig. 3. Antibody dilution studies of anti-GRF antibodies against different concentrations of cold GRF.

107

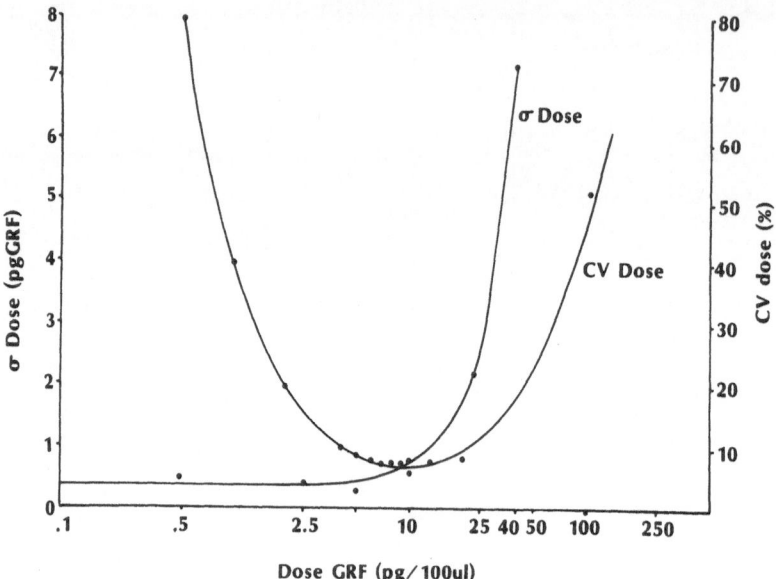

Fig. 4. Precision profile of the GRF chemilu-
minescence assay.

production of GRF (19,20). It is noteworthy, however, that a significant
number of acromegalic patients have fasting GRF levels which fall above
the fasting normal range (19,20). The reason for this observation is
presently unknown. In measuring circulating levels of GRF in normal and
disease states, it is important that fasting specimens be analyzed since
food stimulation can cause a rise in plasma GRF levels (25) (Table 1).

Using our own chemiluminescent assay for GRF, we have detected
immunoreactive GRF in normal, fasting individuals as well as very high
circulating levels of peptide in patients with the ectopic GRF syndrome.
Extraction and characterization studies of the various forms of circulating immunoreactive GRF in a patient with acromegaly due to the ectopic
GRF syndrome indicate that the dominant circulating peptide is GRF 1-40
with lesser contributions from GRF 1-44 and GRF 1-37 (30).

ALTERATIONS IN CIRCULATING GRF LEVELS IN NORMAL SUBJECTS

We are presently investigating the relationship between circulating
GH and GRF levels during the slow wave sleep-related GH surge in normal
individuals (Fig. 5). Normal slow wave sleep-related GH release is
accompanied by pulses of immunoreactive GRF release. The episodes of
immunoreactive GRF release clearly are not related to EEG sleep stages.
Abolition of nocturnal slow wave sleep-related GH release by cholinergic
muscarinic receptor blockade with pirenzepine (Fig. 5) does not affect the
occurrence of the nocturnal pulses of GRF release (Fig. 6). Since we do
not yet have adequate data on GRF release throughout the 24-hour period,
we have not been able to determine whether this pulsatile phenomenon is
strictly a nocturnal event. However, if this nocturnal GRF release is in
any way hypothalamic in origin, it is not influenced by cholinergic muscarinic receptor blockade while GH release can be abolished by cholinergic
antagonism without influencing immunoreactive GRF levels. These data are
quite compatible with the view that cholinergic muscarinic blockade produces its effects on GH release by modulating the release of hypothalamic
somatostatin (22-24).

Table 1. Plasma and CSF GRF levels in normal and pathological conditions
and during pharmacological and physiological manipulations.

Normal Subjects	Plasma GRF	CSF GRF
Adults	<10-60 pg/ml (19,20)	10-54 pg/ml (16)
Children	8-148 pg/ml (17)	
Disease States		
Acromegaly	Normal or increased* (19,20)	Normal (16)
Idiopathic GH deficiency (IGH)	Normal (25)	Reduced (16)
Hypothalamic germinoma		Undetectable (16) Reduced
Stimulators and Inhibitors		
Mixed meal	Increased** (26)	
Glucose	Increased (27)	
Hypoglycemia	Increased*** (27,28)	
L-dopa	Increased (17,28)	
Ornithine/Arginine	Reduced or no effect (17,28)	
Cholinergic blockade	Normal (Fig. 5 and 6)	
Somatostatin	Reduced (29)	

*4/80 patients with ectopic GRF (19); 6/177 with ectopic GRF (20).

**Blocked by somatostatin infusion (29).

***No effect on patients with IGH deficiency (27).

Several groups have studied the relationship between circulating immunoreactive GRF and GH levels following the administration of GH secretagogues and inhibitors (Table 1). The GH response to L-dopa stimulation is preceded by a rise in circulating immunoreactive GRF levels (17,28) whereas ornithine (17) or arginine (28) stimulation of GH release is associated with a fall in GRF immunoreactivity. It appears also that there is a direct relationship between peak circulating GRF and GH levels in response to L-dopa (17). Taken together with other available data that dopaminergic stimulation of GH release is mediated by hypothalamic GRF, it is possible that the rise in circulating GRF following L-dopa administration is a reflection of the release of hypothalamic GRF into the hypophyseal portal circulation.

A mixed meal stimulus causes a significant rise in circulating immunoreactive GRF levels which is still observed in patients with presumed hypothalamic GRF deficiency (25,26). Sopwith et al. suggest that the increased GRF levels in this instance are likely a reflection of gastrointestinal release. More recently it has been shown that the GRF response to meal stimulation in normal individuals can be abolished by somatostatin infusion (29). Others have found that glucose loading produced a biphasic rise in immunoreactive GRF levels (27). The first phase occurred within 60 min whereas the second phase was delayed for 2-3 hours but preceded the late GH response to glucose loading. The authors concluded that the first phase of GRF release was gastrointestinal in origin whereas the second phase reflected increased hypothalamic activity leading to the late peak of growth hormone release (27). Recent reports also indicate a clear rise in circulating GRF levels following insulin-induced hypoglycemia in association with the increase in GH levels in normal subjects but not in patients with idiopathic growth hormone deficiency (27,28). It remains to be established whether the increase in circulating GRF levels following oral glucose administration and insulin-induced hypoglycemia is due to GRF release from the gut or the hypothalamus, respectively.

Further studies are required to clarify these points of conflict and to delineate further physiological changes in GRF levels in normal individuals. From the data published thus far, however, it is reasonable to conclude that total circulating GRF is probably a reflection of both hypothalamic and gastrointestinal GRF release. Moreover, the observed variations in circulating GRF levels are likely due to alterations in GRF synthesis and release at these two sites in relation to different physiological signals.

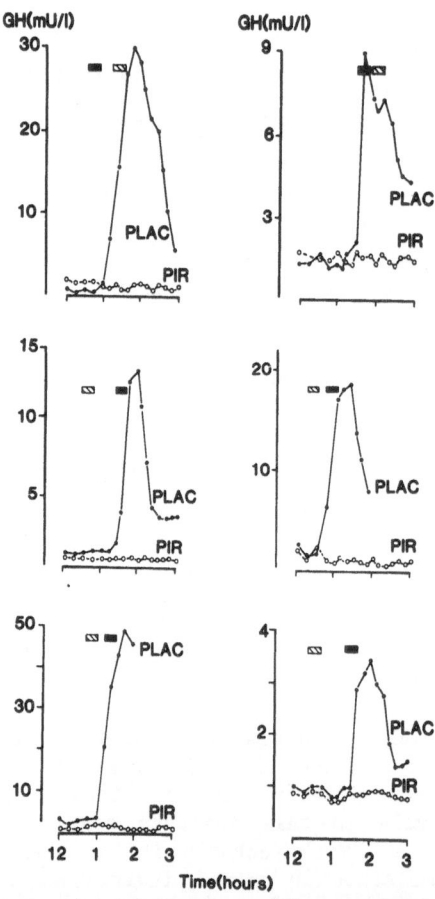

Fig. 5. GH levels in normal males during treatment with placebo (PLAC) or pirenzepine (PIR). Solid and hatched bars indicate episodes of slow wave sleep on PLAC and PIR nights respectively.

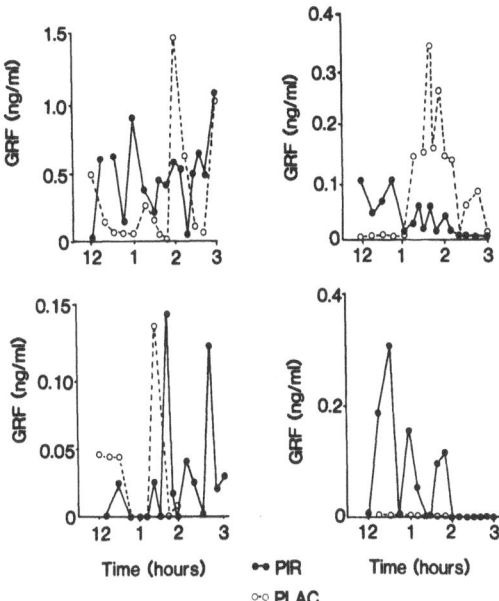

Fig. 6. GRF levels in 4/6 subjects represented in Figure 5.

ACKNOWLEDGMENTS

We would like to thank Professor A. V. Schally for the kind supply of GRF antibodies. This study was supported by grants from the CAICYT (84/1210 to Dr. C. Dieguez) and the Medical Research Council of Great Britain (Dr. M. F. Scanlon). Dr. M. D. Page is a Wellcome Trust Medical Graduate Fellow.

REFERENCES

1. Bohlen P, Brazeau P, Bloch B, Ling N, Gaillard R, Guillemin R. Human hypothalamic growth hormone releasing factor (GRF): evidence for two forms identical to tumour derived GRF-44-NH$_2$ and GRF-40. Biochem Biophys Res Commun 1983; 114:930.
2. Christofides NO, Stephanou AS, Suzuki H, Yiangou Y, Bloom SR. Distribution of immunoreactive growth hormone-releasing hormone in the human brain and intestine and its production by tumours. J Clin Endocrinol Metab 1984; 59:747.
3. Bloch B, Brazeau P, Ling N, et al. Immunohistochemical detection of growth hormone-releasing factor in brain. Nature 1983; 301:607.
4. Rivier J, Spiess J, Thorner M, Vale W. Characterization of a growth hormone-releasing factor from a human pancreatic islet tumour. Nature 1982; 300:276.
5. Guillemin R, Brazeau P, Bohlen P, Esch F, Ling N, Wehrenberg W. Growth hormone-releasing factor from a human pancreatic tumor that caused acromegaly. Science 1982; 218:585.
6. Thorner MO, Perryman RL, Cronin MJ, et al. Somatotroph hyperplasia: successful treatment of acromegaly by removal of a pancreatic islet tumor secreting a growth hormone releasing factor. J Clin Invest 1982; 70:965.
7. Asa SL, Kovacs K, Thorner MO, Leong DA, Rivier J, Vale W. Immuno-histochemical localisation of growth hormone releasing hormone in human tumors. J Clin Endocrinol Metab 1985; 60:3:423.

8. Shalet SM, Beardwell CG, MacFarlane IA, et al. Acromegaly due to production of a growth hormone releasing factor by a bronchial carcinoid tumour. Clin Endocrinol (Oxf) 1979; 10:61.

9. Saeed uz Zafar M, Mellinger RC, Fine G, Szabo M, Frohman LA. Acromegaly associated with a bronchial carcinoid tumor: evidence for ectopic production of growth hormone-releasing activity. J Clin Endocrinol Metab 1979; 48:66-71.

10. Scheithauer BW, Carpenter PC, Bloch B, Brazeau P. Ectopic secretion of growth hormone-releasing factor. Report of a case of acromegaly with bronchial carcinoid tumor. Am J Med 1984; 76:605.

11. Leveston SA, McKeel DW Jr, Buckley PJ, et al. Acromegaly and Cushing's syndrome associated with a foregut carcinoid tumor. J Clin Endocrinol Metab 1981; 53:682.

12. Asa SL, Scheithauer BW, Bilbao JM, et al. A case for hypothalamic acromegaly: a clinicopathological study of six patients with hypothalamic gangliocytomas producing growth hormone-releasing factor. J Clin Endocrinol Metab 1984; 58:796.

13. Chihara K, Kashio Y, Abe H, et al. Idiopathic growth hormone (GH) deficiency and GH deficiency secondary to hypothalamic germinoma: effect of single and repeated administration of human GH-releasing factor (hGRF) on plasma GH level and endogenous hGRF-like immunoreactivity level in cerebrospinal fluid. J Clin Endocrinol Metab 1985; 60:269.

14. Sassolas G, Biot-Laporte S, Cohen R, Elm-Charfi A, Ferry S, Borson F. Effects on growth hormone secretion following intravenous and subcutaneous injections of growth hormone-releasing factor (hGRF-44 NH$_2$): comparison of immunoreactive plasma GRF levels. Clin Endocrinol (Oxf) 1985; 22:645.

15. Shibasaki T, Kiyosawa Y, Masuda A, et al. Distribution of growth hormone-releasing hormone like immunoreactivity in human tissue extracts. J Clin Endocrinol Metab 1984; 59:263.

16. Kashio Y, Chihara K, Kaji H, et al. Presence of growth hormone-releasing factor-like immunoreactivity in human cerebrospinal fluid. J Clin Endocrinol Metab 1985; 60:396.

17. Donnadieu M, Evain-Brion D, Tonon MC, Vaudry H, Job JC. Variations of plasma growth hormone (GH)-releasing factor levels during GH stimulation tests in children. J Clin Endocrinol Metab 1985; 60:1132.

18. Losa M, Bock L, Schopohl J, Stalla GK, Muller OA, von Werder K. Growth hormone releasing factor infusion does not sustain elevated GH levels in normal subjects. Acta Endocrinol (Copenh) 1984; 107:462.

19. Penny ES, Penman E, Price J, et al. Circulating growth hormone releasing factor concentrations in normal subjects and patients with acromegaly. Br Med J 1984; 289:453.

20. Thorner M, Frohman LA, Leong DA, et al. Extrahypothalamic GRF secretion is a rare cause of acromegaly; plasma GRF levels in 177 patients. J Clin Endocrinol Metab 1984; 59:846.

21. Frohman LA, Thominet JL, Webb CB, et al. Metabolic clearance and plasma disappearance rates of human pancreatic tumour growth hormone releasing factor in man. J Clin Invest 1984; 73:1304.

22. Massara F, Ghigo E, Goffi S, Molinatti GM, Mueller EE, Camanni F. Blockade of hp-GRF 40 induced growth hormone release in normal men by a cholinergic muscarinic antagonist. J Clin Endocrinol Metab 1984; 58:1025.

23. Jordan V, Dieguez C, Lafaffian I, et al. Influence of dopaminergic, adrenergic and cholinergic blockade and TRH administration on GH response to GRF 1-29. Clin Endocrinol (Oxf) 1986; 24:291.

24. Casanueva FF, Villanueva L, Dieguez C, et al. Atropine blockade of growth hormone (GH)-releasing hormone-induced GH secretion in man is not exerted at pituitary level. J Clin Endocrinol Metab 1986; 62:186.

25. Sopwith AM, Penny E, Grossman A, Savage MO, Besser BM, Rees LH. Normal circulating immunoreactive growth hormone releasing factor (hGRF) concentrations in patients with functional hypothalamic hGRF deficiency. Clin Endocrinol (Oxf) 1986; 24:395.

26. Sopwith AM, Penny ES, Besser GM, Rees LH. Stimulation by food of peripheral plasma immunoreactive growth hormone releasing factor. Clin Endocrinol (Oxf) 1985; 22:337.

27. Kashio Y, Chihara K, Kita T, et al. Effect of oral glucose administration on plasma growth hormone-releasing hormone-like immunoreactivity levels in healthy subjects and patients with idiopathic growth hormone deficiency [Abstract 740]. 68th annual meeting of the Endocrine Society, Anaheim, CA, 1986.

28. Masuda A, Shibasaki T, Imaki T, Demura H, Shizume K. The manner of GHRH involvement in GH stimulation test in man [Abstract 186]. First International Congress of Neuroendocrinology, San Francisco, CA, 1986.

29. Sopwith AM, Penny ES, Besser GM, Rees LH. Secretion of circulating immunoreactive human growth hormone releasing factor is inhibited by somatostatin [Abstract 260]. J Endocrinol 1986; 106(5).

30. Penny ES, Patience RL, Sopwith AM, Wass JAH, Besser GM, Rees LH. Characterisation by high performance liquid chromatography of circulating growth hormone releasing factors in a human plasma. J Endocrinol 1985; 105:R1-4.

12

ECTOPIC GRH SYNDROMES

Lawrence A. Frohman, Thomas R. Downs

Division of Endocrinology and Metabolism
University of Cincinnati College of Medicine
Cincinnati, Ohio

Although the occasion for this symposium is the commemoration of the centennial of the first description of acromegaly, it has been only 27 years since a patient with an extrapituitary cause for acromegaly was described. In 1959, Altmann and Schutz described a patient with acromegaly of 12 years' duration who did not respond to a course of pituitary irradiation, but who experienced a marked regression of the features of GH hypersecretion following excision of a bronchial carcinoid tumor (1). This report in the German literature was overlooked by the numerous authors who, during the next two decades, described patients with coexisting acromegaly and carcinoid tumors of various types (see references 2 and 3 for reviews). Fifteen years later, Dabek reported a similar case history (4) and two years after that, Sonksen added an additional case report of regression of GH hypersecretion after removal of a carcinoid tumor (5). In 1979, we had an opportunity to study a tumor removed from a patient whose history was remarkably similar to that of the original patient described (1), and reported that it stimulated GH release by rat pituitary cell cultures (6). In another report, Shalet et al. (7) described similar findings using a perifusion system. Within the next few years, several other patients with the syndrome were recognized (8) and finally, identification of two patients prior to surgical removal of the extrapituitary tumor resulted in the preservation of two pancreatic islet tumors from which GH-releasing hormone (GRH) was eventually isolated and sequenced (9,10).

Patients with the ectopic GRH syndrome have been recognized with greater frequency prior to surgical exploration of the pituitary subsequent to increased awareness of this disease entity. This presentation will focus on the clinical features of the syndrome, the spectrum of tumors involved, potential utility of various diagnostic procedures, circulating immunoreactive GRH levels, characterization of the form(s) of GH secreted by the tumors, and possible modes of therapy.

TUMOR TYPES ASSOCIATED WITH GRH PRODUCTION

GRH secretion has been reported in association with only a limited number of tumor types (Table 1). In the 29 well-documented reports of ectopic GRH secretion (excluding tumors of the hypothalamic-pituitary region), 59% of the tumors were carcinoids, with the majority being of bronchial origin and the remainder derived from the GI tract or pancreas. Approximately 20% originated in the pancreatic islets. Nearly 60% of the carcinoid and pancreatic islet tumors were malignant, although this was not always evident at the time of original diagnosis. Whereas the majority of bronchial carcinoid tumors were benign, nearly all of the tumors derived from the GI tract were malignant. The first information suggesting tumor recurrence in these patients was frequently the return of elevated GH levels after a period of normal GH secretion. Nearly all of the malignant tumors exhibited a slow growth rate, compatible with prolonged survival of the patient. This appears to be important for the development of the syndrome, since the features of acromegaly require a considerable period of time for development.

A wider spectrum of tumor types from patients without the ectopic GRH syndrome has been found to contain GRH (3,12,13). Three different methods have been utilized to identify these tumors: bioactivity of tumor tissue, immunohistochemical staining with anti-GRH serum, and measurement of immunoreactive GRH levels. In addition to being very time consuming, measurement of bioactivity is somewhat insensitive and many GRH-containing tumors may be overlooked, since only the net bioactivity is measured and tumor tissue also frequently contains factors that inhibit GH release. The most common of these is somatostatin, which has been found in nearly every GRH-containing tumor we have examined (3,8), and in some was present in sufficient concentration to inhibit the GH-releasing effects of GRH. Inhibitory factors other than somatostatin, many of which remain to be identified, may also be present. Immunohistochemical studies have identified GRH in pancreatic endocrine tumors, carcinoids, medullary thyroid carcinomas, small-cell lung carcinomas, and pheochromocytomas (12,13). This technique has also been used for identifying GRH-containing tumors of the hypothalamus (hamartomas) and the pituitary (gangliocytomas) (14; B. W. Scheithauer, unpublished observations). Although the sensitivity of immunohistochemistry is excellent, the percentage of tumors found to contain GRH (20% or less) was less than that reported using RIA; nearly 60% of tumors with similar histology contain immunoreactive GRH (3,15). In addition, we have detected GRH immunoreactivity in a wide variety of neural crest tumors, and in 15 endometrial carcinomas (3), a tumor type

Table 1. Tumor types associated with the ectopic GRH syndrome.

Tumor type	Primary site	No.	Malignant	Benign	?
Carcinoid	Bronchus	11	4	6	1
	GI tract/ pancreas	5	3	1	1
	Undetermined	4	4		
(Total)		(20)	(11)	(7)	(2)
Pancreatic islet		6	4	2	
Small-cell carcinoma	Lung	2	2		
Adenoma	Adrenal	1		1	
TOTAL		29	17	10	2

Notes: For details of individual reports see, in addition, references 2, 8, 11. This summary is restricted to tumors with venous drainage into the systemic circulation.

not generally associated with ectopic hormone secretion. Whether this finding is responsible for the paradoxical rises in GH levels in response to glucose seen in patients with endometrial carcinoma (16) remains to be clarified. It must be emphasized that in most tumors with low levels of immunoreactive GRH, there is limited documentation of the validation of the measurement and the true identity of the bioactivity or immunoreactivity of GRH remains unproven.

LABORATORY STUDIES

Efforts to diagnose the ectopic GRH syndrome by laboratory methods have been focused on three areas: imaging procedures, GH responses to provocative stimuli, and measurement of plasma GRH immunoreactivity. The use of imaging techniques, in particular, computed tomography (CT), has received the greatest attention. Although several of the tumors responsible for ectopic secretion of GRH have been identified by CT, the cost effectiveness of this procedure is very questionable, given the extremely low prevalence of GRH-secreting tumors among the population of acromegalics. In addition, the relative limitations of CT in the region of the pancreas raises the possibility of unnecessary surgical procedures for scan defects of uncertain significance. This is not to deny that interesting findings may result from such studies. For example, the first report of a patient with a GH-secreting pancreatic islet tumor was based on CT identification of a presumed GRH-secreting tumor (17).

Measurement of GH responses to agents such as TRH, glucose, and dopaminergic agonists has also failed to be of much help in identifying those acromegalics with GRH-secreting tumors. As shown in Table 2, GH secretion in nearly all patients with GRH-secreting tumors is increased by TRH, fails to suppress with glucose and decreases in response to dopaminergic agonists. The same findings, however, are observed in most acromegalics and, therefore, the procedures are not of particular value. It has been suggested that the development of GH responsiveness to TRH is induced by excessive GRH secretion since successful removal of the extrapituitary tumor is associated with loss of the response (18). If valid, the extremely high percentage of patients with acromegaly who exhibit positive responses to TRH raises implications for a role of GRH in the pathogenesis of acromegaly (see below).

Information is currently available concerning the GH responses to exogenous GRH in 4 patients with ectopic GRH secretion (Table 2). A single intravenous injection of GRH was ineffective in increasing GH levels in 3 patients, and in one the response was restored after removal of the GRH-secreting tumor. A fourth patient, however, was responsive to GRH. Thus, the diagnosis of ectopic GRH secretion cannot be excluded by a

Table 2. Plasma growth hormone responses to stimuli in patients with ectopic GRH secretion.

Stimulus	No. Tested	No. of Responses
TRH	13	12 (stimulation)
Glucose	5	4 (absence of suppression)
Dopaminergic agonists	6	5 (suppression)
GRH	4	1 (stimulation)

positive response. The basis for the absent GH response to GRH in these patients, in contrast to other patients with acromegaly, where the response is almost invariably positive, deserves comment. Among the suggested possible explanations are receptor downregulation and saturation of receptors or defects in the postreceptor mechanisms. Either of these explanations would imply a cellular mechanism in somatotrophs subjected to chronic GRH stimulation that differs from that in the common variety of acromegaly. Recent measurements, however, suggest another and perhaps less complicated explanation. The levels of circulating immunoreactive GRH (IR-GRH) achieved after the intravenous injection of a single dose of GRH (1 μg/kg) only transiently reach the low ng/ml range and within 10 minutes are less than 1 ng/ml (26). Considering the levels of IR-GRH present in patients with GRH-secreting tumors, the small and temporary incremental rise in circulating IR-GRH levels may be insufficient to stimulate further the already supranormal GH secretion.

The levels of plasma IR-GRH in patients with ectopic GRH secretion are summarized in Table 3. Values range from 0.39 to 50 ng/ml with a mean of 11 ng/ml. These values are not, however, truly comparable since they are based on assays unique to individual laboratories, employing different standards and antisera with varying degrees of cross-reactivity with the different forms of GRH. Nevertheless, the values are clearly distinguishable from those in normals, where IR-GRH levels are < 50 pg/ml in most assays and < 20 pg/ml in several (see below). Thus, the diagnosis of ectopic GRH secretion would be quite unlikely in a patient with a plasma IR-GRH level of < 350 pg/ml. We have suggested that a single measurement of plasma IR-GRH in newly-diagnosed patients with acromegaly is a cost-effective method of excluding the diagnosis of ectopic GRH secretion (27,28). Despite the low prevalence of this disease, the implications for therapy are sufficient to justify such an approach.

CHARACTERIZATION OF GRH IN TUMOR TISSUE AND PLASMA

Tumor Tissue

Several forms of GRH have been identified in tumor tissue by various investigators (Table 3). In the original characterization of pancreatic islet tumor GRH, two patterns were found. In one tumor, only GRH(1-40)-OH was present (10) while in the other, two additional forms, GRH(1-44)-NH$_2$ and GRH(1-37)-OH were found (9). Subsequent reports of other tumors have described various combinations of these three forms. Although there has been no consistent pattern, GRH(1-40)-OH has been present in each of the tumors. Since there is only a single copy of the GRH gene (29) and the single amino acid difference in the two forms of the GRH precursor (due to differential processing of the GRH mRNA) is in the region of the carboxy-terminal extension (30,31), the various forms of GRH found in tumor tissue must be attributed to differential enzymatic processing of the GRH precursor or of GRH(1-44)-NH$_2$ itself. To date, however, it has not been possible to demonstrate the conversion of GRH(1-44)-NH$_2$ to either GRH (1-40)-OH or GRH(1-37)-OH by tissue extracts.

Plasma

The reports of plasma IR-GRH characterization have been less precise than those of tumor tissue and, because of the lower levels of GRH present, have relied primarily on the use of radioimmunoassay in conjunction with a chromatographic technique. One report utilized differential cross-reactivity with several anti-GRH sera to infer the forms of circulating IR-GRH (22). The most discriminating technique has been high performance liquid chromatography (HPLC). All three forms of GRH have

Table 3. Characterization of plasma and tissue GRH
in patients with GRH-secreting tumors.

Ref	Site	Age/Sex	IR-GRH ng/ml	GRH Form[a]	GH ng/ml	Dx Test Response	Other Features
19	Carcinoid met to liver	17/M	.39[b]	40/44[b]	170		Tumor also contained GH
20	Bronchial carcinoid met	32/F	25	40	42	GRH-	Sephadex G-50
18	Panc islet	21/F	5[b]	40	150	TRH+	Turner's syndrome
21	Panc islet	55/M	50	44/40/-37	40-60	TRH+ Bromo+	
11	Bronchial carcinoid	56/F		37/40	160		
22	Panc islet tumor	25/F	5.6	40/37[c]	480	TRH+	Based on RIA parallelism Poor response to SMS
23	Panc carcinoid	54/F	0.6-1.1		10-12	TRH+ GRH- Ins+	Acute response to GRH+ after tumor removal
24	Panc tumor met to liver	58/F	10-13		15-25	TRH+ GRH-	No response to bromocriptine; Mod. response to SMS
25	Carcinoid met to bone/lung	26/M	2-8		50-100	TRH+ GRH+	Partial response to bromocriptine
--	Carcinoid met to bone[d]	69/M	2-4[b]	37/40[b,c]	10-15	TRH+	Partial response to SMS
--	Carcinoid met to bone[e]	57/F	5-10[b]	40/44[b,c]	15-25	GRH-	Minimal response to bromocriptine

[a] Determined by HPLC in tumor tissue except as noted.

[b] Determined in author's laboratory.

[c] Plasma

[d] M. L. Vance, L. A. Frohman, D. L. Kaiser, M. O. Thorner, unpublished observations.

[e] S. Melmed, T. R. Downs, L. A. Frohman, unpublished observations.

met = metastatic

SMS = SMS 201-995 (Sandoz), long-acting somatostatin analog

been found in plasma, though not necessarily in the same proportions as present in tumor tissue (32).

We have recently reported that exogenous GRH(1-44)-NH$_2$, after intravenous administration, is rapidly converted to a biologically inactive metabolite by removal of an amino-terminal dipeptide (26) and have subsequently found that GRH(1-40)-OH is metabolized in a similar manner. In contrast to native GRH, the metabolite is relatively stable and exhibits a more prolonged half-life in plasma. With further modifications of the HPLC conditions, we have now observed that the major form of plasma IR-GRH in one patient with ectopic GRH secretion is GRH(3-40)-NH$_2$ (Fig. 1). Since none of the antisera used for GRH radioimmunoassays have been reported to be sensitive to changes in the amino-terminal end of the molecule, this metabolite would be expected to exhibit full immunoreactivity in all of the assays. Thus, the levels of true biologically active GRH in plasma of patients with ectopic GRH secretion may be considerably lower than those shown in Table 3.

ECTOPIC GRH SECRETION IN HYPOTHALAMIC PITUITARY DISEASE

The accumulated information concerning the effects of ectopic GRH secretion into the systemic circulation has led to questions concerning ectopic or excessive GRH secretion associated with hypothalamic-pituitary disorders. Three separate areas of investigation have been pursued: GRH-secreting tumors of the hypothalamus or pituitary, McCune-Albright syndrome, and classical acromegaly.

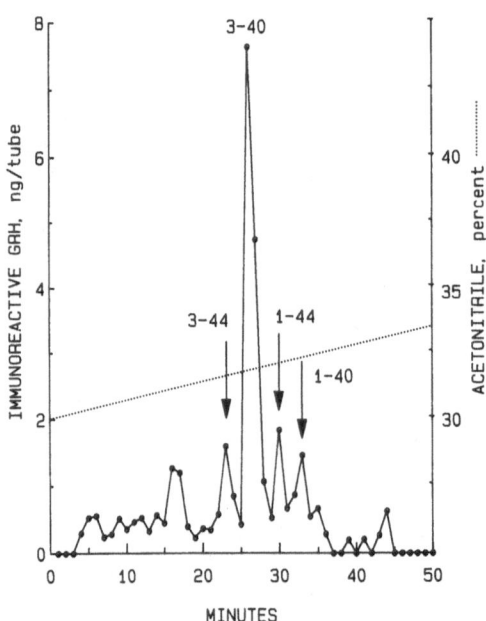

Fig. 1. HPLC elution pattern of plasma IR-GRH from a patient with ectopic GRH secretion. Details of HPLC conditions were as previously described (26). The location of the different forms and metabolites of GRH are indicated by the labels and arrows. The patient's tumor contained both GRH(1-44)-NH$_2$ and GRH(1-40)-OH.

A series of patients has recently been reported with coexisting GH-secreting pituitary tumors and pituitary gangliocytomas that have been shown by immunohistochemical staining to contain GRH (14). These tumors were discovered at the time of surgical removal of the GH-secreting tumor and it is believed that the excessive GRH secretion in these patients exerted its effects by a paracrine mechanism in the adjacent somatotrophs. In addition, there is at least one well-documented case of a coexisting hypothalamic hamartoma in a patient with acromegaly (33) that was subsequently shown to contain GRH (B. W. Scheithauer, unpublished observations). In this patient, GRH would have been secreted into the portal vascular system with a route of delivery to the pituitary similar to that of normal endogenous GRH. These patients did not exhibit clinically distinguishing characteristics and, although no measurements of peripheral IR-GRH levels were reported, one would not expect elevated levels in the peripheral circulation.

There have been several reports of acromegaly in patients with the McCune-Albright syndrome. This disorder, as originally described, consists of the combination of polyostotic fibrous dysplasia, cutaneous pigmentation, and endocrine dysfunction leading to precocious puberty. Included in the list of other endocrine disorders often associated with this syndrome is acromegaly (34,35). In several of the reported patients, and those we have studied, GH hypersecretion, at least initially, was unassociated with any pituitary abnormalities on radiographic studies. We have examined the GH responses to GRH in 2 patients with McCune-Albright syndrome associated with acromegaly and have found them to be normal (36). Endogenous plasma IR-GRH levels in 3 patients with the syndrome have ranged from 20 to 40 pg/ml, considerably lower than in patients with ectopic GRH secretion, but higher than in normal subjects (see below). Consequently, the possibility of excessive GRH secretion in these patients remains likely.

Considerable debate exists concerning the etiology of acromegaly, as has been presented at this symposium. The absence of diffuse somatotroph hyperplasia and the restoration of normal GH secretory responses after successful removal of the pituitary tumor in many acromegalic patients constitute the strongest arguments for a primary pituitary disorder. Recent observations on plasma IR-GRH levels in acromegaly, however, may warrant a reexamination of this question. A few years ago, we measured plasma IR-GRH levels in a series of acromegalic patients in a collaborative effort to determine the frequency of ectopic GRH secretion in acromegalics unsuspected of having the syndrome (28). With the exception of previously diagnosed patients with ectopic GRH secretion, none of the levels were > 90 pg/ml. The relatively insensitive assays used at that time (1983) and the limited quantity of plasma available for analysis may have contributed to our inability to distinguish between levels in acromegalics and those in normal controls. With further refinements in our assay, and the use of a plasma concentrating procedure, we have consistently found levels of < 20 pg/ml during the last 2½ years (37). Our mean sensitivity in the 21 assays in which plasma from acromegalics has been measured during this period has been 12 pg/ml with no evidence of a downward trend. The plasma IR-GRH levels in 11 normal and 45 acromegalic patients are shown in Figure 2. Seventy-eight percent of acromegalics had detectable IR-GRH levels ranging from 10 to 191 pg/ml with a mean ± SE of 33 ± 7 pg/ml. In contrast, no normal subject exhibited a detectable value of > 10 pg/ml. Among detectable values, there was no overlap between normal and acromegalic subjects. The results indicate that, at least in a subgroup of acromegalic subjects, plasma IR-GRH levels are significantly greater than in normals. They also imply that levels in portal-hypophyseal plasma may be considerably greater and could exert a potential pathogenic role in the development of acromegaly. The interpretation of these results, however, requires some caution, since validation studies remain to be performed. It still remains to be shown that the measured immunoreactivity exhibits the characteristics of one of the native GRH forms rather than a metabolite or another cross-reacting substance.

THERAPY OF GRH-SECRETING TUMORS

Optimal therapy for the ectopic GRH syndrome is the excision of the extrapituitary tumor. This will remove the stimulus for GH hypersecretion and plasma GH levels will rapidly return to normal. However, the high frequency of malignant tumors, recognized either at the time of initial diagnosis or at a later date, necessitates the need for other therapeutic options. Total hypophysectomy should be an effective therapy, though this may not always be possible and even small amounts of residual tissue can become hyperactive in the continued presence of high circulating GRH levels. Since many of the tumors exhibit a slow growth rate, relatively long periods of survival occur, even in the presence of widespread metastatic disease. Therefore, pharmacologic attempts to control GH hypersecretion are necessary. Two categories of drugs have been tried: bromocriptine, a dopamine agonist, and SMS 201-995, a somatostatin agonist. The results are still fragmentary, but suggest that bromocriptine is not very effective in most patients while SMS 201-995 may have greater potential. With both agents, the primary site of action is the somatotroph rather than the extrapituitary tumor. Additional experience with these agents is needed to determine whether the effects in ectopic GRH secretion will be comparable to those in the more common form of acromegaly. At this time, successful chemotherapy of the extrapituitary tumor has yet to be reported.

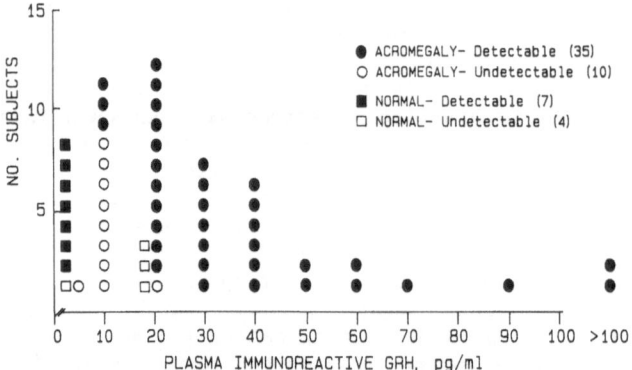

Fig. 2. Frequency histogram of plasma IR-GRH levels in patients with acromegaly and normal controls measured during the period January 1984 through June 1986 in 21 separate assays with a sensitivity of < 20 pg/ml (adjusted for plasma concentration). Each symbol represents a separate patient or control. Solid symbols represent detectable values while open symbols represent undetectable values that have been assigned the least detectable value of the assay. Numbers in parentheses indicate the number of patients tested in each group.

ACKNOWLEDGMENTS

The studies in the authors' laboratory were supported, in part, by USPHS Grant AM-30667.

REFERENCES

1. Altmann H-W, Schutz W. Uber ein knochen haltiges Bronchuscarcinoid (Morphologische und klinische Beobachtungen bei einer akromegalen Patientin). Beitr Pathol Anat 1959; 120:455.
2. Frohman LA. Ectopic hormone production by tumors: growth hormone releasing factor. Neuroendocrine Perspectives 1984; 3:201.
3. Frohman LA, Thominet JL, Szabo M. Ectopic growth hormone releasing factor syndromes. In: Raiti S, Tolman R, eds. Human growth hormone. New York: Plenum Publishing, 1986:347.
4. Dabek JT. Bronchial carcinoid tumor with acromegaly in two patients. J Clin Endocrinol Metab 1974; 38:329.
5. Sonksen PH, Ayres AB, Braimbridge M, et al. Acromegaly caused by pulmonary carcinoid tumours. Clin Endocrinol (Oxf) 1976; 5:503.
6. Zafar MS, Mellinger RC, Fine G, Szabo M, Frohman, LA. Acromegaly associated with a bronchial carcinoid tumor: evidence for ectopic production of growth hormone-releasing activity. J Clin Endocrinol Metab 1979; 48:66.
7. Shalet SM, Beardwell CG, MacFarlane IA, et al. Acromegaly due to production of a growth hormone releasing factor by a bronchial carcinoid tumor. Clin Endocrinol (Oxf) 1979; 10:61.
8. Frohman LA, Szabo M, Berelowitz M, Stachura ME. Partial purification and characterization of a peptide with growth hormone-releasing activity from extrapituitary tumors in patients with acromegaly. J Clin Invest 1980; 65:43.
9. Guillemin R, Brazeau P, Bohlen P, Esch F, Ling N, Wehrenberg WB. Growth hormone releasing factor from a human pancreatic tumor that caused acromegaly. Science 1982; 218:585.
10. Rivier J, Spiess J, Thorner M, Vale W. Characterization of a growth hormone releasing factor from a human pancreatic islet tumor. Nature 1982; 300:276.
11. Scheithauer BW, Carpenter PC, Bloch B, Brazeau P. Ectopic secretion of a growth hormone-releasing factor. Am J Med 1984; 76:605.
12. Asa SL, Kovacs K, Thorner MO, Leong DA, Rivier J, Vale W. Immunohistochemical localization of growth hormone-releasing hormone in human tumors. J Clin Endocrinol Metab 1985; 60:423.
13. Dayal Y, Lin HD, Tallberg K, Reichlin S, DeLellis RA, Wolfe HJ. Immunocytochemical demonstration of growth hormone-releasing factor in gastrointestinal and pancreatic endocrine tumors. Am J Clin Pathol 1986; 85:13.
14. Asa SL, Scheithauer BW, Bilbao JM, et al. A case for hypothalamic acromegaly: a clinicopathological study of six patients with hypothalamic gangliocytomas producing growth hormone releasing factor. J Clin Endocrinol Metab 1984; 58:796.
15. Frohman LA. Growth hormone releasing factor—a neuroendocrine perspective. J Lab Clin Med 1984; 103:819.
16. Benjamin F, Casper DJ, Sherman L, Kolodny HD. Growth-hormone secretion in patients with endometrial carcinoma. N Engl J Med 1969; 281:1448.
17. Melmed S, Ezrin C, Kovacs K, Goodman RS, Frohman LA. Acromegaly due to secretion of growth hormone by an ectopic pancreatic islet-cell tumor. N Engl J Med 1985; 312:9.
18. Thorner MO, Perryman RL, Cronin MJ, et al. Somatotroph hyperplasia. Successful treatment of acromegaly by removal of a pancreatic islet tumor secreting a growth hormone-releasing factor. J Clin Invest

1982; 70:965.

19. Leveston SA, McKeel DW Jr, Buckley PJ, et al. Acromegaly and Cushing's syndrome associated with a foregut carcinoid tumor. J Clin Endocrinol Metab 1981; 53:682.

20. Penny ES, Penman E, Sopwith, et al. Measurement and characterisation of GH-releasing factor in human plasma [Abstract 1790]. Program, 7th Int Congr Endocrinology. Amsterdam: Elsevier, 1981.

21. Sassolas G, Chayvialle JA, Partensky C, et al. Acromegalie, expression clinique de la production de facteurs de liberation de l'hormone de croissance (G.R.F.) par une tumeur pancreatique. Ann Endocrinol (Paris) 1983; 44:347.

22. Wilson DM, Ceda GP, Bostwick DG, et al. Acromegaly and Zollinger-Ellison syndrome secondary to an islet cell tumor: characterization and quantification of plasma and tumor human growth hormone-releasing factor. J Clin Endocrinol Metab 1984; 59:1002.

23. Schulte HM, Benker G, Windeck R, Olbright T, Reinwein D. Failure to respond to growth hormone releasing hormone (GHRH) in acromegaly due to a GHRH secreting pancreatic tumor: dynamics of multiple endocrine testing. J Clin Endocrinol Metab 1985; 61:585.

24. Ch'ng JLC, Christofides ND, Kraenzlin ME, et al. Growth hormone secretion dynamics in a patient with ectopic growth hormone-releasing factor production. Am J Med 1985; 79:135.

25. Barkan A, Jolley D, Beals T, Lloyd R. Acromegaly due to ectopic growth hormone-releasing hormone secretion [Abstract 487]. Program, Annual Meeting, Endocrine Society, 1985.

26. Frohman LA, Downs TR, Williams TC, Heimer EP, Pay Y-CE, Felix AM. Rapid enzymatic degradation of growth hormone-releasing hormone by plasma in vitro and in vivo to a biologically inactive, N-terminally cleaved product. J Clin Invest 1986; 78(4)906-13.

27. Frohman LA, Thominet J, Downs T. Secretion of growth hormone releasing factor (GRF) by tumors. In: Labrie F, Proulx L, eds. Endocrinology. Amsterdam: Elsevier, 1984:73.

28. Thorner MO, Frohman LA, Leong DA, et al. Extra-hypothalamic growth hormone-releasing factor (GRF) secretion is a rare cause of acromegaly: plasma GRF levels in 177 acromegalic patients. J Clin Endocrinol Metab 1984; 59:846.

29. Mayo KE, Vale W, Rivier J, Rosenfeld MG, Evans RM. Expression-cloning and sequence of a cDNA encoding human growth hormone-releasing factor. Nature 1983; 306:86.

30. Gubler U, Monahan JJ, Lomedico PT, et al. Cloning and sequence analysis of cDNA for the precursor of human growth hormone-releasing factor, somatocrinin. Proc Natl Acad Sci USA 1983; 80:4311.

31. Mayo KE, Cerelli GM, Lebo RV, Bruce BD, Rosenfeld MG, Evans RM. Gene encoding human growth hormone-releasing factor precursor: structure, sequence, and chromosomal assignment. Proc Natl Acad Sci USA 1985; 82:63.

32. Asa SL, Bilbao JM, Kovacs K, Linfoot JA. Hypothalamic neuronal hamartoma associated with pituitary growth hormone cell adenoma and acromegaly. Acta Neuropathol (Berl) 1980; 52:231.

33. Frohman LA, Jansson J-O. Growth hormone releasing hormone. Endocr Rev 1986 (in press).

34. Lightner ES, Penny R, Frasier SD. Growth hormone excess and sexual precocity in polyostotic fibrous dysplasia (McCune-Albright syndrome): evidence for abnormal hypothalamic function. J Pediatr 1975; 87:922.

35. Lipson A, Hsu T-H. The Albright syndrome associated with acromegaly: report of a case and review of the literature. Johns Hopkins Med J 1981; 149:10.

36. Cuttler L, Levitsky LL, Zafar MS, Mellinger RC, Frohman LA. Hypersecretion of growth hormone and prolactin in McCune-Albright syndrome [Abstract]. Progr Soc Ped Res 1986.

37. Frohman LA, Downs TR. Measurement of growth hormone releasing factor. In: Conn PM, ed. Neuroendocrine peptides (methods in enzymology). 2nd ed. New York: Academic Press, 1986:371-89.

III. DIAGNOSIS OF ACROMEGALY

13

CLINICAL DEVELOPMENTS OVER THE PAST 100 YEARS OF ACROMEGALY

William H. Daughaday

Metabolism Division, Department of Medicine
Washington University School of Medicine
St. Louis, MO

INTRODUCTION

I propose to trace the development of our current concepts of the cause and consequences of growth hormone excess in man. I will not address the parasellar manifestations of pituitary tumors, ectopic GHRH acromegaly, or the therapy of hypersomatotropism. These aspects have been well covered in other chapters.

ASSOCIATION WITH PITUITARY TUMORS

As we heard from Dr. Roger Guillemin, Pierre Marie in 1886 provided the first definition of the clinical syndrome of acromegaly based on personal observations of two patients and his recognition of five similar cases reported earlier by other authors (1). His proposal of the name "acromegaly" found immediate acceptance and led to recognition of similar cases by many authors and aroused intense interest in the pathophysiology of the condition.

The relation of the pituitary to this syndrome was not immediately apparent. One of the earlier cases collected from the literature by Marie (i.e., that of Henrot [2]), was found at autopsy to have a pituitary tumor. In 1891, in a paper with Marinesco, Marie described a pituitary tumor in one of his patients at necropsy (3). Soon, many other authors confirmed these findings. Nevertheless, the significance of the association was not immediately recognized and was a subject of widespread speculation. Even as late as 1911, Marie wrote to Harvey Cushing:

"After, having passed from one hypothesis to another, I find myself in no definite position regarding this question (i.e., hypo or hyper pituitarism). I wonder if the solution does not lie in a somewhat different direction. That is to say, that the important fact concerns itself less, perhaps, with the quantitative function of the hypophysis than with the modification and alterations of its secretions." (4)

The suggestion that pituitary hyperfunction occurred in acromegaly is generally attributed to Massalongo (5) who described in 1892 the granular cytoplasm of the cells of a pituitary tumor from an acromegalic patient. He attributed the pituitary tumor to excess thymic stimulation.

Further refinements in histologic stain technology allowed Benda (6) to recognize the frequent presence of eosinophilic cells in pituitary adenomas from acromegalic patients. Since eosinophil cells are prominent in the pituitaries of young, rapidly growing individuals, hyperfunction of the adenomatous cells was proposed. Support for the secretory activity of eosinophilic adenomas was provided by Cushing (4) and other early neurosurgeons who observed clinical remissions of soft tissue changes after hypophysectomy.

Experimental evidence accumulated which linked the pituitary with the regulation of growth. A number of partially successful hypophysectomies in immature dogs and other animals led to impaired growth. However, it was not until P. E. Smith (7) developed a practical, reliable method of hypophysectomy in the rat that the way was opened to many investigators to study the growth promoting effects of pituitary extracts. The experimental production of acromegaloid gigantism in the rat by administration of crude pituitary extracts by Evans and Long (8) was an important milestone in our understanding of acromegaly.

SERUM GROWTH FACTORS: THE SOMATOMEDINS

Progress in the isolation and characterization of bovine growth hormone in the 1930s and 1940s led clinical investigators to explore methods which might quantitate the growth hormone excess in acromegalic patients. Kinsell et al. (9) in 1948, and Gemzell (10) eleven years later, attempted to measure serum growth hormone (GH) by measurement of tibial epiphyseal cartilage width of hypophysectomized rats, a relatively sensitive method of GH bioassay developed by Evans et al. (11) in 1941 and later refined by Greenspan et al. (12). While both Kinsell and Gemzell found increased amounts of growth promoting substances in the serum of acromegalic patients, the concentrations detected were orders of magnitude greater than we now know to be present. With the wisdom of retrospection, it is likely that these assays were responding to growth factors other than pituitary growth hormone.

The nature of at least some of these growth factors resulted from work done in my laboratory. Murphy et al. (13) found in 1956 that the defect in the uptake of ^{35}S-sulfate by hypophysectomized rat cartilage was restored within 24 hours by relatively small amounts of GH injected in vivo. Based on these preliminary experiments, a young research fellow, William D. Salmon, Jr., undertook the development of an in vitro bioassay for GH suitable for clinical investigations. We knew from earlier workers that ^{35}S-sulfate incorporation into chondroitin sulfate was a sensitive and quantitative index of cartilage anabolism and that cartilage was easily maintained metabolically intact in simple media for a sufficient time for GH action. Nonetheless, our attempts to stimulate ^{35}S-sulfate uptake by hypophysectomized costal cartilage segments by bovine GH proved totally unsuccessful.

The possibility was then considered that GH might be acting indirectly and that this postulated factor might be present in serum. Support for this hypothesis was rapidly obtained by finding that serum from hypophysectomized rats had little or no ability to stimulate sulfate uptake but serum from normal rats, even in dilutions of 1:50 or 1:100, was markedly active. Since the effects of serum could not be replicated with insulin, thyroxine or adrenal steroids in physiologic concentrations, we postulated in 1957 the existence of a hormonal "sulfation factor" which mediated GH action (14). Sixteen years later, when acceptance of this hypothesis became more widespread, research interest intensified and the less procedurely restrictive name of somatomedin was proposed (15).

Attempts to isolate the somatomedins and the independently recognized nonsuppressible insulin-like growth factors converged and culminated in the structural characterization by Rinderknecht and Humble (16,17) in 1978 of two somatomedins which they called insulin-like growth factor I and II. In retrospect, we were extremely fortunate in our original studies because the serum of adult rats contains high concentrations of IGF I with little IGF II and hypophysectomized rat cartilage is selectively responsive to IGF I. The somatomedin hypothesis remains virtually intact today after the contributions of many workers with the significant modification that, in addition to its possible hormonal role, the somatomedins are produced by some growth hormone target tissues and act locally as paracrine growth factors.

The in vitro bioassay for somatomedins was promptly applied to sera of patients with acromegaly and elevated levels were found (18). This was subsequently confirmed by assays with chick embryo cartilage (19) and immature porcine cartilage (20) in several laboratories. Because the procedures were technically demanding and the presence of somatomedin inhibitors rendered many assays invalid, the sulfation factor bioassays never became a practical diagnostic procedure.

Furlanetto et al. (21) made a major contribution in developing the first radioimmunoassay for SM-C (IGF I). In validating their assay, they clearly showed elevations of serum SM-C in active acromegalic subjects. Two years later, Clemmons et al. (22) were able to report their experience with 57 patients with clinically active acromegaly. All had serum SM-C concentrations which were elevated 2.6 to 21.7 times their normal adult reference serum. Clinical evidences of disease activity correlated better with SM-C levels than with postglucose GH levels. The measurement of SM-C/IGF I is now a widely accepted diagnostic procedure in evaluating acromegalic patients.

RADIOIMMUNOASSAY OF GH

While the study of serum growth factors did lead to new understandings of the mechanism of growth hormone action and eventually provided an important laboratory procedure in evaluating acromegalic patients, it did not provide a direct measure of serum GH. This had to await the isolation of human growth hormone by Raben (23) and the development of the principle of radioimmunoassay as applied to insulin by Yalow and Berson in 1960 (24). While the raising of antisera against GH was easily achieved, the methods of iodination of GH, which were adequate for insulin, resulted in a partially degraded ^{131}I-GH which reacted only partially with antibody. An early RIA for serum GH using this available label, described by Utiger et al. (25) in 1962, required extraction of GH prior to assay. Nevertheless, clearly elevated levels of serum GH in acromegaly were found.

Direct RIA of human serum became a reality when Hunter and Greenwood (26) in 1963 developed a much gentler procedure for radioiodination of GH using Chloramine-T. Glick et al. (27) were quick to exploit this iodination method and reported the first successful RIA for GH in unextracted serum. While elevated levels of GH were found in the sera of acromegalic patients, the clinical application of this method also had problems. First, at intervals, normal individuals have peaks of serum GH comparable to serum GH levels of acromegalic patients. It was learned that these secretory surges could be inhibited by glucose administration. Also, many acromegalic patients secreted GH in a highly inconsistent manner so that single assays might on occasion be normal and not representative of the mean serum level. Also, acute alterations of serum growth hormone after glucose, arginine, and adrenergic agents were observed by Beck et al. (28)

and Cryer et al. (29) suggested residual hypothalamic modulation of GH secretion. When GH secretion is only slightly elevated, it is often necessary to measure the mean serum GH repeatedly over a 24-hour period.

CONSEQUENCES OF GH EXCESS

Skeletal Growth

The relationship between gigantism and acromegaly was not recognized initially by Marie because "in gigantism the extremities are in proportion to stature, that the face is not elongated, that the jaw especially presents neither the hypertrophy nor the prognathism so characteristic of acromegaly" (30). Credit is given by Cushing to Massalongo (5) in 1892 for recognizing that acromegaly was delayed gigantism. Brissaud and Meige (31) later expressed it: "L'acromégalie est le gigantisme de l'adulte, le gigantisme est l'acromégalie de l'adolescent." This was later rephrased by Launois and Roy (32) in 1904 to: "Le gigantisme est l'acromégalie des sujets aux cartilages epiphisaires non ossifiés, quelque soit leur age."

Giants have always attracted public and professional interest. Unfortunately, much of the popular information about the height of giants is grossly inflated as reviewed in a delightful essay by Al Hayles of the Mayo Clinic (33). The tallest of the medically documented giants was carefully observed over a number of years in the Washington University Medical Center. Robert Wadlow, the Alton giant, was born of parents of average height in Alton, Illinois. It is likely that he was born with a somatotroph tumor because he grew at the remarkable rate of 45 cm for the first year (34-36). Accelerated growth velocity continued until his fifth year. Thereafter, he maintained an essentially normal growth velocity. An abortive and incomplete puberty failed to fuse his epiphyses and he continued to grow until his death at age 22. Shortly before his death, his height was meticulously measured at 272.0 cm by Dr. Cecil Charles, a physician expert in physical anthropology. As is common in untreated pituitary giants, Wadlow developed severe peripheral neuropathy with a drop foot and a Charcot ankle. His death resulted from and excoriation from a brace with resulting bacteremia.

After closure of the epiphyses, growth in the length is still possible in the mandible with resulting prognathism and the ribs with the acquisition of a barrel chest. Deforming overgrowth occurs at the ends of many bones, most evident in X-rays of the terminal phalanges and at sites of tendon insertion. These changes may be sufficiently severe to limit joint motion. Overgrowth in the bones of skull and vertebrae are common.

Bone and Joint Disorders

Changes in the density of bones are variable. Early in the disease normal or increased density is common but later osteopenia may supervene. Vertebral collapse with the development of kyphos is particularly common among pituitary giants (37).

Articular cartilage participates in the general overgrowth of acromegaly. Definitive studies of these changes were carried out by Waine, Bennett and Bauer (38) in 1945 and by Kellgren et al. (39) in 1952. At first, thickening of the articular cartilage occurs. Later, degeneration and erosion of cartilage may supervene with resulting acromegalic arthropathy, a condition some authors have distinguished from osteoarthropathy. Effusions and synovial thickening are secondary to chronic arthropathy.

Connective Tissue

Soft tissue swelling contributes as much or more to the acromegalic appearance than do bony changes. This was recognized by Marie and other early clinicians and histologists who described its mucinous character. Ikkos, Luft, and Sjogren (40) in 1954 found the volume of extracellular water in acromegaly exceeded normal levels by 41 percent. Obviously the expansion of this connective tissue space occurs in visceral as well as dermal tissues.

Neurologic Complications

Neuromuscular complaints are common in acromegaly. These were noted by Marie and Marinescro (3) in 1891 in discussing the autopsy findings in one of their original patients. A number of subsequent authors have made important contributions including Kellgren et al. (39) in 1952, Lewis (41) in 1972, and Low et al. (42) in 1974. Entrapment of the median nerve at the carpal tunnel with sensory and motor defects is very common. Entrapment of other peripheral nerves occurs at other sites.

A more diffuse proliferative neuropathy with palpably enlarged peripheral nerves and functional defects can be recognized clinically. The pathologic changes were carefully correlated with functional changes by Low et al. (42). They found an increase in fascicular size with a reduction in the density of myelinated and unmyelinated fibers. There was subperineurial and endoneurial tissue proliferation. As already mentioned, peripheral neuropathy can be particularly severe and disabling in pituitary giants.

Diabetes Mellitus and Insulin Resistance

The occurrence of diabetes in acromegaly was clearly recognized by Marie (29) who wrote in 1890: "I shall point out the almost insatiable appetite observed in certain patients, and also the no less excessive thirst. I have observed them several times, and other authors have also recorded them. . . . Must we attribute the polyphagia and polydipsia to the diabetes or to the acromegaly alone? I cannot say."

In a comprehensive description of the clinical manifestations of 100 cases of acromegaly observed by Harvey Cushing, Davidoff (43) found that diabetes and abnormal glucose tolerance were present in 25% of the cases, a figure which corresponds to experience of subsequent authors (44). When insulin became available, Davidoff and Cushing (45) showed that the hyperglycemia of acromegalic patients would respond to sufficient doses of insulin. This eliminated one of the major causes of mortality existing prior to that time. Improvement in diabetes and occasionally its disappearance followed successful hypophysectomy.

The experimental production of permanent diabetes in adult dogs with crude extracts of bovine pituitaries was achieved by F. G. Young (46) in 1937. Degenerative lesions were found in the islets of Langerhans. Diabetes was also produced in cats but with typical British understatement Young wrote: "Cats did not take kindly to the experimental conditions or to the administration of extract, and were not considered suitable as test animals."

It was recognized early that GH reduced the insulin responsiveness of several experimental animals. This led to a series of experiments in the late 1940s and 1950s in the laboratory of Carl F. Cori, and elsewhere, to study this resistance in isolated tissue. GH treatment of hypophysecto-mized rats reduced the glucose uptake of the rat diaphragm (47). Studies were continued by Kipnis with the intact rat diaphragm, a preparation which allowed him to demonstrate that GH both inhibited glucose transport and phosphorylation (48). Parallel experiments with the isolated rat heart by Park and his collaborators showed similar results (49). In both muscle preparations, direct addition of GH had the paradoxical effect of stimulation of glucose uptake. Randle et al. (50) proposed that the indirect inhibition of insulin action in muscle was secondary to an increase in free fatty acids provoked by GH. Recent studies by Muggeo et al. (51) have suggested that insulin resistance in acromegaly is associated with a decrease in the number of insulin receptors and in some cases in receptor affinity as studied in circulating monocytes.

Insulin resistance occurs in clinical acromegaly, even in patients with normal glucose tolerance. Cerasi and Luft (52) and Beck et al. (53) found elevated serum insulin responses to intravenous and oral glucose.

Cardiorespiratory Complications

While diabetes is no longer a major cause of death in acromegaly, accounting for less than 2% of the deaths recorded by Wright et al. (54), cardiovascular and respiratory diseases account for the twofold excess mortality of acromegalic patients. The causes of the increased cardiovascular and respiratory deaths in this condition are multiple and complex. Hypertension occurs more frequently in acromegalic patients perhaps contributed to by growth hormone induced arterial medical hypertrophy. The increased severity of coronary atherosclerosis is attributable in part to the diabetes which occurred in 20% of Wright's series. In addition, there are many reports of mural and septal myocardial hypertrophy detected by sonography in acromegaly independent of hypertension which could have detrimental effects on cardiac function.

Upper airway and lower airway changes have been reported in acromegaly which could have a bearing on morbidity and mortality. Upper airway obstruction sufficient to lead to symptoms was first noted in 1869 by Chappell (55). It is of interest that his patient died in an attack of acute severe dyspnea several days before he was to be presented to a meeting of laryngologists. There have been many recent papers describing the occurrence of incapacitating sleep apnea in acromegalic patients. In one particularly impressive study by Cadieux et al. (56), the upper airway obstruction was observed endoscopically to result from invagination of the redundant soft tissues of the posterior and lateral hypopharynx into the laryngeal vestibule. Others have suggested that obstruction could be attributed to macroglossia and hypertrophied soft palate. While sleep apnea is a recognized cause of insomnia, daytime sleepiness, psychological and intellectual impairment, it can also trigger cardiac arrhythmias which may be fatal.

Impairment in lung function in acromegaly can have multiple causes. Chest wall movements may be abnormal from the distorted rib cage and from kyphosis. Total lung capacity is usually increased and with chronic acromegaly there is small airway obstruction due to mural hypertrophy (57). All these changes probably contribute to the morbidity and mortality of the condition.

SUMMARY

The 100 years which have passed since Marie's original paper have established that somatotroph pituitary tumors are the overwhelmingly predominant, but not exclusive, cause of acromegaly. The ultimate mediator of growth hormone action, the somatomedins, have been recognized.

Practical radioimmunoassays for somatomedin-C provide important information about disease activities. Likewise, radioimmunoassays of growth hormone permit assessment of the secretory activity of the pituitary, but linkage between growth hormone secretion and somatomedin levels is variable.

While the obvious manifestations of connective tissue swelling and bony overgrowth are distressing to the patients, morbidity and mortality result from diabetes, peripheral neuropathy, cardiovascular and respiratory pathology. Fortunately, the advent of insulin therapy has largely prevented death in diabetic coma, but failure to maintain normal blood glucose levels may be contributing to cardiovascular complications. With earlier recognition, improved neurosurgical and medical treatment, the outlook for acromegalic patients for the next century is much brighter.

REFERENCES

1. Marie P. Sur deux cas d'acromegalie; hypertrophie singuliere non congenitale des extremities superieures, inferieures et cephalique. Ref de Med (Paris) 1886; 6:297.
2. Henrot H. Notes de clinique medicale, Reims 1877 and notes de clinique medicale, des lesions anatomiques et de la nature myxoedema. Reims, France, 1882 [cited by Marie, reference 1].
3. Marie P, Marinesco G. Sur l'anatomie pathologique de l'acromegalie. Arch Med Exp Anat Path 1891; 3:539.
4. Cushing H. The pituitary body and its disorders. Philadelphia: JB Lippincott, 1912.
5. Massalongo R. Sull'acromegalia. Riforma Med (Napoli) 1892; 8:74 [cited by Cushing, reference 4].
6. Benda C. Beitrage zur normalen und pathologischen histologie der menschlichen hypophysis cerebri. Klin Wochenschr (Berlin) 1900; 36: 1205.
7. Smith PE. The disabilities caused by hypophysectomy and their repair. JAMA 1927; 83:158.
8a Evans HM, Long JA. Characteristic effects upon growth, oestrus and ovulation induced by the intraperitoneal administration of fresh anterior hypophysial substance. Anat Rec 1921; 21:62.
8b Evans HM. The function of the anterior hypophysis. Harvey lectures 1924; 19:212.
9. Kinsell LW, Michaels GD, Li CH, Larsen WE. Studies in growth. I. Interrelationship between pituitary growth factor and growth-promoting androgens in acromegaly and gigantism. J Clin Endocrinol 1948; 8:1013.
10. Gemzell CA. Demonstration of growth hormone in human plasma. J Clin Endocrinol 1959; 19:1049.
11. Evans HM, Simpson ME, Marx W, Kibrick E. Bioassay of the pituitary growth hormone width of the proximal epiphysial cartilage of the tibia in hypophysectomized rats. Endocrinology 1943; 32:13.
12. Greenspan FS, Li CH, Simpson ME, Evans HM. Bioassay of hypophysial growth hormone: the tibia test. Endocrinology 1949; 45:455.
13. Murphy WR, Daughaday WH, Hartnett C. The effect of hypophysectomy and growth hormone on the incorporation of labeled sulfate into tibial epiphyseal and nasal cartilage of the rat. J Lab Clin Med 1956; 47:715.
14. Salmon WD Jr, Daughaday WH. A hormonally controlled serum factor which stimulates sulfate incorporation by cartilage in vitro. J Lab Clin Med 1957; 49:825.
15. Daughaday WH, Hall K, Raben MS, Salmon WD Jr, Brande JL van den, Wyk JJ van. Somatomedin: proposed designation for sulphation factor. Nature 1972; 235:107.

16. Rinderknecht E, Humbel RE. The amino acid sequence of human insulin-like growth factor I and its structural homology with proinsulin. J Biol Chem 1978; 253:2769.

17. Rinderknecht E, Humbel RE. Primary structure of human insulin-like growth factor II. FEBS Lett 1978; 89:283.

18. Daughaday WH, Salmon WD Jr, Alexander F. Sulfation factor activity of sera from patients with pituitary disorders. J Clin Endocrinol 1959; 19:743.

19. Hall K. Quantitative determination of the sulfation factor activity in human serum. Acta Endocrinol (Copenh) 1970; 63:338.

20. Van den Brande JL, Du Caju MVL. An improved technique for measuring somatomedin activity in vitro. Acta Endocrinol (Copenh) 1974; 75:233.

21. Furlanetto RW, Underwood L, Van Wyk JJ, D'Ercole AJ. Estimation of somatomedin-C levels in normals and patients with pituitary disease by radioimmunoassay. J Clin Invest 1977; 60:648.

22. Clemmons DR, Van Wyk JJ, Ridgway EC, Kliman B, Kjellberg RN, Underwood LE. Evaluation of acromegaly by radioimmunoassay of somatomedin-C. N Engl J Med 1979; 302:1138.

23. Raben MS. Preparation of growth hormone from pituitaries of man and monkey. Science 1957; 125:883.

24. Yalow RS, Berson SA. Immunoassay of endogenous plasma insulin in man. J Clin Invest 1960; 39:1157.

25. Utiger RD, Parker ML, Daughaday WH. Studies on human growth hormone. I. A radioimmunoassay for human growth hormone. J Clin Invest 1962; 41:254.

26. Hunter WM, Greenwood FC. Preparation of iodine-^{131}I labelled human growth hormone in plasma. Nature 1962; 194:495.

27. Glick SM, Roth J, Yalow RS, Berson SA. Immunoassay of human growth hormone in plasma. Nature 1963; 199:784.

28. Beck P, Schalch D, Parker ML, Kipnis DM, Daughaday WH. Correlative studies of growth hormone and plasma insulin concentration with metabolic abnormalities in acromegaly. J Lab Clin Med 1965; 66:366.

29. Cryer PE, Jacobs LS, Daughaday WH. Regulation of growth hormone and prolactin secretion in patients with acromegaly and/or excessive prolactin secretion. Mt Sinai J Med (NY) 1973; 40:402.

30. Marie P. Acromegaly. Brain 1890; 12:59.

31. Brissaud E, Meige H. Gigantisme et acromegalie. Rev Scient (Paris) 1895; 3:330.

32. Launois P-E, Roy P. Etude biologique sur les geante. (Paris) 1904.

33. Hayles AB. Gigantism. Pediatr Ann 1980; 9:163.

34. Behrens LH, Barr DP. Hyperpituitarism beginning in infancy: the Alton giant. Endocrinology 1932; 16:120.

35. Humberd CD. Gigantism, report of a case. JAMA 1937; 108:544.

36. Daughaday WH. Extreme gigantism. N Engl J Med 1977; 297:1267.

37. Whitehead EM, Shalet SM, Davies D, Enoch BA, Price DA, Beardwell CG. Pituitary gigantism: a disabling condition. Clin Endocrinol (Oxf) 1982; 17:271.

38. Waine H, Bennett GA, Bauer W. Joint disease associated with acromegaly. Am J Med Sci 1945; 209:671.

39. Kellgren JH, Ball J, Tutton GK. The articular and other limb changes in acromegaly. Q J Med 1952; 21:405.

40. Ikkos D, Luft R, Sjogren B. Body water and sodium in patients with acromegaly. J Clin Invest 1954; 33:989.

41. Lewis PD. Neuromuscular involvement in pituitary gigantism. Br Med J 1972; 1:499.

42. Low PA, McCleod JG, Turtle JR, Donnely P, Wright RG. Peripheral neuropathy in acromegaly. Brain 1974; 97:139.

43. Davidoff LM. Studies in acromegaly. III. The anemnesis and symptom etiology in one hundred cases. Endocrinology 1926; 10:461.

44. Jadresic A, Banks LM, Child DF, et al. The acromegaly syndrome—

relation between clinical features, growth hormone values and radiological characteristics of the pituitary tumours. Q J Med 1982; 51:189.

45. Davidoff LM, Cushing H. Studies in acromegaly. The disturbances of carbohydrate metabolism. Arch Intern Med 1927; 39:751.

46. Young FG. Permanent experimental diabetes produced by pituitary (anterior lobe) injections. Lancet 1937; II:372.

47. Park CR, Brown DH, Cornblath M, Daughaday WH, Krahl ME. Effect of growth hormone on glucose uptake by isolated rat diaphragm. J Biol Chem 1952; 197:151.

48. Riddick FA Jr, Reisler DM, Kipnis DM. The sugar transport system in striated muscle. Effect of growth hormone, hydrocortisone and alloxan diabetes. Diabetes 1962; 11:171.

49. Park CR, Morgan HE, Henderson MJ, Regen DM, Adenas EC, Post RL. The regulation of glucose uptake in muscle as studied in the perfused rat heart. Recent Prog Horm Res 1961; 17:493.

50. Randle PJ, Garland PB, Hales CN, Nesholme EA. The glucose fatty-acid cycle. Its role in insulin sensitivity and the metabolic disturbances of diabetes mellitus. Lancet 1963; I:785.

51. Muggeo M, Bar RS, Roth J, Kahn CR, Gorden P. The insulin resistance of acromegaly: evidence for two alterations in the insulin receptor on circulating monocytes. J Clin Endocrinol Metab 1979; 48:17.

52. Cerasi E, Luft R. Insulin response to glucose loading in acromegaly. Lancet 1964; II:769.

53. Beck P, Schalch D, Park ML, Kipnis DM, Daughaday WH. Correlative studies of growth hormone and insulin plasma concentration with metabolic abnormalities in acromegaly. J Lab Clin Med 1965; 66:366.

54. Wright AD, Hill DM, Lowy C, Fraser TR. Mortality in acromegaly. Q J Med 1970; 39:1.

55. Chappel WF. A case of acromegaly with laryngeal and pharyngeal symptoms. J Laryngol Rhinol Otol 1896; 10:142.

56. Cadieux RJ, Kales A, Santen RJ, Bixler EO, Gordon R. Endoscopic findings in sleep apnea associated with acromegaly. J Clin Endocrinol Metab 1982; 55:18.

57. Harrison BDW, Millhouse KA, Harrington M, Nabarro JDN. Lung function in acromegaly. Q J Med 1978; 47:517.

14

GONADAL STEROID MODULATION OF GROWTH HORMONE SECRETORY PATTERNS IN THE RAT

William J. Millard,* Thomas O. Fox,[2] Thomas M. Badger,[3] and Joseph B. Martin[2]

*Department of Pharmacodynamics, College of Pharmacy, University of Florida, Gainesville, FL 32610; [2]Neurology Service, Massachusetts General Hospital, Boston, MA 02114 [3]Department of Pediatrics, University of Arkansas for Medical Sciences, Little Rock, AR 72205

INTRODUCTION

Growth hormone (GH) secretory patterns are governed principally by two peptides, somatostatin and growth hormone-releasing factor (GRF) whose centers are located within the medial preoptic/anterior periventricular and the ventromedial/arcuate region of the hypothalamus, respectively (1-3). Somatostatin, which inhibits GH secretion, is primarily responsible for the GH trough periods while GRF mediates the GH secretory episodes. The release of these two regulatory peptides is, in turn, modulated by a number of neurotransmitters and neuropeptides (1,2). Recent studies have indicated that gonadal steroids may also be an important determinant of the GH secretory patterns in male and female rats (4-9).

This chapter reviews our current knowledge of GH secretory patterns in male and female rats with emphasis on the modulatory actions of the gonadal steroids in maintaining sex-dependent GH secretion.

SEX-DEPENDENT PATTERNS OF GH SECRETION

Frequent sampling of blood has permitted researchers to identify spontaneous fluctuations in GH in a variety of species including man, primates, sheep, dogs and rats (1,2). In rats, episodic GH secretion first occurs prior to puberty, between 25 and 30 days of age (10), is maximal during early adulthood (5,10,11), and decreases with age (11), similar to reports in humans (1,2).

In adult rats sampled at 15 min intervals, plasma GH levels fluctuate dramatically throughout the day with males displaying GH secretory patterns which are distinct from those of females (2,4-10,12,13). Adult male rats display a low-frequency, high-amplitude pattern of GH secretion (left side, Fig. 1), whereas females exhibit a high-frequency, low-amplitude GH profile (right side, Fig. 1). Differences in parameters of the GH secretory pattern (pulse frequency, interpulse interval, peak concentration, baseline level and baseline duration) have been quantitatively evaluated in male and female rats using PULSAR analysis (14, see Table 1).

Adult Sprague-Dawley female rats display twice as many GH pulses (5.9 ± 0.5 pulses/8 hours) as Sprague-Dawley males (2.9 ± 0.2 pulses/8 hours). GH pulses occur approximately every hour in females and every 2.5-3 hours in males. Individual GH peak levels are higher in males than in females (870.0 ± 123.5 ng/ml vs. 296.2 ± 50.0 ng/ml). GH trough periods are substantially longer in males (77.8 ± 3.9 min) than females (38.0 ± 4.9 min) and mean GH basal or trough levels are 3-4 times lower than those observed in females.

We find that this sex-dependent pattern of GH secretion occurs across rat strains. Adult animals derived from either the King-Holtzman (15) or Zucker (16) lines show the same low-frequency, high-amplitude GH secretory pattern in males and high-frequency low-amplitude GH profile in females as Sprague-Dawley rats (described above).

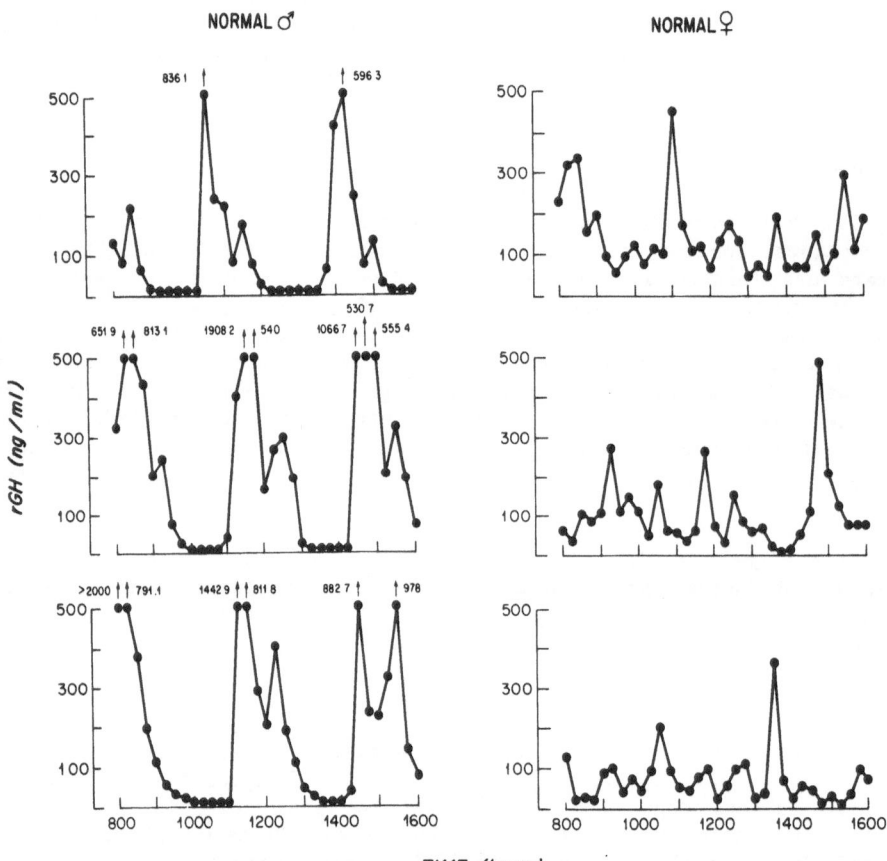

Fig. 1. GH secretory profiles of 3 male and 3 female rats. Plasma GH values greater than 500 ng/ml are indicated at the top of their respective panel (arrows and numbers). Male animals were sampled between 90 and 100 days of age and females between 130 and 140 days of age. As determined by vaginal lavage, these females were in late estrus, early diestrus (upper right panel), proestrus (middle right panel) or estrus (bottom right panel). A clear low-frequency, high-amplitude GH secretory pattern is evident in males (left side of figure), whereas females display a high-frequency, low-amplitude pattern of GH secretion.

Table 1. Comparison of growth hormone secretory pattern parameters using PULSAR analysis.

Group	peaks/8hr	peak amplitude (ng/ml)	inter-peak interval (min)	baseline levels (ng/ml)	baseline duration (min)
MALES:					
control[*] (11)	2.9±0.2	870.0±123.5	168.1±18.2	6.8±0.7	77.8±3.9
day 1 cast (9)	4.6±0.4[a]	453.7±100.6[a]	100.0±15.5[a]	14.7±1.8[a,b]	44.7±5.2[a]
day 7 cast (7)	3.9±0.3[b]	485.3±62.7[a]	114.6±6.7[b]	12.3±2.2[a,b]	64.3±6.3[b]
FEMALES:					
control[*] (16)	5.9±0.5	296.2±50.0	72.7±4.9	28.9±6.1	38.0±4.9
day 1 TP (7)	5.1±0.3[a]	190.3±35.6[a]	84.8±4.4[a]	34.4±8.4[a]	45.9±2.7[a]
day 7 TP (5)	5.6±0.9[a]	181.4±26.0[a]	69.5±3.5[a]	50.4±16.1[a]	34.5±4.5[a]

values are mean ± SE; Numbers in parentheses indicate the sample size. Statistical analysis was performed by the Kruskal-Wallis nonparmetric one way ANOVA and multiple comparison test. Significance was set at $p \geq 0.05$.

[*] = values in all categories were significantly different between male and female controls.
a = values significantly different from male controls.
b = values significantly different from female controls.

We have not been able to correlate changes in the GH secretory profile with the stages of the estrous cycle. It is possible that differences in the GH secretory pattern throughout the estrous cycle are subtle and that a 15-min sampling interval may not be sufficient to detect pulse frequency or amplitude changes (13).

GONADAL STEROID MODULATION OF GH SECRETION

Since GH secretory patterns are sexually dimorphic, both qualitatively and quantitatively we investigated the underlying cause of these GH pattern differences, thus turning our attention to gonadal steroid influences on GH secretory patterns. Gonadal steroids, by virtue of their ability to modulate gene expression, neurogenesis, and basic cellular processes, have long been known to have both long-term and short-term effects on a number of sex-dependent physiological processes (17-19). The long-term or organizational actions of steroids are generally permanent and occur during a critical phase in development encompassing both pre- and early postnatal (perinatal) development. Short-term or activational effects of steroids are immediate, dose-dependent, reversible and occur throughout the life of the individual.

Our first series of experiments have focused on the possible organizational effects of androgens on the expression of the sex dependent GH secretory pattern, using the neonatally androgenized (administered 500 μg testosterone propionate on either day 1 or 7 of life) female rat and castrated male rat as our models. If androgens act to organize GH secretory patterns, then it would be expected that androgen treatment of females should result in masculinized/defeminized GH secretory patterns as adults and castration of males should result in demasculinized/feminized GH secretory patterns. We found that except for higher baseline levels, androgenized females (left side, Figure 2; Table 1), show GH patterns which are indistinguishable from those of normal adult females (right side, Figure 1; Table 1). Male rats castrated at 7 days of age (right side, Figure 2; Table 1) show a predominant male-like GH pattern, although their GH trough levels are higher and peak GH concentrations lower than their male controls (left side, Figure 1; Table 1). Males castrated on day 1 of life display a GH secretory pattern somewhat intermediate between males and females (Table 1). Day 1 castrate males demonstrate a higher GH pulse frequency and basal secretion, lower peak concentrations and prolonged periods of basal GH secretion. Thus, neonatal castration alters the GH pulse frequency, peak concentration and basal secretion, but the effects on frequency are more pronounced when castration occurs earlier in postnatal life.

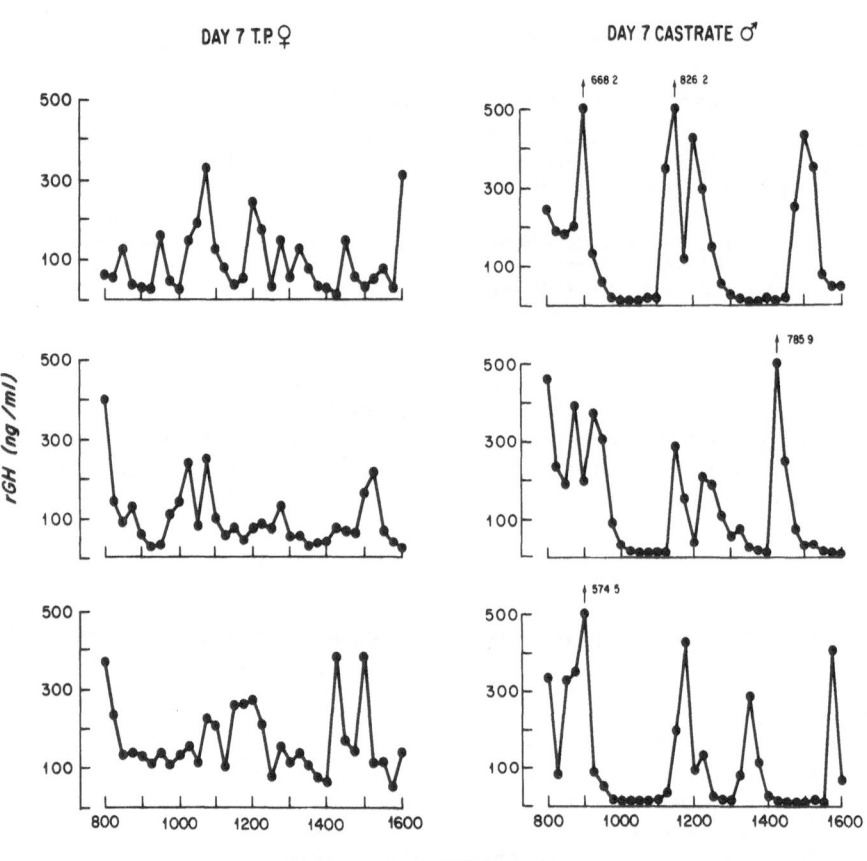

Fig. 2. GH secretory profiles of 3 female rats administered 500 μg testosterone propionate (TP) and 3 males castrated on day 7 of age. Plasma GH values greater than 500 ng/ml are indicated at the top of their respective panel (arrows and numbers). Androgenization of female pups was evidenced in both the delay in vaginal opening and the persistence of cornified epithelial cells in the vaginal smear. GH secretory patterns in these animals were not different from normal females (compare Figure 1, right side). Except for reduced GH peak levels and elevated GH baseline levels, day 7 castrate males had GH secretory patterns that closely resembled those of intact males (compare Figure 1, left side).

From these data it is difficult to determine if androgens "organize" GH secretory patterns. On the one hand, we find that neonatal androgen treatment does not masculinize/defeminize the female GH secretory pattern, whereas castration of males results in somewhat feminized/demasculinized GH secretory patterns. One interpretation of these data is that early postnatal development may be a period of submaximal sensitivity to the organizing effects of androgens. Perhaps androgens act during both pre- and postnatal development to permanently influence GH secretory patterns. Further experiments are needed to determine this.

As a second possible mechanism, regulation of GH patterns by steroids might involve both early development effects, as displayed in the males castrated on day 1, and activational effects during adulthood. The lack of an effect on GH release patterns of androgenized females might have been caused by adult feminizing effects of estrogen. Two results are consistent with this explanation. First, estrogen suppresses peak amplitudes and elevates basal GH levels in adult gonadectomized females and in both intact and gonadectomized males (5-9). Second, Jansson et al. (6) have recently demonstrated that testosterone propionate administered to neonatal ovariectomized female rats results in increased peak amplitudes and suppressed basal GH levels. These data were taken to imply that neonatal androgen imprints the brain with a masculine pattern of GH release. The testosterone propionate-treated females in our study were androgenized with regard to vaginal opening and reproductive acyclicity, but did not display GH patterns typical of males. However, these animals were not ovariectomized and a recent study has shown that androgenized females have measurable levels of estrogen in the plasma (20). Thus, our data could be in keeping with the imprinting hypothesis if estrogen from the adult ovaries was acting to prevent expression of masculine GH release patterns.

A third mechanism by which gonadal steroids affect GH secretory patterns is via a continued modulation of GH secretion throughout the life of the animal. Thus, steroids may act by means of an activational and not an organizational effect. Recent evidence indicates that the expression of the GH secretory pattern in adult male and female rats is continuously modulated by gonadal steroids. Gonadectomy during early postnatal development results in decreased GH pulse amplitudes and elevated GH basal levels in males (4-6, see above), and is without an effect in females (6). After adult or prepubertal castration, only a slight elevation in GH trough levels is observed in males (4-6,8,9, Fig. 3). No effect on pulse amplitude or pulse frequency has been found. Adult or prepubertal ovariectomy in females results in a slight diminution of baseline GH values (4-6,8,9, Fig. 4). However, the effects of ovariectomy on pulse amplitude are variable and depend upon the time of life in which ovariectomy occurs. GH pulse amplitudes are increased after prepubertal ovariectomy (4,5) but, following adult ovariectomy, no effect has been found on either GH pulse amplitudes (4,5,8,9, Fig. 4) or pulse frequency (Fig. 4).

Gonadal steroid replacement studies in adult animals have also been used to demonstrate modulatory actions of gonadal steroids on GH secretory patterns. Estrogen given to adult male and female rats has been shown to elevate baseline plasma GH levels and suppress GH pulse amplitudes (4,5, 8,9, Fig. 3,4). Testosterone replacement lowers elevated GH trough levels in castrated males indicating that the continued presence of testosterone is necessary to maintain low baseline GH levels (4-6,8, Fig. 3). Furthermore, androgen-resistant testicular feminized animals, which have reduced numbers of androgen receptors, exhibit a female GH secretory pattern suggesting that a functional androgen receptor is necessary for expression of the male GH secretory pattern (15).

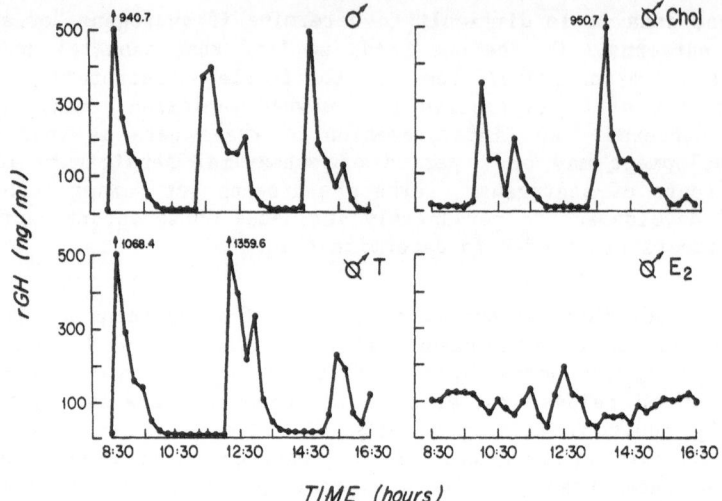

Fig. 3. Effects of long-term steroid replacement on GH secretory patterns in individual male rats. Animals were castrated at 45 days of age and immediately given either a Silastic 30 mm testosterone (T) implant, 30 mm cholesterol (CHOL) implant, or 5 mm estradiol (E$_2$) implant. Implants were repositioned every 2 weeks to prevent encapsulation and maintain constant levels of gonadal steroids within their respective physiological ranges. Animals were exposed to the steroids for 6-8 weeks. The low-frequency, high-amplitude GH secretory pattern was evident in intact rats, and castrate males given testosterone or cholesterol implants. Estrogen-treated castrate males displayed elevated baseline levels and diminished GH peak levels.

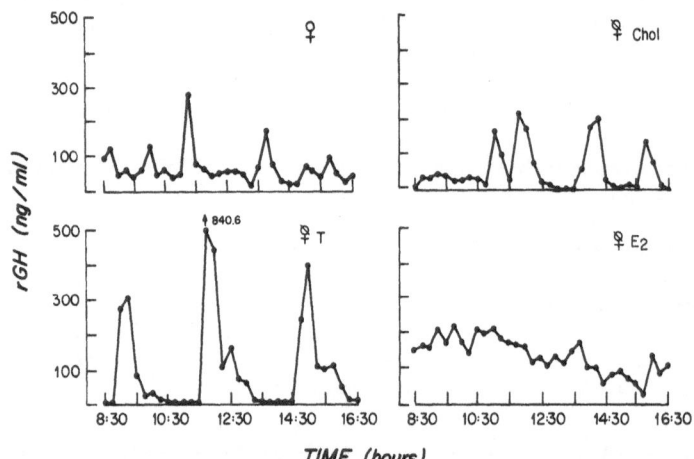

Fig. 4. GH secretory patterns in individual female rats given long-term steroid replacement therapy. Experimental protocols are described in Figure 3. Except for a lowering of baseline GH levels, ovariectomy did not affect GH secretory patterns in females. Estrogen replacement elevated basal GH levels and diminished GH peak levels. However, testosterone-treated ovariectomized females displayed a low-frequency, high-amplitude GH secretory pattern typical of males.

144

We have recently found that both intact and ovariectomized female rats given subcutaneous implants of testosterone display the low-frequency, high-amplitude GH secretory pattern characteristic of males (Fig. 4,5). Basal GH levels are reduced and GH pulse amplitudes increased in testosterone-treated females. More importantly, we have found that testosterone treatment reduces the GH pulse frequency to that of normal males (Fig. 4). Further, we have found that the conversion of female GH secretory patterns to the male pattern occurs within one week of testosterone treatment (Fig. 5). One week after removal of the testosterone implants, female GH secretory patterns are again observed in intact female animals (Fig. 5). A similar sex reversal of the GH secretory pattern is observed in intact males given estrogen replacement (data not shown).

These data indicate that GH pulse frequency, peak concentrations and baseline levels can be affected in opposing directions rather quickly (within one week) by elevating endogenous levels of the opposite sex steroid. There is a high degree of plasticity in the hypothalamic-pituitary unit which would not be expected if the system were "hard-wired" or organized by gonadal steroids. Thus, our results indicate that GH secretory patterns are not the result of the organizational effects classically ascribed to gonadal steroids and do not agree with previous reports on androgen modulation of GH secretion (4-6).

The reversibility of the gonadal steroid effects along with the observations that gonadal steroids act rather quickly to modulate GH secretion, imply an activational mode of action of gonadal steroids in regulating GH secretion. However, not all modulatory actions of steroids can be classified as activational in the classical sense. Removal of the gonads in adult animals of either sex produces only slight alterations in basal GH levels. Very little change is seen in the GH secretory pattern parameters (pulse frequency, interpulse interval, pulse amplitude or baseline duration) in either male or female rats following gonadectomy as adults. This implies that gonadal steroids (except for basal GH levels) are not necessary to maintain continually the masculine or feminine GH secretory profile. It may be that the GH secretory pattern persists in gonadectomized animals simply because steroid levels are not completely eliminated by gonadectomy.

Perhaps a more interesting interpretation of these data is that gonadal steroids may act through a novel mechanism, a steroid-sensitive "switch." This switch is not activational in the classic meaning, but instead is dependent upon or responsive to the last steroid to activate or trigger the switch. Once the switch has been activated, it will remain in that position until exposed to the other gonadal steroid, thus acting like an electronic switch to set the pattern of GH secretion in the male or female mode.

Such a mechanism would explain why intact animals reverted to pre-treatment GH profiles, since the gonad produced the appropriate steroid to trigger the switch to its native position once exogenous steroids were removed. Adult gonadectomized animals maintain their respective homotypic GH secretory patterns because they are not exposed to the opposite steroid in large enough amounts to cause significant alteration of the GH patterns. This steroid-sensitive switch mechanism may help explain why we found that male rats castrated early in development display predominant masculine GH secretory patterns. Perhaps prenatal exposure to androgens is all that is necessary to trigger the switch for the low-frequency, high-amplitude male pattern. Furthermore, testicular feminized animals display feminine GH secretory patterns because these animals have a normal complement of estrogen receptors (21), and thus may have been exposed to estrogens either prenatally or perhaps throughout life.

Since we have argued that the two major components (GH pulse frequency and amplitude) which distinguish male from female patterns are controlled centrally, the major site of this proposed steroid-sensitive switch is likely within the hypothalamus. The most likely sites would be in either the preoptic/anterior periventricular region, the ventromedial/arcuate region, or both, since these two hypothalamic centers are those principally involved in GH regulation (1,2).

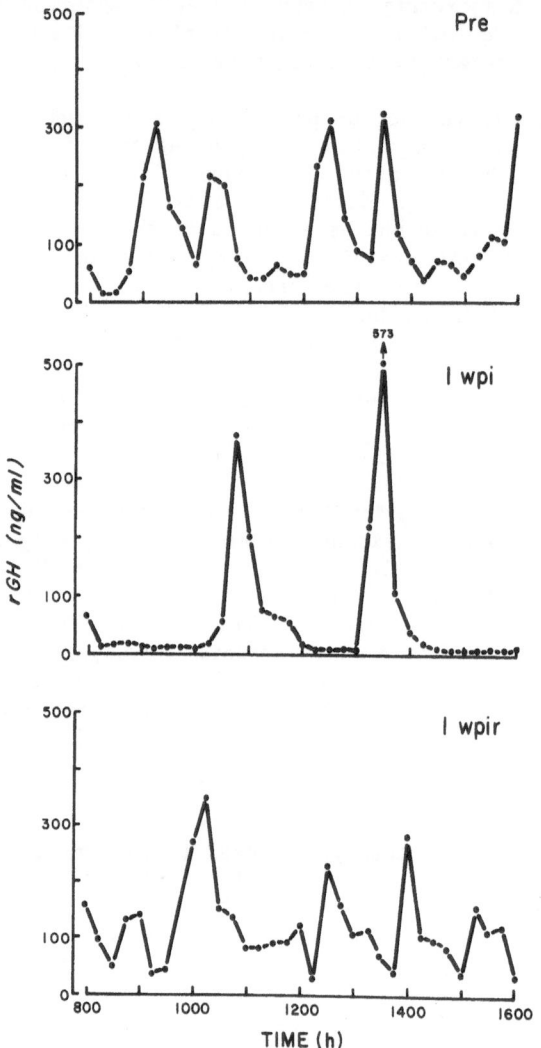

Fig. 5. Example of the inherent plasticity of the GH secretory pattern in an intact adult female rat. Immediately following the first sampling period, the animal was given a 15 mm testosterone-filled Silastic implant. The testosterone implant remained in the animal for 2 weeks at which time the testosterone capsule was removed and the animal sampled one week later. Within one week the female displayed a low-frequency, high-amplitude GH secretory pattern characteristic of males. When the steroid was removed, the GH pattern reverted back to the basic female pattern of GH secretion. Pre = preimplant; 1 wpi = 1 week post testosterone-implant; and 1 wpir = 1 week after the testosterone implant was removed.

In addition to a proposed central effect of gonadal steroids on GH secretion in the rat, there is increasing evidence that gonadal steroids also act at the pituitary level to regulate GH secretion. No difference in the GH content of the pituitary is found in male and female rats until puberty, after which pituitary content is increased in males compared to females (22,23). Using the hemolytic plaque assay, Leong et al. (24) and Ho et al. (25) have demonstrated that there is a significantly greater number of somatotropes in the male pituitary. Furthermore, testosterone administration has been found to increase and estrogen to decrease pituitary GH content (23). Both the synthesis of GH and its release appears to be higher in males than females (26-28).

Although estrogen has been shown to increase GH secretion in higher primates and man (22), the effects of estrogen in rats is less clear. In earlier studies the administration of estrogen and progesterone has been found to sensitize the pituitary to GH-releasing activity of hypothalamic extracts (22,29). Wehrenberg et al. (30) found that estrogen does not affect GRF-induced GH secretion. However, there is recent evidence that estrogen reduces GRF-induced GH release (31,32). Testosterone, on the other hand, has been associated with an enhanced GRF-stimulated GH release (25,30-32). Furthermore, GRF-induced GH secretion in vitro was greater in male rat pituitaries than in female (25,31,33).

Although the pituitary and hypothalamus are implicated as the anatomical sites of gonadal steroid modulation of GH secretory patterns, peripheral organs may also be key factors. For example, there is evidence that GH causes the induction of both hepatic GH and prolactin receptors (34-39). Some biological actions of GH are mediated through the liver via the production of somatomedins (1,2,36), and both estrogen and testosterone can influence somatomedin-C release through alterations in GH secretion (40). The patterns of spontaneous GH secretion observed in female rats result in reduced amounts of GH release which appears to correlate with the differences of the pattern of certain hepatic enzymes and liver functions that are known to be GH-dependent.

Apparently, differences in GH output between males and females are critical factors in determining the sex differences in adult body size and body length (36). GH replacement regimens resembling male GH secretory patterns to hypophysectomized rats enhances both longitudinal bone growth and body weight gain (41,42). Recently, the administration of 1 µg of GRF every 3 hours to normal female rats was found to accelerate body growth and increase pituitary GH content (43). Thus, a better appreciation of the effects that steroids exert on GH, and of the sites of action and the mechanisms by which these effects occur would greatly improve our understanding of the physiology and pathophysiology of growth.

ACKNOWLEDGMENTS

This work was supported by NIH grants AM26252, HD10818 and HD17364 and by a biomedical research support grant from the College of Pharmacy, University of Florida.

REFERENCES

1. Martin JB. Neuroendocrine regulation of growth hormone secretion. In: Laron Z, Butenandt O, eds. Evaluation of growth hormone secretion. Basel: S Kargar, 1983:1.
2. Martin JB, Millard WJ. Brain regulation of growth hormone secretion. J Anim Sci 1985 (in press).

3. Tannenbaum GS, Ling N. The interrelationship of growth hormone (GH)-releasing factor and somatostatin in generation of the ultradian rhythm of GH secretion. Endocrinology 1984; 115:1952.

4. Jansson JO, Ekberg S, Isaksson OGP, Eden S. Influence of gonadal steroids on age- and sex-related secretory patterns of growth hormone in the rat. Endocrinology 1984; 114:1287.

5. Jansson JO, Eden S, Isaksson O. Sexual dimorphism in the control of growth hormone secretion. Endocr Rev 1985; 6:128.

6. Jansson JO, Ekberg S, Isaksson O, Mode A, Gustafsson JA. Imprinting of growth hormone secretion, body growth, and hepatic steroid metabolism by neonatal testosterone. Endocrinology 1985; 117:1881.

7. Mode A, Gustafsson JA, Jansson JO, Eden S, Isaksson O. Association between plasma level of growth hormone and sex differentiation of hepatic steroid metabolism in the rat. Endocrinology 1982; 111:1692.

8. Millard WJ, Badger TM, Fox TO, Martin JB. Gonadal steroid modulation of growth hormone (GH) secretory patterns in adult male and female rats [Abstract]. Program 67th annual meeting, Endocrine Society, 1985:194.

9. Millard WJ, Badger TM, Fox TO, Martin JB. Effects of short-term exposure to gonadal steroids on growth hormone (GH) secretory patterns in adult male and female rats [Abstract]. Program 15th annual meeting, Society of Neuroscience, 1985:1299.

10. Eden S. Age- and sex-related differences in episodic growth hormone secretion in the rat. Endocrinology 1979; 105:555.

11. Sonntag WE, Steger RW, Forman LJ, Meites J. Decreased pulsatile release of growth hormone in old male rats. Endocrinology 1980; 107:1875.

12. Terry LC, Saunders A, Audet J, Willoughby JO, Brazeau P, Martin JB. Physiologic secretion of growth hormone and prolactin in male and female rats. Clin Endocrinol (Oxf) 1977; 6:19s.

13. Millard WJ, O'Sullivan DM, Fox TO, Martin JB. Sexually dimorphic patterns of growth hormone secretion in the rat. In: Crowley WF Jr, ed. Episodic hormone secretion, methods of analysis and normative data. Orlando, FL: Academic Press (in press).

14. Merriam GR, Wachter KW. Algorithms for the study of episodic hormone secretion. Am J Physiol 1982; 243:E310.

15. Millard WJ, Politch JA, Martin JB, Fox TO. Growth hormone secretory patterns in androgen-resistant (testicular feminized) rats. Endocrinology 1986; 119(6):2655.

16. O'Sullivan DM, Millard WJ, Badger TM, Martin JB, Martin RJ. Growth hormone secretion in genetic large (LL) and small (SS) rats. Endocrinology 1986; 119(5):1948-53.

17. Goy RW, McEwen BS. Sexual differentiation of the brain. Cambridge: MIT Press, 1980.

18. Gorski RA. Sexual differentiation of brain structure in rodents. In: Serio M, Motta M, Zanisi M, Martini L, eds. Sexual differentiation: basic and clinical aspects, vol 11. New York: Raven Press, 1984:65.

19. McEwen BS, Bigon A, Fischette T, Luine V, Parsons B, Rainbow TC. Toward a neurochemical basis of steroid hormone action. In: Martini L, Ganong WF, eds. Frontiers in neuroendocrinology; vol 8. New York: Raven Press, 1984:153.

20. Grady RR. Effect of neonatal treatment with the sex-opposite steroid on gonadotropin responsiveness in rats. Neuroendocrinology 1986; 43:322.

21. Krey LC, Lieberburg I, Maclusky NJ, Davis PG, Robbins R. Testosterone increases cell nuclear estrogen receptor levels in the brain of the Stanley-Gumbreck pseudohermaphrodite male rat: implications for testosterone modulation of neuroendocrine activity. Endocrinology 1982; 110:2168.

22. Reichlin S. Regulation of somatotropic hormone secretion. In:

Greep RO, Astwood EB, eds. Handbook of physiology; sect 7, vol 4. Baltimore: Williams and Wilkins, 1974:405.

23. Birge CA, Peake GT, Mariz IK, Daughaday WH. Radioimmunoassayable growth hormone in the rat pituitary gland: effects of age, sex and hormonal state. Endocrinology 1967; 81:195.

24. Leong DA, Kau SK, Sinha YN, Kaiser DL, Thorner MO. Enumeration of lactotropes and somatotropes among male and female pituitary cells in culture: evidence in favor of a mammosomatotrope subpopulation in the rat. Endocrinology 1985; 116:1371.

25. Ho KY, Leong DA, Sinha YN, Johnson ML, Evans WS, Thorner MO. Sex-related differences in GH secretion in rat using reverse hemolytic plaque assay. Am J Physiol 1986; 250:E650.

26. MacLeod RM, Abad A, Eidson LL. In vivo effect of sex hormones on the in vitro synthesis of prolactin and growth hormone in normal and pituitary tumor-bearing rats. Endocrinology 1969; 84:1475.

27. Yamamoto K, Taylor LM, Cole FE. Synthesis and release of GH and prolactin from the rat anterior pituitary in vitro as functions of age and sex. Endocrinology 1970; 87:21.

28. Burek CL, Frohman LA. Growth hormone synthesis by rat pituitaries in vitro: effect of age and sex. Endocrinology 1970; 86:1361.

29. Malacara JM, Valverde R, Reichlin S. Elevation of plasma radio-immunoassayable growth hormone in the rat induced by porcine hypo-thalamic extract. Endocrinology 1972; 91:1189.

30. Wehrenberg WB, Baird A, Ying SY, Ling N. The effects of testosterone and estrogen on the pituitary growth hormone response to growth hormone-releasing factor. Biol Reprod 1985; 32:369.

31. Evans WS, Krieg RJ, Limber ER, Kaiser DL, Thorner MO. Effects of in vivo gonadal hormone environment on the in vitro hGRF-40-stimulated GH release. Am J Physiol 1985; 249:E276.

32. McCormick GF, Millard WJ, Badger TM, Martin JB. Gonadal steroid modulation of growth hormone-releasing factor-stimulated growth hormone secretion [Abstract]. Program 14th annual meeting, Society of Neuroscience, 1984:1214.

33. Cronin MJ, Rogol AD. Sex differences in the cyclic adenosine 3':5'-monophosphate and growth hormone response to growth hormone-releasing factor in vitro. Biol Reprod 1984; 31:984.

34. Baxter RC, Zaltsman Z, Turtle JR. Rat growth hormone (GH) but not prolactin (PRL) induces both GH and PRL receptors in female rat liver. Endocrinology 1984; 114:1893.

35. Norstedt G, Andersson G, Gustafsson JA. Growth hormone induction of lactogenic receptors at intracellular sites in male rat liver. Endocrinology 1984; 115:672.

36. Isaksson OGP, Eden S, Jansson JO. Mode of action of pituitary growth hormone on target cells. Annu Rev Physiol 1985; 47:483.

37. Mode A, Norstedt G, Simic B, Eneroth P, Gustafsson JA. Continuous infusion of growth hormone feminizes hepatic steroid metabolism in the rat. Endocrinology 1981; 108:2103.

38. Gustafsson JA, Eden S, Eneroth P, et al. Regulation of sexually dimorphic hepatic steroid metabolism by the somatostatin-growth hormone axis. J Steroid Biochem 1983; 19:691.

39. Norstedt G, Palmiter R. Secretory rhythm of growth hormone regulates sexual differentiation of mouse liver. Cell 1984; 36:805.

40. Copeland KC, Johnson DM, Kuehl TJ, Castracane VD. Estrogen stimu-lates growth hormone and somatomedin-C in castrate and intact female baboons. J Clin Endocrinol Metab 1984; 58:698.

41. Jansson JO, Albertsson-Wikland K, Eden S, Thorngren KG, Isaksson O. Circumstantial evidence for a role of the secretory pattern of growth hormone in control of body growth. Acta Endocrinol (Copenh) 1982; 99:24.

42. Clark RG, Jansson JO, Isaksson O, Robinson ICAF. Intravenous growth hormone: growth hormone to patterned infusions in hypophysectomized

149

rats. J Endocrinol 1985; 104:53.

43. Clark RG, Robinson ICAF. Growth induced by pulsatile infusion of amidated fragment of human growth hormone-releasing factor in normal and GHRF-deficient rats. Nature 1985; 314:281.

15

PATHOGENESIS OF ACROMEGALY

Mark E. Molitch

Center for Endocrinology, Metabolism and Nutrition
Northwestern University Medical School
Chicago, Illinois 60611

INTRODUCTION AND HISTORICAL PERSPECTIVE

In his initial description of acromegaly as a distinct disorder, Marie speculated on three possible etiologies: (1) a primary rheumatologic disease; (2) a sympathetic nervous system disorder; and, (3) a developmental disorder (1). After some early uncertainty about the precise nature of the pituitary pathology, it soon became clear that most, if not all, cases were associated with eosinophilic adenomas (2,3). Initially it was not clear whether the pituitary enlargement was just another manifestation of the syndrome or whether it was in some way causative. Lewis summarized the popular theories current in 1905 (3):

(1) Nervous theory. The disease is supposed to be dependent upon changes in the nervous system.

(2) Theory of growth anomaly. Acromegaly is not to be regarded as a disease proper but as an anomaly of growth; the whole appearance suggests a reversion to the anthropoid ape type.

(3) Thymus theory. This theory suggests that an increase in vascular canals of a large and persistent thymus is the etiologic factor.

(4) Genital theory. Acromegaly is accompanied in the majority of females by an early menopause, and in males by impotence; hence the assumption that by the loss of function of the organs of generation an excess of blood is diverted to the extremities, resulting in their hypertrophy.

(5) Thyroid theory. Diseased conditions of the thyroid gland, which are occasionally found in acromegaly, are regarded as the causative factor.

(6) Hypophysis theory. Acromegaly is caused by excessive function of the cellular elements of the anterior lobe of the hypophysis.

Proof that the eosinophilic adenomas were etiologic in acromegaly and not just another manifestation of organ hyperplasia was obtained with the documented clinical improvement in two patients following partial resection of adenomas by Cushing (4) and by Hochenegg (see reference 5) and the later finding by Evans and Long in the 1920s that injections of anterior pituitary extract caused gigantism in rats (6).

The role of the hypothalamus in the pathogenesis of the pituitary hyperfunction in acromegaly was first questioned by Severi (7) in 1938 at a time when the concept of the hypothalamic regulation of pituitary was only just being formulated by Harris and others. This question lay dormant only to be cogently brought to the fore again by Leszynsky in 1960 (8) at the same time as Reichlin's definitive demonstration in the rat of the hypothalamic control of growth (9). As the etiology of acromegaly in her patient in 1960, Leszynsky (8) postulated ". . . whether . . . a primary hypothalamic process causing a disturbance of pituitary function, may possibly be the underlying pathogenetic lesion." Subsequently, Reichlin (10), Cryer and Daughaday (11), and Lawrence et al. (12) again raised the possibility that acromegaly may arise as a result of a defect in the hypothalamic regulation of GH secretion.

A number of recent developments permit new insights into an understanding of the role of the hypothalamus in the pathogenesis of growth hormone (GH)-secreting tumors in acromegaly. These developments include the characterization of the GH-releasing hormones (GRH), detailed descriptions of GH secretory dynamics in patients with GRH-secreting tumors as well as GH-secreting tumors, new immunohistochemical techniques for documenting the hormone content of pituitary cells, and the careful characterization of GH secretory dynamics before and after transsphenoidal selective adenomectomy in a large number of patients with acromegaly.

The primary question is whether such tumors arise spontaneously within the pituitary or are due to prolonged stimulation from hypothalamic dysfunction, such as excessive GRH (Fig. 1) or decreased somatostatin secretion. Decreased somatostatin is quite unlikely in view of the normal thyroid function and blunted thyrotropin (TSH) response to TSH releasing hormone (TRH) found in most patients (13). An exaggerated TSH response to TRH would be expected if somatostatin were decreased. Excessive stimulation by GRH may occur either because of an actual increased GRH secretion into the hypothalamic-pituitary portal vessels or because of increased sensitivity of somatotroph cells to normal GRH levels. Such an excess of GRH could arise because of altered catecholaminergic regulation. If tumors are due to excessive stimulation by GRH, it is likely that a two-stage process is needed, as formulated by Melmed et al. (14), involving initially excessive stimulation and subsequently neoplastic transformation by a specific cell type in response to such stimulation.

IS ACROMEGALY DUE TO UNDERLYING HYPOTHALAMIC DYSFUNCTION?

Four areas can be examined to determine whether acromegaly is due to an underlying hypothalamic disorder: (1) Can excess GRH explain the various types of tumors seen, including prolactin (PRL)- and GH-secreting tumors? (2) Is there hyperplasia of the somatotrophs in the nonneoplastic portions of the pituitary, as would be expected if GRH excess exists? (3) Can excessive GRH alone explain the abnormal GH secretory dynamics, or are these abnormal dynamics secondary to the tumor and thus resolve with pituitary tumor resection? (4) Can the acromegaly be permanently cured by pituitary tumor resection or does hypothalamic dysfunction cause recurrent tumor formation?

Can Excess GRH Explain the Various Tumor Types Found in Acromegaly?

There are at least six different tumor cell types that are associated with GH hypersecretion. Since cell types ranging from the primitive stem cell to the mature somatotroph are found in GH-secreting tumors, it is obvious that neoplastic transformation may occur at any stage of development of these cells, regardless of whether the initiating factor was GRH or some unknown cellular phenomenon. The finding of different cell types in these tumors, therefore, does not provide evidence for or against a hypothalamic role in the pathogenesis of these tumors.

The fact that 20-40% of tumors secrete both GH and PRL has been regarded as evidence against the hypothalamic theory of pathogenesis, since GRH has not been regarded as a PRL releasing factor (15). However, we (16) and others (17,18) have found that GRH can stimulate both GH and PRL release in both normal individuals and acromegalic patients.

Although in most reports there was no rise in PRL in response to the acute injection of GRH (15), we (16) have found small but significant elevations of PRL after such injection (Fig. 2). Furthermore, in our studies of 6-hour GRH infusions, the PRL response to an acute injection of GRH toward the end of the infusion was not attenuated as the GH response was (Fig. 2), suggesting either a different receptor or other pathway of PRL release or simply the fact that there was no depletion of the rapidly releasable PRL pool (16). In other studies, Borges et al. (17) have shown that very large single boluses (10 μg/kg) of GRH (1-40) could elevate PRL

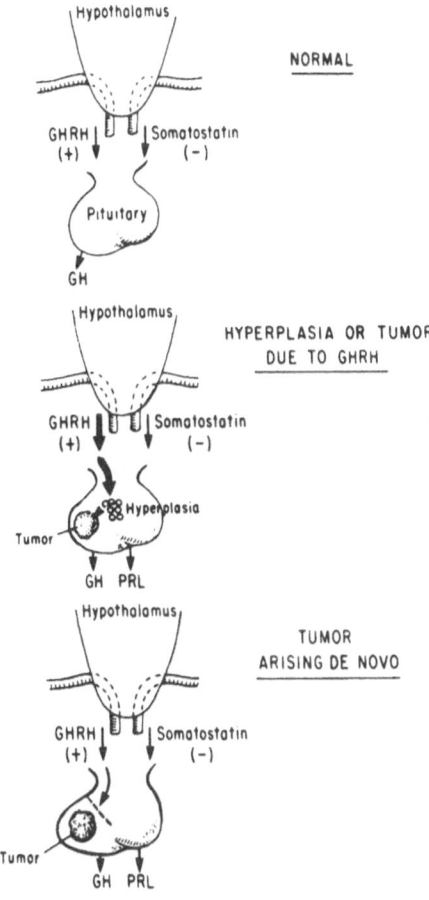

Fig. 1. Possible mechanisms leading to the formation of GH-secreting pituitary tumors in acromegaly. Reprinted with permission from Human Growth Hormone, S. Raiti, R. A. Tolman, eds., Plenum Medical Book Co., New York, 1986.

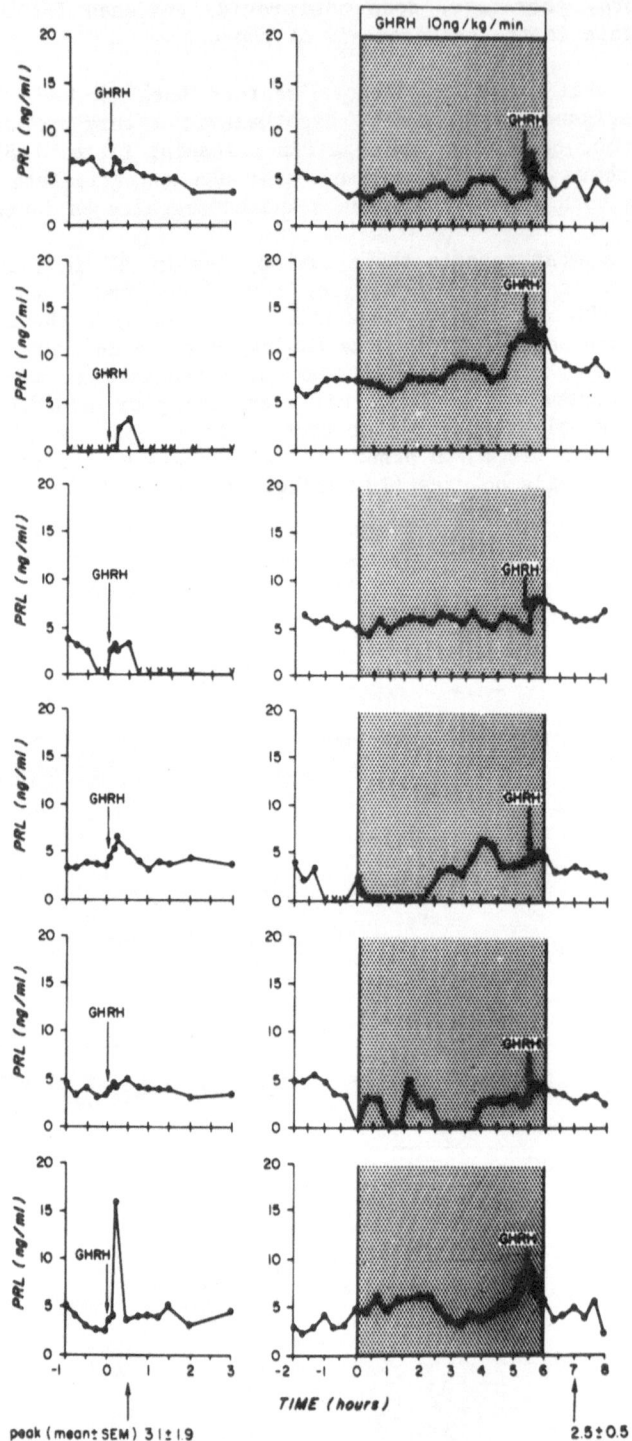

Fig. 2. Prolactin secretory responses to bolus injections of GRH, 3.3 mcg/kg, to continued infusions of GRH, and to second bolus injections in 6 patients. Note that small but significant responses were present both before and after infusions and that PRL levels did not rise during the infusions.

in 3 of 6 normal subjects and in all 11 subjects with idiopathic GH
deficiency. Sassolas et al. have shown similar results (18). Whether the
PRL release in these subjects is due to PRL release from GRH-stimulated
lactotrophs or somatotrophs is unknown.

It is possible that the release of PRL is mediated by GRH acting on
the VIP receptor rather than the GRH receptor, as shown in the recent
studies of Laburthe et al. (19). The physiological significance of such
GRH-induced PRL release is not certain, but given the concomitant release
of GH and PRL in a variety of circumstances (e.g., hypoglycemia, exercise,
stress, cirrhosis, renal failure), the possibility of dual hormone release
by GRH is intriguing.

Whereas GH has been shown to respond to GRH in patients with acromegaly in vivo (20,21), we have also found that in most acromegalic
patients there is a parallel release of GH and PRL in response to GRH
regardless of whether there was basal hyperprolactinemia (Fig. 3). In 6
of 8 patients studied, GH and PRL levels were highly correlated following
GRH injection. PRL and GH levels were also highly correlated in 4 of the
8 patients even during placebo administration (Table 1). Furthermore,
Webb et al. (22) have demonstrated the release of GH and PRL in vitro in
response to GRH from an adenoma from a patient with acromegaly and hyperprolactinemia. Six of the 7 patients with acromegaly secondary to ectopic
GRH secretion, in whom PRL levels were measured, had hyperprolactinemia
(23-29). In the patient with acromegaly and somatotroph hyperplasia
caused by a GRH-secreting tumor described by Thorner et al. (25), there
was a parallel fall of GH and PRL following resection of the GRH-producing
pancreatic tumor. Thus, stimulation of both GH and PRL by GRH may explain
the development of bihormonal tumors, depending on the initial cell type
that is stimulated, according to the hypothalamic theory of tumor pathogenesis.

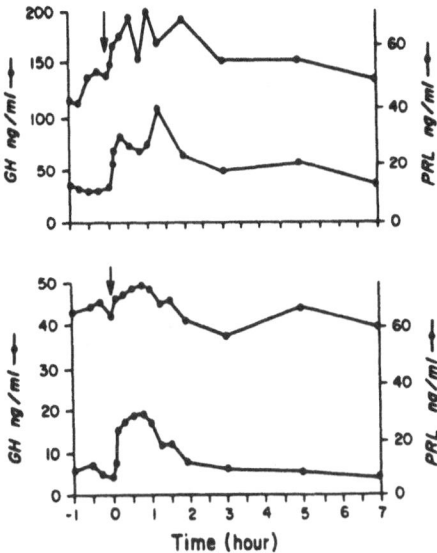

Fig. 3. GH and PRL secretory
responses to GRH, 3.3 mcg/kg or
1 mcg/kg, IV as bolus injections
in 2 patients with acromegaly with
elevated basal PRL levels. Arrow
indicates time of injection.

Table 1. Correlation between serum PRL and GH
in patients with acromegaly after placebo
or GRH 1-40-OH injection.

		r-Value	
Subject	Dose	Placebo	GRH
1	3.3	.655+	.704++
2	3.3	NA	.308
3	3.3	.628++	.666++
4	1.0	.193	.810+
5	1.0	-.599	.358
6	1.0	.180	.872+++
7*	3.3	.639++	.726+++
8*	3.3	.575+	.798+++

NA = not available; * = basal hyperprolactinemia; + = P < 0.05; ++ = P < 0.01; +++ = P < 0.001

Is There Hyperplasia of the Nonneoplastic Somatotrophs in Patients with Acromegaly?

If excessive hypothalamic stimulation were to cause acromegaly, the pituitary should show diffuse somatotroph hyperplasia, or at least some evidence of somatotroph hyperplasia in nonneoplastic portions of the gland. Such is not the case, however. In virtually all cases in which systemic GRH secreting tumors are not implicated, discrete pituitary adenomas have been found (14). In two series of patients with pituitary tumors in whom immunohistochemical techniques were used to study the para-adenomatous "normal" pituitary tissue, there was no evidence of such hyperplasia (30,31). If anything, the numbers of GH secreting cells in the adjacent "normal" pituitary were decreased (30,31), possibly due to negative feedback by the increased somatomedin levels.

For comparison, we now have descriptions of the pituitary abnormal-ities in several patients in whom the acromegaly was clearly due to ectopic GRH secreting tumors. Diffuse somatotroph hyperplasia was found in all cases of ectopic GRH secretion when there was adequate pituitary tissue for histologic examination using immunohistochemical techniques (25,26,32).

In contrast to these cases, however, are the findings in 5 patients in whom acromegaly and increased GH levels occurred in association with GRH producing hypothalamic gangliocytomas (33). In 4 of these 5 cases, distinct pituitary somatotroph adenomas, and not diffuse somatotroph hyperplasia, were found (33); no pituitary abnormalities were found in the fifth case. In 3 of these cases, both the GRH- and GH-producing tumors were removed surgically with amelioration of the acromegaly. Only in the one case in which no pituitary abnormality was found was the GRH-producing gangliocytoma removed alone. In this latter case, postoperative basal GH levels (8.7 ng/ml) were similar to preoperative levels (11.8 ng/ml) and these elevated levels remained nonsuppressible by glucose (33). Thus, these cases have not provided evidence to prove that the GRH-producing tumors caused the elevated GRH levels or the somatotroph adenomas. It is quite possible, however, that the excess GRH caused the adenoma which then was relatively autonomous. This would be contrary to evidence provided by the patients with systemic GRH-secreting tumors in whom adenomas were not found.

In summary, patients with the common variety of acromegaly do not show para-adenomatous hyperplasia. However, based on evidence from cases with ectopic tumors and hypothalamic gangliocytomas secreting GRH, there is strong but not conclusive evidence against excessive GRH secretion being etiologic.

Can the Abnormal GH Secretory Dynamics in Acromegaly be Explained by Excessive GRH Stimulation or Are They Due to the Tumor Itself?

One argument used in favor of a hypothalamic etiology for acromegaly is that in patients with acromegaly there often appears to be some measure of hypothalamic influence over GH secretion. In patients with acromegaly, one of the hallmarks is the nonsuppressibility of GH by glucose. Indeed, this lack of response to glucose is used as a diagnostic criterion. In our own series of 18 patients whose GH responses to an oral glucose load were evaluated prior to any therapy (Fig. 4), 5 showed a paradoxical increment (defined as being greater than 50% of baseline values) of GH, 12 did not suppress, and one patient showed suppression of GH levels but not to < 2 ng/ml; these results are similar to those reported by others (11,12,34-36). Of 12 of our patients whose GH responses to insulin-induced hypoglycemia were measured prior to therapy, 9 had an increment in GH values of > 50% of basal values (a normal response would be an increment of > 100% of basal values) while only 3 did not respond to hypoglycemia. Therefore, many patients with acromegaly continue to display some response to changing glucose levels, although the response may be paradoxical. Since it is thought that at least the response to hypoglycemia is mediated through hypothalamic mechanisms, this hypothesis implies retention of hypothalamic influence over GH secretion (56).

A number of studies have recently demonstrated that the tumors in most acromegalic patients retain the ability to release GH in response to

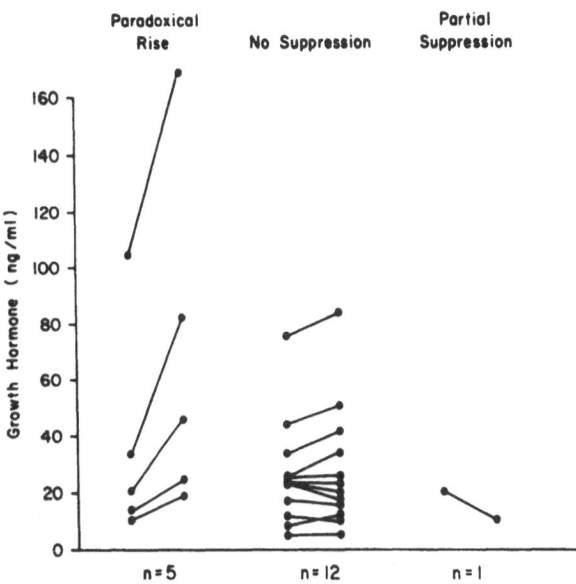

Fig. 4. GH responses to hyperglycemia achieved by an oral glucose load in 18 patients with acromegaly prior to therapy. Reprinted with permission from Human Growth Hormone, S. Raiti, R. A. Tolman, eds., Plenum Medical Book Co., New York, 1986.

GRH both in vivo (20,21) and in vitro (22). Figure 3 demonstrates the parallel between GH and PRL responses to GRH in subjects with acromegaly. Similarly, somatostatin had previously been found to suppress GH secretion from adenomas in most acromegalic patients in vivo (37) and in vitro (22). Thus, qualitatively and quantitatively normal responses to GRH and somato-statin are found in most patients with acromegaly, although there is a great deal of variability of such responses, and a similar variability is also found in normal individuals.

Adrenergic influence over GH secretion is also qualitatively normal in patients with acromegaly (38). Dopamine, however, inhibits rather than stimulates GH secretion in most subjects with acromegaly (39). Dopamine directly inhibits GH release by the adenomatous pituitaries in vitro from subjects whose GH levels were also decreased by dopamine in vivo (39). Such inhibition is mediated by specific membrane dopaminergic receptors (39).

TRH was initially demonstrated to release GH in the majority of acromegalic patients by Irie and Tsushima (40). In our own series, of 17 patients given TRH prior to therapy, 10 responded with an increment of GH (> 50% increment over basal values) and 7 did not have a response; these proportions are similar to those reported by others (34,35,40). In vitro studies indicate this effect is mediated directly at the level of the pituitary (41). The common explanation given for this response to TRH in patients with acromegaly is that in this abnormal, neoplastic tissue there is an "unmasking" of TRH receptors.

Thus, there remains at least some hypothalamic influence over GH secretion in most patients with acromegaly, albeit the GH responses may not be the same as those in normal individuals. Moreover, the response to GRH is retained and even exaggerated in some individuals.

Recent evidence suggests that some of these abnormal responses can be explained by postulating prior stimulation of the cells by GRH. All of the cases of acromegaly due to ectopic GRH secretion had abnormal GH secretory dynamics when tested, including a paradoxical increase in response to an oral glucose load (25,26,28,29,32,42-45). When complete GRH tumor resection was performed, these abnormal responses returned to normal in most cases (23,25,26,29,32,42-44). Interestingly, in the patient reported by Sassolas et al. (30), the GH response to TRH normal-ized following the GRH secreting tumor resection but again became abnormal concomitant with tumor recurrence. Thus, in these cases, the excess GRH was likely responsible for these abnormal responses rather than a tumor cell which had become altered or "dedifferentiated." In studies of rat pituitary cells in vitro, Borges et al. (46) have shown that the GH response to TRH is greatly augmented after prior infusion of GRH.

Thus, these data derived from experiments with GRH administration, and from the patients with ectopic GRH secretion, provide new support for the hypothesis that excess secretion of GRH by the hypothalamus, or hypersensitivity of the pituitary to normal levels of GRH, may play a primary role in the pathogenesis of these tumors. An alternative explana-tion to the hypothalamic etiology is that these tumors, like so many endocrine tumors, remain partially responsive to normal stimuli and may show aberrant responses to a variety of secretagogues.

On the other hand, the return of GH secretory dynamics to normal following selective tumor resection has been the strongest evidence against the hypothesis that the hypothalamus plays a primary role in the pathogenesis of these tumors. Figure 5 shows that the lack of suppression by glucose and the response to TRH found preoperatively in 2 of our patients have been reversed by surgery. To date, there is no evidence of recurrence in these 2 patients after 2 and 8 years of follow-up. A number of similar patients have been reported by other investigators (34,35,47-50). In all of these series, however, a large number of patients were reported to have basal GH levels persistently below 5 ng/ml, but had abnormal responses to glucose or TRH. Whether such patients have residual tumor tissue or underlying hypothalamic dysregulation is unknown.

Can the Acromegaly be Permanently Cured by Pituitary Tumor Resection or Does Hypothalamic Dysfunction Cause Recurrent Tumor Formation?

If hypothalamic dysregulation caused the development of GH secreting tumors, there should be a high rate of tumor recurrence following apparently "curative" selective tumor resection and this rate should increase over time. In 11 reported studies totaling 282 cases, only 8 incidences of tumor recurrence were documented (2.8%) (34-36,47-54). These data were derived from patients who were deemed clinically and biochemically "cured" postoperatively, as evidenced by basal GH levels < 5 ng/ml to loss of responsiveness to TRH, suppressibility by glucose and normalization of SM-C levels. Although the follow-up periods were not very long (ranging from 2-4 years), most of the recurrences were observed within 1-2 years of surgery (35,49-51). No late recurrences were found.

Recently, long-term (5-11 years) follow-up data were reported on 21 cured (GH levels < 5 ng/ml) surgical patients followed by Dr. Hardy (55). Within this group there was a clinical recurrence in 3 patients (14%) which occurred within 6 years of surgery. In one other patient there was no clinical evidence of recurrence; however, basal GH levels were not fully suppressible by glucose. Given the probable long time frame necessary for the initial development of these tumors, it is likely that the tumor recurrences represented regrowth of tumor remnants left at the time

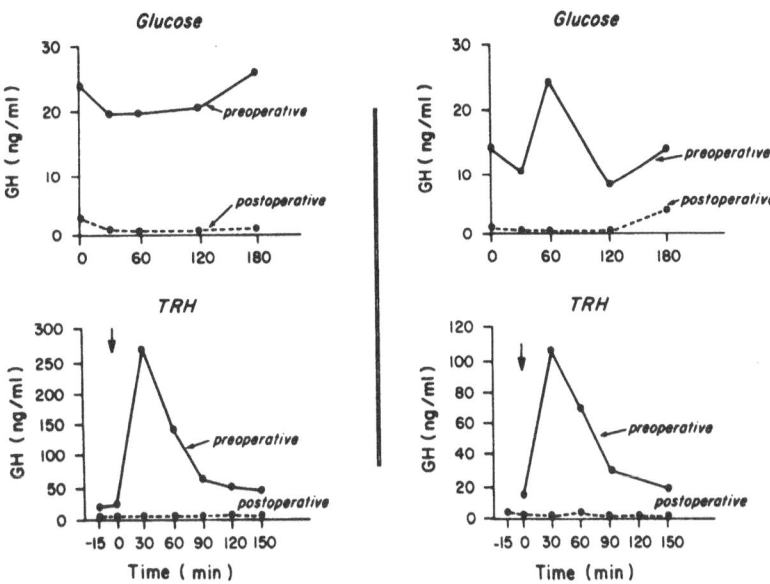

Fig. 5. Resolution of abnormal GH secretory dynamics in two patients following transsphenoidal selective resection of GH secreting pituitary adenomas. Arrows indicate time of TRH injection. Reprinted with permission from Human Growth Hormone, S. Raiti, R. A. Tolman, eds., Plenum Medical Book Co., New York, 1986.

of the original surgery rather than the de novo formation of new tumors. Thus, these data provide evidence against underlying hypothalamic dysregulation, since a higher rate of new tumor formation would be expected and this rate would likely increase with time.

CONCLUSIONS

The role of the hypothalamus in the pathogenesis of GH-secreting tumors remains controversial. Excessive secretion of GRH as the cause for acromegaly has only been proven for the small number of patients with ectopic and hypothalamic GRH-secreting tumors. Although increased GRH secretion by the hypothalamus, or increased pituitary sensitivity to GRH, may play a primary role in the pathogenesis of the more common GH-secreting pituitary tumor, this theory has not yet been proven. Evidence in favor of a hypothalamic etiology includes: (1) retention of hypothalamic influence on GH secretion; (2) retention of GH responsivity to GRH; (3) explanation of the nonsuppressibility by glucose and the abnormal response to TRH by prior exposure to GRH, as shown experimentally and in the patients with ectopic GRH secretion; and, (4) explanation of the occurrence of GH and PRL secreting tumors by finding PRL release in response to GRH.

However, none of this is evidence against tumors arising de novo in the pituitary. On the other hand, evidence against tumors arising because of hypothalamic dysregulation, and in favor of such tumors arising de novo in the pituitary include: (1) the pituitary tissue surrounding the GH-secreting adenoma does not show hyperplasia, as it should if there were excess GRH; and, (2) the fact that many patients cured by surgery remain cured for long periods of observation and have a return of secretory dynamics to normal.

It is quite possible that there is more than one etiology for the pituitary tumors of patients with acromegaly. In some patients the tumors may arise because of hypothalamic dysfunction but, in most, the weight of evidence suggests that the tumors arise spontaneously.

REFERENCES

1. Marie P. Sur deux cas d'acromegalie. Hypertrophie singuliere non congenitale des extremites superieures, inferieures et cephalique. Rev de Med 1886; 6:297-333.
2. Benda C. Beitrage zur normalen und pathologischen histologie der menschlichen hypophysis cerebri. Berl Klin Wchnschr 1900; 37: 1205-10.
3. Lewis DD. Hyperplasia of the chromophile cells of the hypophysis as the cause of acromegaly, with report of a case. Bull Johns Hopkins Hosp 1905; 16:157-64.
4. Cushing H. Partial hypophysectomy for acromegaly. Ann Surg 1909; 1:1002-18.
5. Stumme E. Akromegalie und hypophyse. Arch I Klin Chir 1908; 87: 437-66.
6. Evans HM, Long JA. The effect of the anterior lobe administered intraperitoneally upon growth, maturity, and oestrus cycles of the rat. Anat Rec 1921; 21:62-3.
7. Severi L. L'ipothalamo nella patogenesis dell'acromegalia. Arch "de Vecchi" per Anat Pat Med Clin 1938; 1:74-107.
8. Leszynsky HE. Acromegaly of suspected hypothalamic origin without pituitary tumor. Is Med J 1960; 19:146-51.

9. Reichlin S. Growth and the hypothalamus. Endocrinology 1960; 67:760-73.
10. Reichlin S. Regulation of somatotrophic hormone secretion. In: Harris GW, Donovan BT, eds. The pituitary gland. London: Butterworths, 1966:270-98.
11. Cryer PE, Daughaday WR. Regulation of growth hormone secretion in acromegaly. J Clin Endocrinol 1969; 29:386-93.
12. Lawrence AM, Goldfine ID, Kirsteins L. Growth hormone dynamics in acromegaly. J Clin Endocrinol Metab 1970; 31:239-47.
13. Lamberg B-A, Pelkonen R, Aro A, Grahne B. Thyroid function in acromegaly before and after transsphenoidal hypophysectomy followed by cryoapplication. Acta Endocrinol (Copenh) 1976; 82:254-66.
14. Melmed S, Braunstein GD, Horvath E, Ezrin C, Kovacs K. Pathophysiology of acromegaly. Endocr Rev 1983; 4:271-90.
15. Thorner MO, Spiess J, Vance ML, et al. Human pancreatic growth-hormone releasing factor selectively stimulates growth-hormone secretion in man. Lancet 1983; 1:24-8.
16. Goldman JA, Molitch ME, Thorner MO, Vale W, Rivier J, Reichlin S. Growth hormone and prolactin responses to bolus and sustained infusions of GRH-1-40-OH in man (submitted for publication).
17. Borges JLC, Blizzard RM, Gelato MC, et al. Effects of human pancreatic tumour growth hormone releasing factor on growth hormone and somatomedin C levels in patients with idiopathic growth hormone deficiency. Lancet 1983; 2:119-24.
18. Sassolas G, Chatelain P, Cohen R, et al. Effects of human pancreatic tumor growth hormone-releasing hormone (hpGRH1-44-NH$_2$) on immunoreactive and bioactive plasma growth hormone in normal young men. J Clin Endocrinol Metab 1984; 59:705-9.
19. Laburthe M, Amiranoff B, Boige N, Royer-Fessard C, Tatemoto N, Moroder L. Interaction of GRF with VIP receptors and stimulation of adenyl cyclase in rat and human intestinal epithelial membranes. FEBS Lett 1983; 159:89-92.
20. Wood SM, Ch'ng JLC, Adams EF, et al. Abnormalities of growth hormone release in response to human pancreatic growth hormone releasing factor (GRF (1-44) in acromegaly and hypopituitarism. Br Med J 1983; 286:6379-83.
21. Gelato MC, Merriam GR, Vance ML, et al. Effects of growth hormone-releasing factor on growth hormone secretion in acromegaly. J Clin Endocrinol Metab 1985; 60:251-7.
22. Webb CB, Thominet JL, Frohman LA. Ectopic growth hormone releasing factor stimulates growth hormone release from human somatotroph adenomas in vitro. J Clin Endocrinol Metab 1983; 56:417-9.
23. Saeed uz Zafar M, Mellinger RC, Fine G, Szabo M, Frohman A. Acromegaly associated with a bronchial carcinoid tumor: evidence for ectopic production of growth hormone-releasing activity. J Clin Endocrinol Metab 1979; 48:66-71.
24. Leveston SA, McReel DW Jr, Buckley PJ, et al. Acromegaly and Cushing's syndrome associated with a foregut carcinoid tumor. J Clin Endocrinol Metab 1981; 53:682-9.
25. Thorner MO, Perryman RL, Cronin MJ, et al. Somatotroph hyperplasia. Successful treatment of acromegaly by removal of a pancreatic islet tumor secreting a growth hormone-releasing factor. J Clin Invest 1982; 70:965-77.
26. Sassolas G, Chayvialle JA, Partensky C, et al. Acromegalie, expression clinique de la production de facteurs de liberation de l'hormone de croissance (G.R.F.) par une tumeur pancreatique. Ann Endocrinol (Paris) 1983; 44:347-54.
27. Scheithauer BW, Carpenter PC, Bloch B, Brazeau P. Ectopic secretion of a growth hormone-releasing factor. Report of a case of acromegaly with bronchial carcinoid tumor. Am J Med 1984; 76:605-16.
28. Wilson DM, Ceda GP, Bostwick DG; et al. Acromegaly and Zollinger-

Ellison syndrome secondary to an islet cell tumor: characterization and quantification of plasma and tumor human growth hormone-releasing factor. J Clin Endocrinol Metab 1984; 59:1002-5.

29. Spero M, White EA. Resolution of acromegaly, amenorrhea-galactorrhea syndrome, and hypergastrinemia after resection of jejunal carcinoid. J Clin Endocrinol Metab 1985; 60:392-5.

30. Saeger W, Ludecke DK. Pituitary hyperplasia. Definition, light and electron microscopical structures and significance in surgical specimens. Virchows Arch [A] 1983; 399:277-87.

31. Landolt AM, Minder H. Immunohistochemical examination of the para-adenomatous "normal" pituitary. An evaluation of prolactin cell hyperplasia. Virchows Arch [A] 1984; 403:181-93.

32. Shalet SM, Beardwell CG, MacFarlane A, et al. Acromegaly due to production of a growth hormone releasing factor by a bronchial carcinoid tumour. Clin Endocrinol (Oxf) 1979; 10:61-7.

33. Asa SL, Kovacs K, Thorner MO, Leong DA, Rivier J, Vale W. Immunohistological localization of growth hormone-releasing hormone in human tumors. J Clin Endocrinol Metab 1985; 60:423-7.

34. Arafah BM, Brodkey JS, Kaufman B, Velasco M, Manni A, Pearson OH. Transsphenoidal microsurgery in the treatment of acromegaly and gigantism. J Clin Endocrinol Metab 1980; 50:578-85.

35. Tucker HSG, Grubb SR, Wigand JP, Watlington CO, Blackard WG, Becker DP. The treatment of acromegaly by transsphenoidal surgery. Arch Intern Med 1980; 140:795-802.

36. Schuater LD, Bantle JP, Oppenheimer JH, Seljeskog EL. Acromegaly: reassessment of the long-term therapeutic effectiveness of transsphenoidal pituitary surgery. Ann Intern Med 1981; 95:172-4.

37. Hall R, Besser GM, Schally AV, et al. Action of growth-hormone-release inhibitory hormone in healthy men and in acromegaly. Lancet 1973; 2:581-4.

38. Cryer PE, Daughaday WH. Adrenergic modulation of growth hormone secretion in acromegaly: alpha- and beta-adrenergic blockade produce qualitatively normal responses but no effect on L-dopa suppression. J Clin Endocrinol Metab 1977; 44:977-9.

39. Bression D, Brandi AM, Nousbaum A, Le Dafniet M, Racadot J, Peillon F. Evidence of dopamine receptors in human growth hormone (GH)-secreting adenomas with concomitant study of dopamine inhibition of GH secretion in a perifusion system. J Clin Endocrinol Metab 1982; 55:589-93.

40. Irie M, Tsushima T. Increase of serum growth hormone concentration following thyrotropin-releasing hormone injection in patients with acromegaly or gigantism. J Clin Endocrinol Metab 1972; 35:97-100.

41. Ishibashi M, Yamaji T. Effect of thyrotropin-releasing hormone and bromocriptine on growth hormone and prolactin secretion in perifused pituitary adenoma tissues of acromegaly. J Clin Endocrinol Metab 1978; 47:1251-6.

42. Dabek JT. Bronchial carcinoid tumour with acromegaly in two patients. J Clin Endocrinol Metab 1974; 38:329-33.

43. Sonksen PH, Ayres AB, Braimbridge M, et al. Acromegaly caused by pulmonary carcinoid tumors. Clin Endocrinol (Oxf) 1976; 5:503-13.

44. Caplan RH, Koob L, Abellera RM, Pagliara AS, Kovacs K, Randall RV. Cure of acromegaly by operative removal of an islet cell tumor of the pancreas. Am J Med 1978; 64:874-81.

45. Ch'ng JLC, Christofides ND, Kraenzlin ME, et al. Growth hormone secretion dynamics in a patient with ectopic growth hormone-releasing factor production. Am J Med 1985; 79:135-8.

46. Borges JLC, Uskavitch DR, Kaiser DL, Cronin MJ, Evans WS, Thorner MO. Human pancreatic growth hormone-releasing factor-40 (hpGRF-40) allows stimulation of GH release by TRH. Endocrinology 1983; 113:1519-21.

47. Arosio M, Giovanelli MA, Riva E, Nava C, Ambrosi B, Faglia G. Clinical use of pre- and postsurgical evaluation of abnormal GH

responses in acromegaly. J Neurosurg 1983; 59:402-8.

48. Leavens ME, Samaan NA, Jesse RH Jr, Byers RM. Clinical and endocri-
     nological evaluation of 16 patients treated by transsphenoidal
     surgery. J Neurosurg 1977; 47:853-60.

49. Jaquet P, Guibout M, Jaquet C, et al. Circadian regulation of growth
     hormone secretion after treatment in acromegaly. J Clin Endocrinol
     Metab 1980; 50:322-8.

50. Baskin DS, Boggan JE, Wilson CB. Transsphenoidal microsurgical
     removal of growth hormone-secreting pituitary adenomas. A review of
     137 cases. J Neurosurg 1982; 56:634-41.

51. Williams RA, Jacobs HS, Kurtz AB, et al. The treatment of acromegaly
     with special reference to trans-sphenoidal hypophysectomy. Q J Med
     1975; 44:79-98.

52. Giovanelli MA, Gaini SM, Tomei G, Motti EDF, Villani R. Acromegaly:
     surgical failures and recurrences. In: Derome PJ, Jedynak CP,
     Peillon F, eds. Pituitary adenomas. Biology, physiopathology and
     treatment. Paris: Asclepios Publishers, 1980:253-62.

53. Schaison G, Couzinet B, Moatti N, Pertuiset B. Critical study of the
     growth hormone response to dynamic tests and the insulin growth
     factor assay in acromegaly after microsurgery. Clin Endocrinol (Oxf)
     1983; 18:541-9.

54. Bynke O, Karlberg BE, Kagedal B, Nilsson OR. Early post-operative
     growth hormone levels predict the result of transsphenoidal tumour
     removal in acromegaly. Acta Endocrinol (Copenh) 1983; 103:158-62.

55. Serri O, Somma M, Comtois R, et al. Acromegaly: biochemical assess-
     ment of cure after long term follow-up of transsphenoidal selective
     adenomectomy. J Clin Endocrinol Metab 1985; 61:1185-9.

56. Molitch ME. Growth hormone hypersecretion syndromes. In: Raiti S,
     Tolman RA, eds. Human growth hormone. New York: Plenum Medical
     Book Co., 1986:29-50.

16

PATHOLOGY OF ACROMEGALY

Kalman Kovacs and Calvin Ezrin

Department of Pathology, St. Michael's Hospital,
University of Toronto, Toronto, Ontario, Canada;
Department of Medicine, Cedars-Sinai Medical Center,
U.C.L.A., Los Angeles, CA, U.S.A.

In 1886, Pierre Marie, the eminent French neurologist, described two patients with acromegaly and created the term for the disease (1). This year, we celebrate the 100th anniversary of this classic publication which dates the beginning of pituitary endocrinology. One can look back on this century with great pride and intellectual satisfaction, since unprecedented progress has been achieved in understanding pituitary structure and function as well as the morphologic, clinical and biochemical aspects of hypophyseal diseases, including pathology and endocrine manifestations of acromegaly.

Although Pierre Marie is credited with the first comprehensive description of the clinical features of acromegaly, it should be noted that acromegaly and gigantism, the two diseases related to GH excess, were known to exist before Marie's publication. The causal link between the pituitary and acromegaly, as well as the role of GH overproduction in the etiology of the disease were substantiated only in the first half of the 20th century.

Early histologic examination of pituitaries in patients with acromegaly or gigantism, claimed that a wide variety of morphologic changes, such as struma, colloid degeneration, hypertrophy, hyperplasia, adenoma, carcinoma, sarcoma, cylindroma, cystic tumor, glioma, teratoma, etc., could account for the clinical abnormality. With the application of sophisticated morphologic techniques and more refined histology, it became evident that the structural findings were often misinterpreted and the most common lesion causing GH oversecretion was an increase in the number of GH-producing adenohypophyseal cells. In early studies, it was uncertain whether cellular accumulation represented hyperplasia or neoplasia. A series of publications by Bailey, Davidoff and Cushing, however, clarified this question (2,3). The study of a large number of surgically-removed or autopsy-obtained pituitaries provided unequivocal proof that a well-defined adenoma is the most frequent abnormality in patients with acromegaly or gigantism.

The assumption that GH-producing adenomas were invariably acidophilic tumors was rather simplistic and cannot be accepted any longer. Progress in biochemical and imaging techniques permitted an earlier and more precise diagnosis of pituitary adenomas. Newly developed microsurgical techniques allowed for their safe removal, even when they were small. The introduction of new morphologic procedures, such as immunohistochemistry, immunoelectron microscopy and morphometry, shed light on structural characteristics of pituitary adenomas and resulted in a novel classification which separates adenomas on the basis of hormone content, fine structural characteristics, cellular composition and cytogenesis (4,5). A better comprehension of hypophyseal cytophysiology and cytopathology emerged from these investigations, and pituitary adenomas producing GH became better known and more clearly defined. It became evident that acidophilic adenomas did not always secrete GH; some of them synthesized PRL or were functionally inactive. Many GH-producing adenomas associated with acromegaly represented chromophobic tumors indicating that chromophobic cells can secrete hormones. This concept was contrary to previously held views which suggested that chromophobic cells were endocrinologically inactive, i.e., incapable of hormone synthesis. Detailed morphologic studies, based on many surgically-removed pituitary adenomas, showed that GH excess may be associated with several morphologically distinct adenoma types (6,7). Although a deeper insight was achieved in the last decade on structure-function correlation, growth rate and biologic behavior of pituitary adenomas, much more work is required, including long-term follow-up of a considerable number of patients to convincingly correlate the morphologic features of adenomas with secretory activity, rate of growth and prognosis.

Grossly, the most characteristic finding in patients with GH excess is a well-demarcated adenoma confined to the adenohypophysis. The adenoma is most often located in one of the lateral wings of the anterior pituitary, which is the main site of GH-producing cells. In some cases, the tumor spreads outside the sella turcica and invades adjacent tissues. In rare cases, the adenoma is ectopic and can be detected in the sphenoid sinus or parapharyngeal region.

Detailed morphologic investigation of a large number of surgically removed or autopsy-obtained pituitaries revealed that, in subjects with GH excess, eight morphologically different lesions can be revealed: (1) densely granulated GH cell adenoma (Fig. 1, 2); (2) sparsely granulated GH cell adenoma (Fig. 3); (3) acidophil stem cell adenoma (Fig. 4); (4) mammosomatotroph cell adenoma (Fig. 5); (5) mixed GH cell-PRL cell adenoma (Fig. 6); (6) GH cell carcinoma; (7) plurihormonal adenoma with GH content (Fig. 7); and, (8) GH cell hyperplasia (Fig. 8). The morphologic differential diagnosis between these 8 well-defined entities may be very difficult in some cases.

The histologic features, immunohistochemical profiles and ultrastructural characteristics of these morphologic entities have been reported in detail in a number of publications (4-7). Thus, there is no need to describe them here; the interested reader can find details and further references in the previously cited papers. The morphologic changes are illustrated in electron micrographs (Figs. 1-10). Three aspects will be discussed here: (1) plurihormonal adenoma; (2) GH cell hyperplasia; and, (3) treatment of GH cell adenomas with SMS 201-995, a long-acting somatostatin analog.

PLURIHORMONAL ADENOMA

Plurihormonal adenomas produce more than one hormone and differ in chemical composition, immunoreactivity and biologic function (8,9). They can be divided into monomorphous and plurimorphous tumors. Monomorphous plurihormonal adenomas consist of one morphologically distinct cell type which synthesizes two or more hormones and may be different in electron

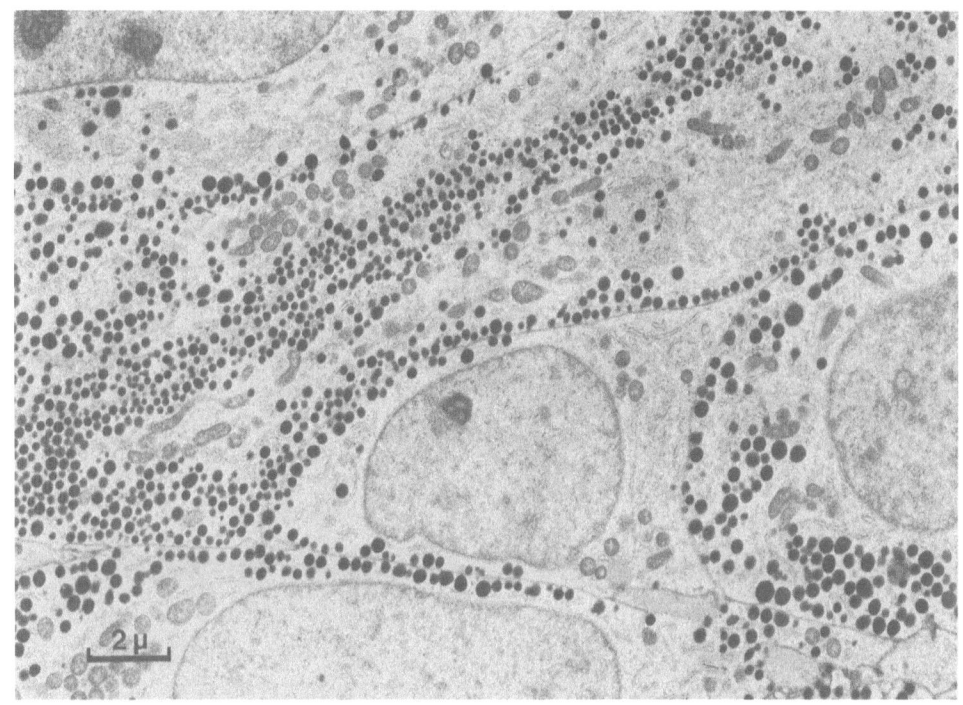

Fig. 1. Densely granulated GH cell adenoma containing numerous large secretory granules.

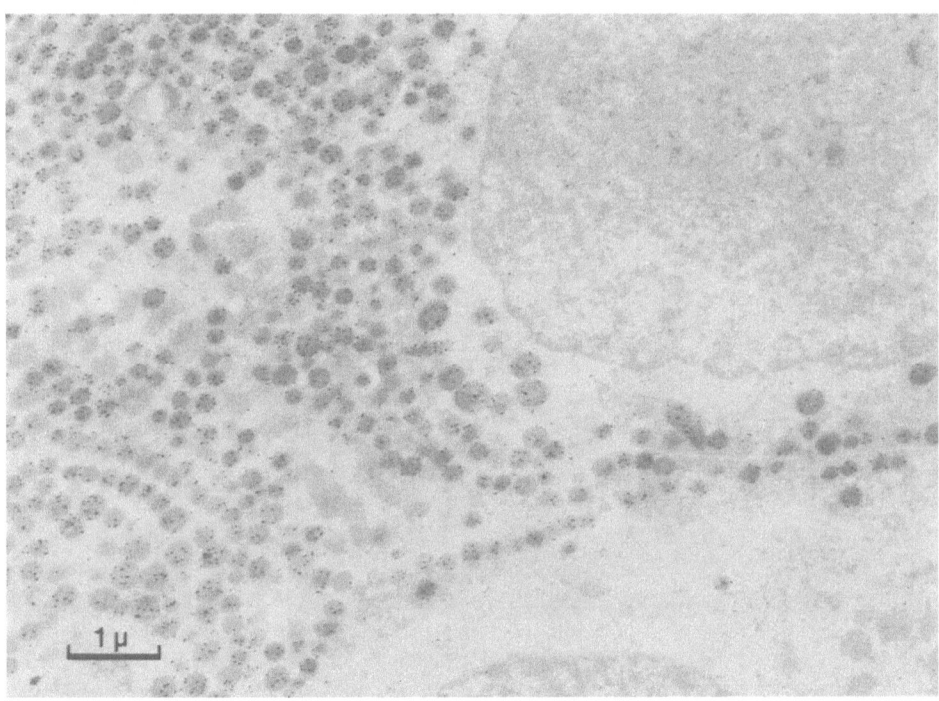

Fig. 2. Densely granulated GH cell adenoma. The secretory granules are heavily labeled with gold particles (immuno-gold technique).

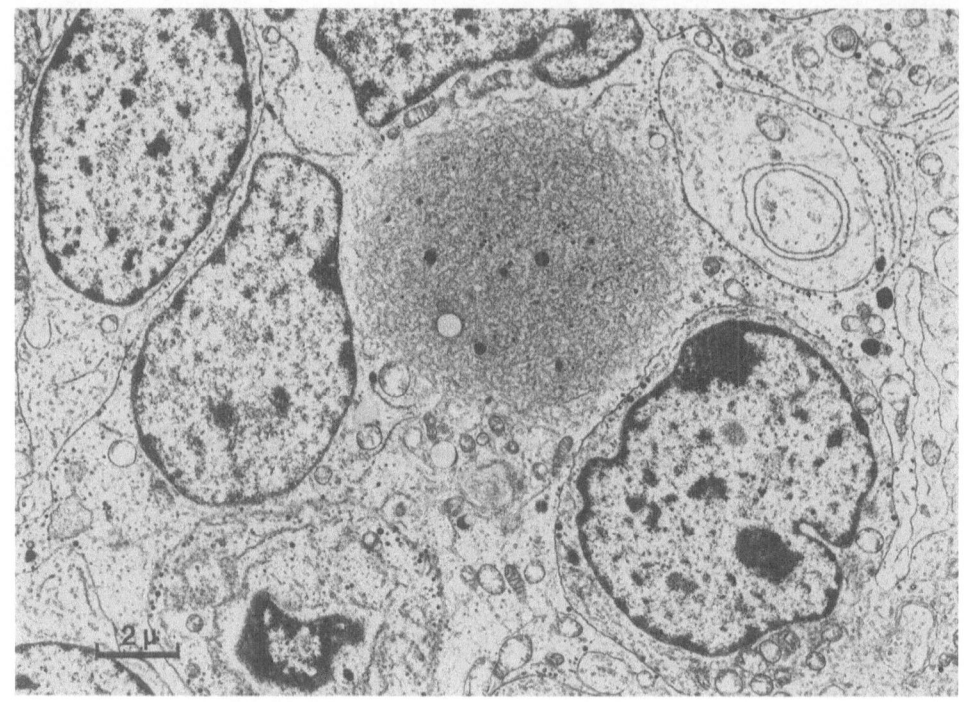

Fig. 3. Sparsely granulated GH cell adenoma. Note the characteristic fibrous body (center).

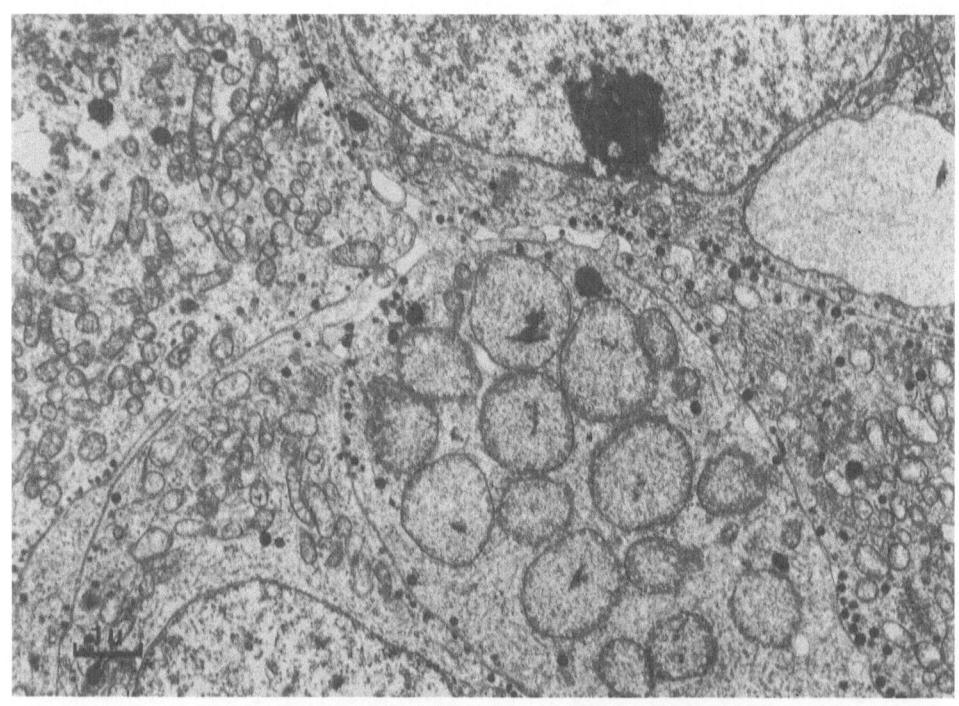

Fig. 4. Acidophil stem cell adenoma exhibiting marked oncocytic transformation. Note giant mitochondria.

microscopic characteristics from known adenohypophyseal cells. Plurimorphous plurihormonal adenomas are composed of two or more morphologically distinct cell types which resemble their nontumorous counterparts. Immunohistochemical procedures have a pivotal role in the diagnosis of plurihormonal adenomas. Electron microscopic study may fail to disclose their cellular derivation, since ultrastructural features may not be specific or the cells constituting the adenoma differ from those of cells in nontumorous adenohypophyses.

In our experience, 16 percent of surgically-removed pituitary adenomas were plurihormonal. The most frequent hormonal combination included the synthesis of GH and PRL. Three morphologically well-defined entities can be recognized with GH and PRL production: acidophil stem cell adenoma, mammosomatotroph adenoma and mixed GH cell-PRL cell adenoma.

Acidophil stem cell adenomas (10) exhibit a rapid rate of growth and frequently spread into neighboring tissues. They are accompanied by a varying degree of hyperprolactinemia. In some patients, clinical features of acromegaly may be evident despite the fact that blood GH levels are not elevated. The correlation between tumor size and blood PRL concentrations, observed in patients with sparsely granulated PRL cell adenoma, is not apparent in many patients with acidophil stem cell adenoma; relatively large adenomas may be accompanied by slight or moderate hyperprolactinemia. Acidophil stem cell adenomas are monomorphous bihormonal tumors, consisting of one cell type which may be the common precursor of GH cells and PRL cells. Immunohistochemical procedures demonstrate positive staining for both PRL and GH in the cytoplasm of the same adenoma cells. Immunoreactivity for GH is often weak or absent. Electron microscopy (Fig. 4) shows closely-apposed elongated adenoma cells with irregular nuclei. The abundant cytoplasm contains dispersed, short RER profiles, poorly developed Golgi complex, fibrous bodies with microfilaments, smooth-walled tubules, multiple centrioles and cilia. The secretory granules are sparse, irregular and measure 100-300 nm. Extrusion of secretory granules is uncommon. Oncocytic change and mitochondrial gigantism can be found in the majority of acidophil stem cell adenomas.

Mammosomatotroph adenomas (11) are slowly growing, benign tumors accompanied by elevated blood GH concentrations, clinical features of acromegaly and, in some patients, slight hyperprolactinemia. They are monomorphous bihormonal tumors, consisting of acidophilic cells. Immunohistochemical methods disclose the presence of GH and PRL in the cytoplasm of the same adenoma cells. By electron microscopy (Fig. 5), the adenoma cells appear to be well differentiated and resemble densely granulated GH cells. The secretory granules are often irregular, evenly electron dense or have a mottled appearance and measure 200-2000 nm. Extrusion of secretory granules and large extracellular deposits of secretory material are characteristic features of this adenoma type.

Mixed GH cell-PRL cell adenomas (12) are associated with high blood GH concentrations, clinical features of acromegaly, hyperprolactinemia and, in some patients, amenorrhea, galactorrhea, infertility, decreased libido and impotence. They are bimorphous bihormonal tumors composed of two distinct cell types, densely or sparsely granulated GH cells and PRL cells. The two cell types are seen in small groups or individually interspersed with other cell populations. Immunohistochemical procedures disclose the presence of GH and PRL in two different cell types. By electron microscopy (Fig. 6), two distinct cell types can be recognized. Every combination can occur; most often, densely granulated GH cells and sparsely granulated PRL cells can be revealed. Recent immunoelectron microscopic studies indicate that distinction between the two cell types may not be easy. In several tumors diagnosed as mixed GH cell-PRL cell

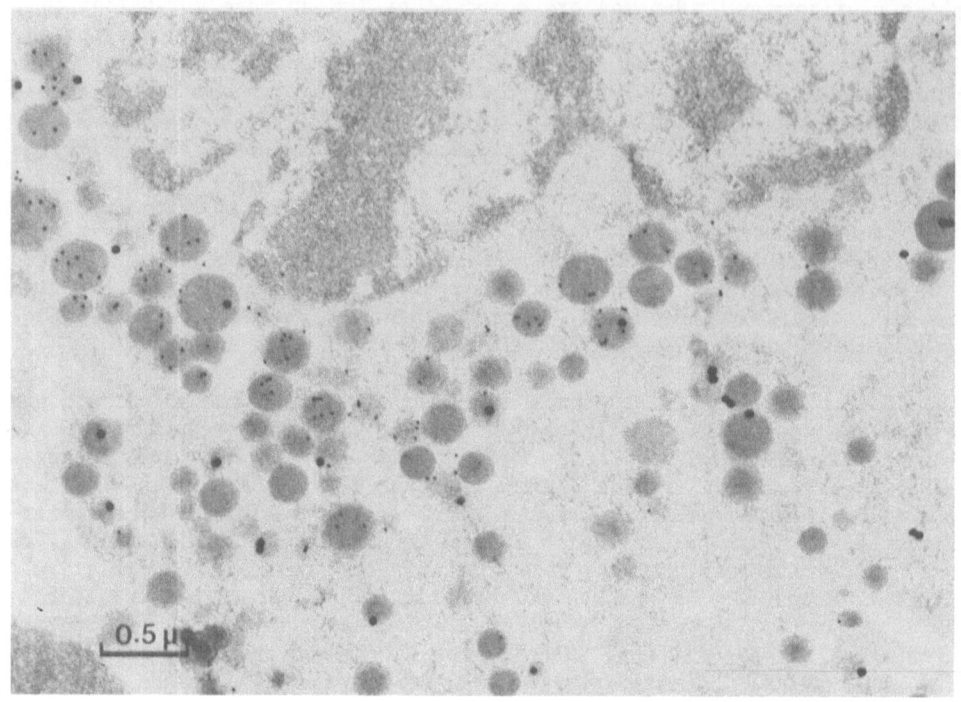

Fig. 5. Mammosomatotroph cell adenoma, GH and PRL are labeled
with 15 nm and 40 nm gold particles (immuno-gold technique).

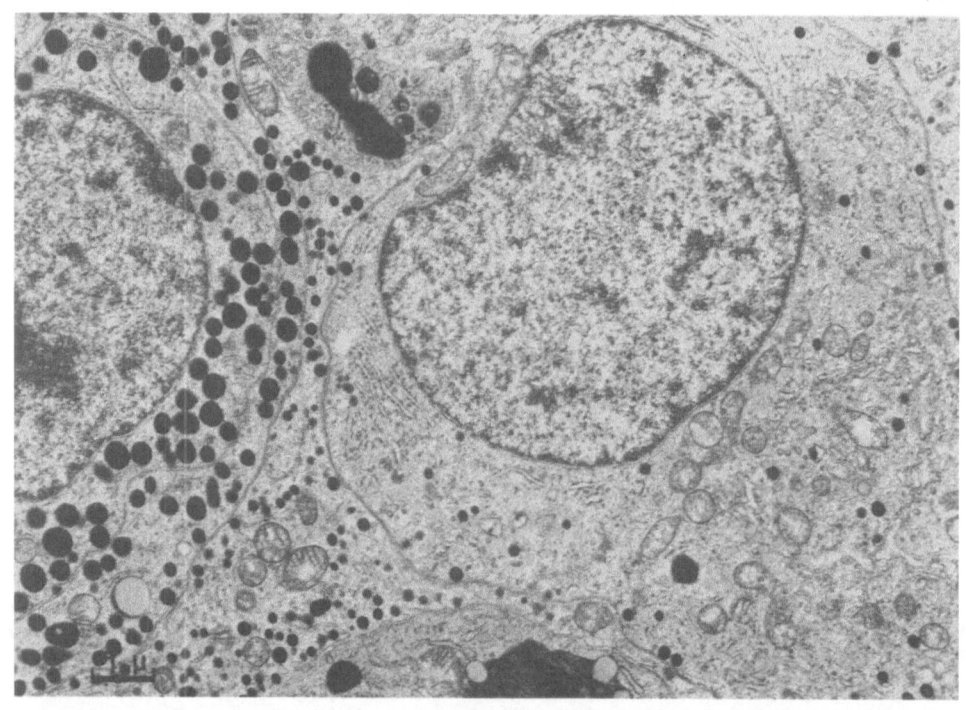

Fig. 6. Mixed adenoma consisting of densely granulated GH
(left) and sparsely granulated PRL cells (right).

adenoma by light microscopic immunohistochemistry, immunoelectron microscopy demonstrates the presence of GH and PRL in the cytoplasm of the same
cells and even in the same secretory granules (13). In some cells, only
GH or only PRL can be confirmed while in others both hormones can be
identified. Despite the different hormone content, these adenoma cells
show the same ultrastructural features, consistent with the view that
different hormones can be synthesized in ultrastructurally identical
cells. Furthermore, the size of the secretory granules and their electron
microscopic appearance cannot identify the endocrine function of adenoma
cells.

Less common types of plurihormonal adenomas produce unusual combinations of two or more hormones, such as GH and TSH; PRL and TSH; GH, PRL
and TSH; occasionally GH, PRL and ACTH; or GH, PRL, FSH/LH and α-subunit.
Such adenomas may be monomorphous or plurimorphous. The cell type or cell
types of these tumors often cannot be identified even by detailed electron
microscopic investigation. In a few adenomas, however, the ultrastructural study discloses two or more distinct cell types similar to their
nontumorous counterparts (Fig. 7). The hormone content and electron
microscopic features of some adenomas cannot be correlated.

By light microscopy, these unusual plurihormonal adenomas consist of
chromophobic, acidophilic or basophilic cells or an admixture of cells
which show affinity for different dyes by histologic staining techniques.
Clinical and biochemical hypersecretion of several hormones has been
associated with these tumors, and patients may show evidence of acromegaly, hyperprolactinemia and hyperthyroidism. The presence of some
hormones can be revealed in the cell cytoplasm by immunohistochemical
methods but hormone release is not manifest clinically and blood hormone
levels are not elevated.

Plurihormonal adenomas are difficult to classify and more work is
needed to determine their endocrine function and cellular derivation.
Occurrence of these intriguing tumors emphasizes the assumption that the
one cell-one hormone theory, which had dominated pituitary cytophysiology
and cytopathology for several decades, is oversimplified and must be
revised.

GH CELL HYPERPLASIA

Hyperplasia is defined as an increase in the number of constituent
cells of an organ. Adenohypophyseal hyperplasia, despite extensive
previous studies, is still controversial and its diagnosis is often
difficult and uncertain. Since the various cell types are unevenly
distributed in the anterior lobe, if only a small piece of pituitary
tissue is available for histologic examination and the pathologist is not
informed of the exact site from which the tissue was removed, the diagnosis of hyperplasia cannot be made convincingly. GH cells predominate in
the two lateral wings of the pars distalis; thus, if the examined tissue
is removed from these areas, misleading conclusions can be made regarding
GH cell hyperplasia.

Hyperplasia involving different cell types has been the subject of
numerous publications. PRL cell hyperplasia occurs in pregnancy, lacta-
tion and following protracted estrogen treatment. Increased numbers of
PRL cells have been documented in the newborn's pituitary and rarely in
the nontumorous portions of the adenohypophysis harboring PRL cell adenoma. ACTH cell hyperplasia has been reported in patients with Addison's
disease, Cushing's disease and in association with GRH-producing primary
hypothalamic and extrahypothalamic tumors. TSH cell hyperplasia occurs in

171

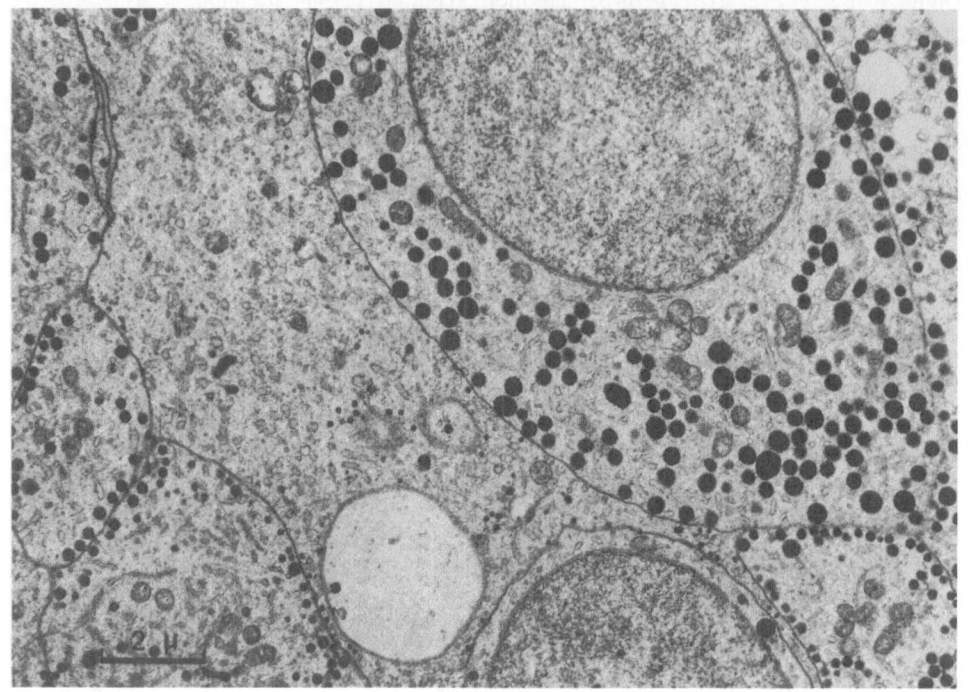

Fig. 7. Plurihormonal, bimorphous adenoma comprised of GH cells
(right) and TSH-like cells (left).

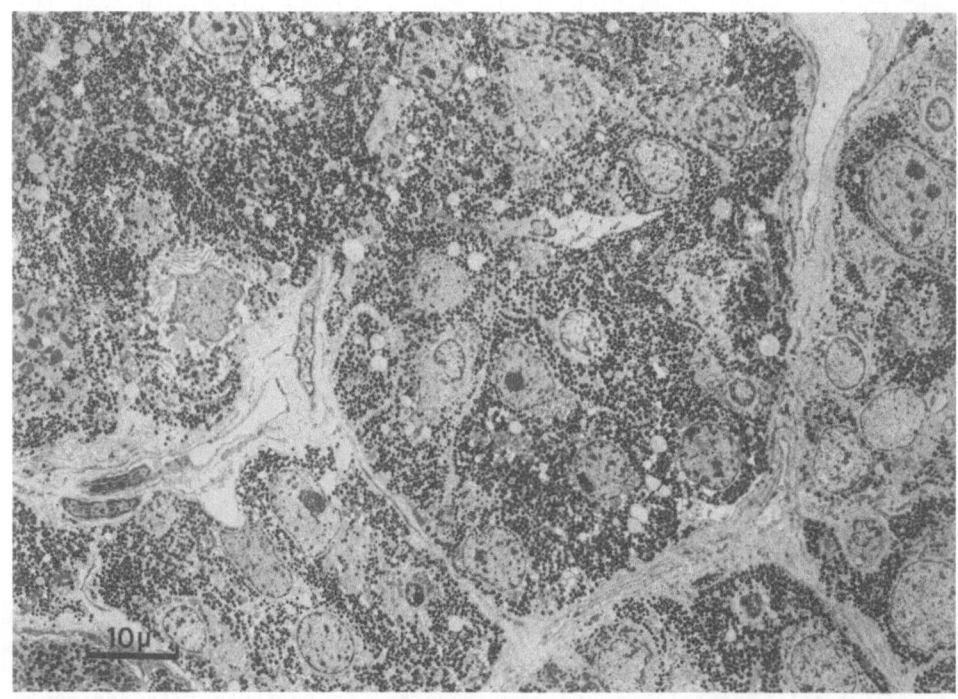

Fig. 8. GH cell hyperplasia. Note the markedly enlarged acini.

patients with long-standing primary hypothyroidism. The enlargement of the pituitary can be documented by various imaging techniques. If the patients are treated with replacement doses of thyroid hormones, the enlarged pituitary regresses indicating that the hyperplastic process is reversible and responds to negative feedback action of peripheral hormones. FSH/LH cell hyperplasia has been reported in patients with long-standing primary hypogonadism.

GH cell hyperplasia (Fig. 8) has only recently been described conclusively as a cause of acromegaly in patients with various growth hormone-releasing hormone (GRH)-producing tumors (14). Such tumors are most frequently represented by pancreatic islet tumors, or bronchial, thymic or gastrointestinal carcinoids. However, hypothalamic gangliocytomas, small cell carcinomas of the lung, medullary carcinomas of the thyroid and pheochromocytomas may also produce GRH. In addition, mammosomatotroph cell hyperplasia has been reported in a patient with McCune-Albright syndrome (15).

The morphologic diagnosis is not easy even if the entire gland is available for study. Accumulation of GH cells might be diffuse or nodular. The former variant has to be distinguished from the normal gland, the latter from adenoma. The distinction between hyperplasia and normal histology can only be made conclusively if several sections have been studied from different areas of the gland. Proliferating GH cells form small groups or are single, interspersed with other cell types. The enlargement of acini is a characteristic finding. They mainly contain GH cells and are surrounded by fibers which can be visualized by the PAS technique or silver impregnation.

In the differential diagnosis between adenoma and nodular hyperplasia, several morphologic features are helpful. The adenomas are well demarcated, there is a sharp border between the adenoma and the nontumorous adenohypophysis. The nontumorous cells, adjacent to the adenoma, are compressed and the reticulin network is condensed. The adenoma, except in plurimorphous adenomas, is composed of one cell type although, in some cases, nontumorous cells can also be recognized, especially at the periphery of the tumor. In contrast, no cell compression and demarcation are evident in hyperplasia and several cell types can be identified. An important differential diagnostic feature is that the reticulin network, which is absent or rudimentary in adenomas, is maintained in hyperplastic and normal glands.

The morphologic differences between adenoma and hyperplasia are clear in the majority of cases; thus, the differential diagnosis can be made conclusively. However, there are intermediary cases in which it is difficult, if not impossible, to determine whether the process represents adenoma or hyperplasia.

We have observed patients with acromegaly due to extrahypophyseal GRH-producing tumors whose pituitaries exhibited GH cell hyperplasia. However, in these glands, there were areas which showed a close resemblance to, and, based on morphologic criteria, were indistinguishable from, GH cell adenoma. In the hyperplastic areas, the reticulin fiber network was irregular but was preserved. In the areas resembling adenoma, the reticulin network was disrupted and only a few irregular, thick reticulin fibers were noticeable adjacent to the capillaries. These morphologic findings seem to suggest that hyperplastic GH cells can transform to adenoma, and GH cell adenomas may arise in hyperplastic cells. However, one must stress that there is no proof that hyperplastic cells are more prone to undergo neoplastic transformation than normal cells. It is also known that in the pituitary of acromegalic patients,

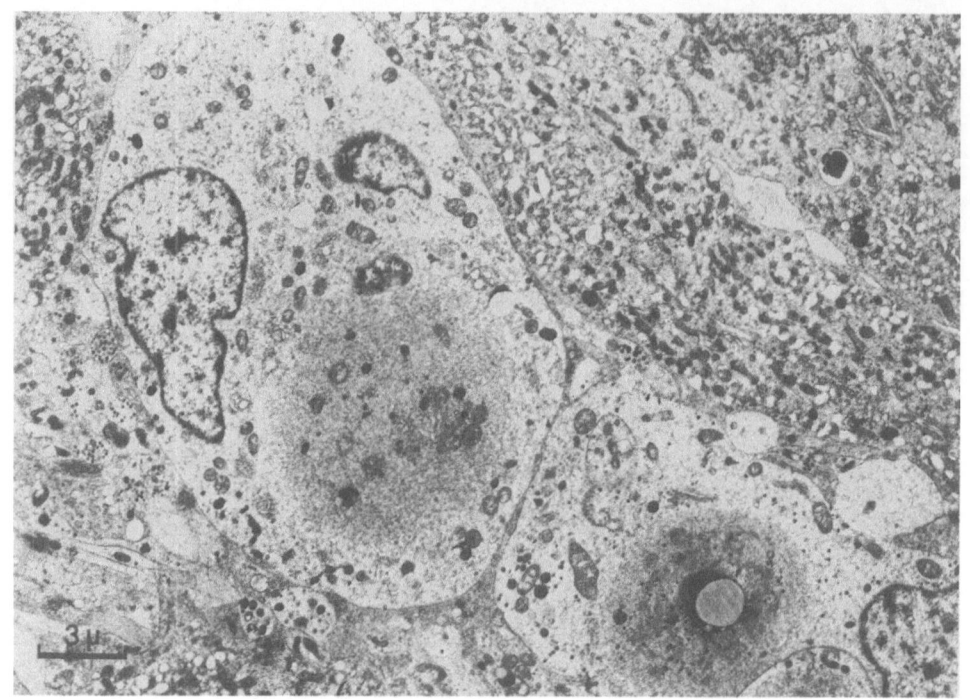

Fig. 9. Combined lesion of hypothalamic gangliocytoma (upper right) and of GH cell adenoma with fibrous bodies.

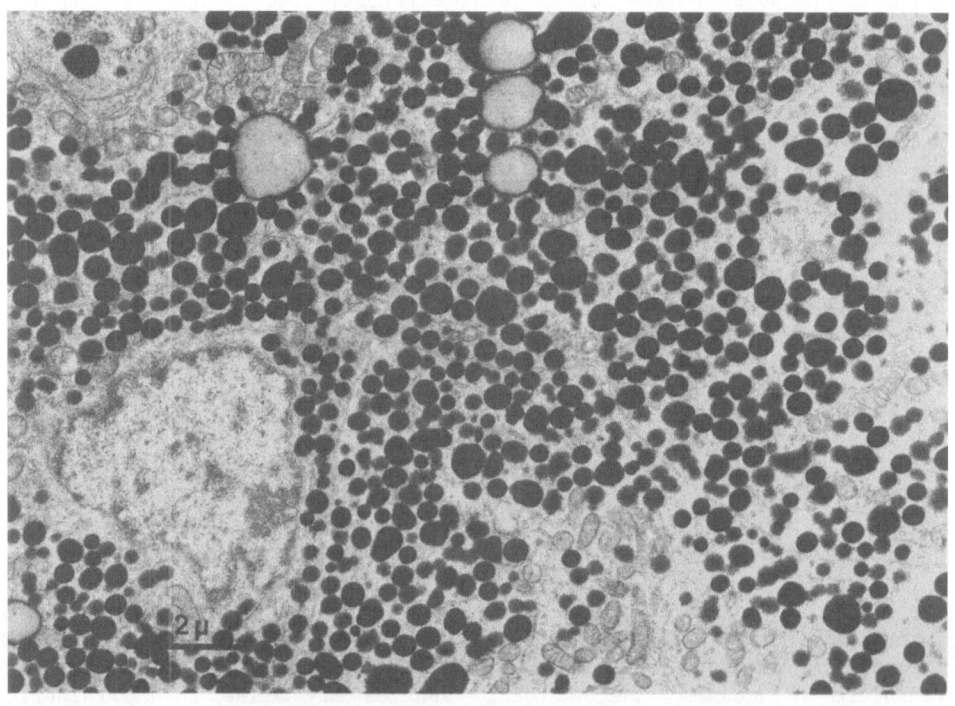

Fig. 10. GH cell adenoma treated with SMS 201-995. Note lysosomes fusing with secretory granules (e.g., upper center).

there is no hyperplasia of GH cells outside the GH cell adenoma, thereby suggesting that adenomas most often arise in nonhyperplastic cells. Thus, the substantial majority of GH cell adenomas represent primary pituitary disease and there is no conclusive evidence that the hypothalamus plays a role in the pathogenesis of GH cell adenoma. The question of whether hypothalamic neuropeptides can initiate adenoma formation, or can promote adenoma growth, requires further study. It may be that the hypothalamic-releasing hormones favor the conditions for neoplastic transformation; they may increase the susceptibility of pituitary cells to oncogenic stimuli or, alternatively, they may promote proliferation of adenoma cells. Prolonged stimulation in the pituitary leads to cellular multiplication. The mechanism whereby a signal, related to increased function, leads to cellular replication is not clearly understood.

EFFECT OF SMS 201-995, A LONG-ACTING SOMATOSTATIN ANALOG, ON PITUITARY GH CELL ADENOMA MORPHOLOGY

Treatment of acromegalic patients with somatostatin (SS), the physiologic inhibitor of GH secretion, is a logical approach since GH cell adenomas possess somatostatin receptors and somatostatin is known to suppress GH release both in vivo and in vitro. Due to the short duration of its action, therapy with natural somatostatin is ineffective in acromegalic patients. It has been shown recently that SMS 201-995 (sandostatin, Sandoz, Basel, Switzerland), a long-acting somatostatin analog, has a potent inhibitory effect on GH secretion and can be used in the treatment of acromegaly (16). It was documented that SMS 201-995 reduces blood GH levels and ameliorates the clinical signs and symptoms in growth hormone excess.

Recently, using histological, immunohistochemical and electron microscopy techniques, we studied a pituitary GH-producing adenoma removed by surgery from a 36-year-old acromegalic woman after 10 days of SMS 201-995 therapy (17). The tumor was an acidophilic adenoma containing GH in many adenoma cells, and TSH and α-subunit in a few adenoma cells. By electron microscopy, we observed that the adenoma was composed of closely-apposed cells possessing oval or irregular nuclei with prominent nucleoli and abundant cytoplasm. The RER consisted of well-organized flat cisternae, and the Golgi apparatus harbored several forming granules and was conspicuous. Mitochondria were spherical or oval, with tubular cristae and a moderately electron dense matrix; their number, size and morphology were within normal range. Lysosomes were numerous (some were unusually large), and crinophagy was evident in the cytoplasm of several adenoma cells. Capillaries were lined by fenestrated endothelium. Cell necrosis, endothelial damage, platelet aggregation or capillary obstruction were not observed. Perivascular spaces were wide and exhibited slight fibrosis.

The tumor was compared by morphometry to 10 GH-secreting adenomas removed by surgery from acromegalic patients not treated with somatostatin. The adenoma cells, after SMS 201-995 administration, were smaller, possessed smaller nuclei and clear cytoplasm and lysosomes occupied more of the cytoplasmic volume than those of the non-SS-treated controls. Nuclear-cytoplasmic ratio, cytoplasmic volume densities of ER, Golgi complexes, mitochondria, secretory granules and secretory granule diameters were within range of control adenomas. In vitro studies showed that the adenoma cells secreted GH and responded to somatostatin suppression.

The effect of SMS 201-995 on adenoma morphology was also investigated by Landolt et al. (18). These authors found amyloid deposits and perivascular necrosis of adenoma cells with no change in secretory apparatus. In our study, somatostatin produced no direct cytotoxic or vasotoxic effects.

Moreover, the ultrastructural and morphometric findings were consistent with functional inhibition of GH release.

Dopaminergic agonists, such as bromocriptine, cause reversible shrinkage and morphologically recognizable cell involution in PRL-producing adenomas (19,20). The structural changes are striking and are characterized by a substantial decrease in overall cell size, as well as nuclear and cytoplasmic areas, an increase in the nuclear/cytoplasmic ratio, and a decrease in cytoplasmic volume densities of ER and Golgi complexes. This severe cell involution is not evident in GH cell adenomas following SMS 201-995 treatment.

ACKNOWLEDGMENT

This work was supported in part by the Medical Research Council of Canada (Grant MT-6349). The authors wish to thank Dr. E. Horvath, Mrs. G. Ilse, Mrs. N. Losinski and Mrs. N. Ryan for their contribution throughout the morphologic study, and Mrs. W. Wlodarski for secretarial work.

REFERENCES

1. Marie P. Sur deux cas d'acromegalie; hypertrophie singuliere, non congenitale, des extremites superieures, inferieures et cephalique. Rev Med 1886; 6:297.
2. Bailey P, Davidoff LM. Concerning the microscopic structure of the hypophysis cerebri in acromegaly (based on a study of tissues removed at operation from 35 patients). Am J Pathol 1925; 1:185.
3. Cushing H, Davidoff LM. The pathological findings in four autopsied cases of acromegaly with a discussion of their significance. New York: Rockefeller Institute, 1927 (monograph 22:1).
4. Horvath E, Kovacs K. Pathology of the pituitary gland. In: Ezrin C, Horvath E, Kaufman B, Kovacs K, Weiss MH, eds. Pituitary Diseases. Boca Raton: CRC Press, 1983.
5. Kovacs K, Horvath E. Morphology of adenohypophyseal cells and pituitary adenomas. In: Imura H, ed. The Pituitary Gland. New York: Raven Press, 1985.
6. Melmed S, Braunstain GD, Horvath E, Ezrin C, Kovacs K. Pathophysiology of acromegaly. Endocr Rev 1983; 4:271.
7. Kovacs K, Horvath E. Pathology of growth hormone-producing tumors of the human pituitary. Semin Diag Pathol 1986; 3:18.
8. Horvath E, Kovacs K, Scheithauer BW, et al. Pituitary adenomas producing growth hormone, prolactin and one or more glycoprotein hormones: a histologic, immunohistochemical and ultrastructural study of four surgically-removed tumors. Ultrastruct Pathol 1983; 5:171.
9. Scheithauer BW, Horvath E, Kovacs K, Laws ER Jr, Randall RV, Ryan N. Plurihormonal pituitary adenomas. Semin Diag Pathol 1986; 3:69.
10. Horvath E, Kovacs K, Singer W, et al. Acidophil stem cell adenoma of the human pituitary. Clinico-pathological analysis of 15 cases. Cancer 1981; 47:761.
11. Horvath E, Kovacs K, Killinger DW, Smyth HS, Weiss MH, Ezrin C. Mammosomatotroph cell adenoma of the human pituitary: a morphologic entity. Virchows Arch [A] 1983; 398:277.
12. Corenblum B, Sirek AMT, Horvath E, Kovacs K, Ezrin C. Human mixed somatotrophic and lactotrophic pituitary adenomas. J Clin Endocrinol Metab 1976; 42:857.
13. Bassetti M, Spada A, Arosio M, Vallar T, Brina M, Giannattasio G. Morphological studies on mixed growth hormone (GH)- and prolactin

(PRL)-secreting human pituitary adenomas. Coexistence of GH and PRL in the same secretory granule. J Clin Endocrinol Metab 1986; 62:1093.

14. Thorner MO, Perryman RL, Cronin MJ, et al. Somatotroph hyperplasia. Successful treatment of acromegaly by removal of a pancreatic islet tumor secreting a growth hormone-releasing factor. J Clin Invest 1982; 70:965.

15. Kovacs K, Horvath E, Thorner MO, Rogol AD. Mammosomatotroph hyperplasia associated with acromegaly and hyperprolactinemia in a patient with the McCune-Albright syndrome. A histologic, immunocytologic and ultrastructural study of the surgically-removed adenohypophysis. Virchows Arch [A] 1984; 403:77.

16. Lamberts SWJ, Uitterlinden P, Verschoor L, Van Dongen KJ, del Pozo E. Long-term treatment of acromegaly with somatostatin analogue SMS 201-995. N Engl J Med 1985; 313:1576.

17. George SR, Kovacs K, Asa SL, Horvath E, Cross EG, Burrow GN. Effect of SMS 201-995, a long-acting somatostatin analog on the secretion and morphology of a pituitary growth hormone cell adenoma (submitted for publication).

18. Landolt AM, Osterwalder V, Stuckmann G. Preoperative treatment of acromegaly with SMS 201-995: surgical and pathological observations. In: Tolis G, Ludecke DK, eds. Growth Hormone. New York: Raven Press (in press).

19. Tindall GT, Kovacs K, Horvath E, Thorner MO. Human prolactin-producing adenomas and bromocriptine: a histologic, immunocytochemical, ultrastructural and morphometric study. J Clin Endocrinol Metab 1982; 55:1178.

20. Horvath E, Kovacs K. Pathology of prolactin cell adenomas of the human pituitary. Semin Diag Pathol 1986; 3:4.

17

ASSOCIATED HYPERSECRETION OF ANTERIOR PITUITARY HORMONES
OTHER THAN GROWTH HORMONE IN ACROMEGALY

G. Faglia, M. Arosio, M. Bassetti,* P. Beck-Peccoz,
L. Guglielmino, A. Spada, G. Medri, G. Piscitelli,
G. Giannattasio,* and B. Ambrosi

Department of Endocrinology, School of Medicine, and *CNR
Center of Cytopharmacology, Department of Pharmacology,
University of Milan, 35 F. Sforza, 20122 Milano, Italy

INTRODUCTION

Although patients showing typical features of acromegaly had been described (Fig. 1) prior to Pierre Marie's report in 1886 (1-3), observations concerning clinical signs and symptoms assumably caused by hypersecretion of growth hormone (GH) and other pituitary hormones were reported only several years later.

The first observations of presumable association of GH and prolactin (PRL) hypersecretion were reported by Fraenkel et al. (4) in 1901, and Roth (5) in 1918, who described acromegalic women complaining of galactor-

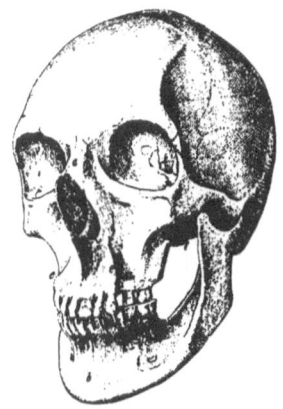 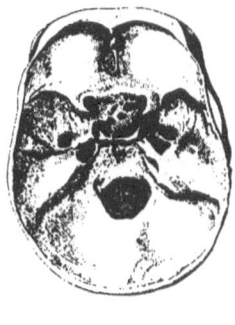

Fig. 1. Skull of an acromegalic patient described in 1864 by the Italian neuropathologist, A. Verga. The author named the disease "Prosopectasia" (from the greek roots "prosopon" = face, and "ectasis" = enlargement). He also described the presence of "a nut-sized intracranial tumor laying in and above the sella turcica, impinging the optic chiasma and mamillary bodies," and suspected that the tumor originated from the pituitary gland. From Verga (1), 1864.

rhea. Soon after the discovery that PRL was a hormone distinct from GH (6) (with which it maintains an ancestral resemblance), it has become widely recognized that PRL hypersecretion is frequently present in acromegalic patients either with or without galactorrhea (7-20).

The association of acromegaly with hyperthyroidism was first described by Davidoff (2) in 1926. Although it is recognized that in the majority of cases the hyperthyroid state results from thyroid autonomy, the possibility that in some patients a concomitant thyrotropin (TSH) hypersecretion may cause hyperthyroidism was documented only in 1969 by Lamberg et al. (21).

The finding that some of the so-called "nonfunctioning" pituitary tumors hypersecreted free alpha-subunit (alpha-sub) of glycoprotein hormones prompted MacFarlane et al. (22) to investigate alpha-sub secretion in acromegaly. This led to the discovery that some acromegalic patients also have high levels of circulating alpha-sub (23).

Clinical evidence suggesting associated pituitary hypersecretion of GH, adrenocorticotropic hormone (ACTH) and/or gonadotropins is a rare event. Although unusual combinations such as GH/ACTH, GH/luteinizing hormone (LH), and GH/follicle stimulating hormone (FSH) have been described in GH-secreting adenomas by immunohistochemical studies (24-26), the high rate of plurihormone content of these adenomas does not usually result in elevated circulating hormone levels.

Associate hormone hypersecretion may result from alterations of the hypothalamic control of anterior pituitary secretion (either primary or secondary to suprasellar extension of the tumor), or from the coexistence of two distinct pituitary adenomas, or from mixed adenomas. In the case of PRL, these possibilities have been documented in different patients (8,18,19,27-29).

The questions of whether in mixed adenomas, PRL (or TSH, or alpha-sub) is secreted along with GH by the same adenomatous cell, or by different cells, and how this is reflected by in vivo hormonal dynamics, have been extensively studied (18,19,30-33). However, these studies provided conflicting results. The discrepancies were most likely due to the varied immunohistochemical methods utilized by different investigators.

This chapter will report our recent findings obtained by comparing hormonal secretory dynamic and morphological studies carried out by a double immunocytochemical labeling in several cases of acromegaly with associate hypersecretion of PRL, TSH, or alpha-sub.

ASSOCIATED GROWTH HORMONE AND PROLACTIN HYPERSECRETION

Frequency of Hyperprolactinemia

The frequency of PRL hypersecretion in acromegaly could not be extensively assessed until specific radioimmunoassay for PRL became available (7). After reviewing a large series of acromegalic patients (7,9-20), we calculated that the overall rate of hyperprolactinemia was 31% (254 of 809 cases, including our series). It is generally accepted that hyperprolactinemia is not related either to sex or to GH basal levels. In our series, high PRL levels (i.e., > 15 ng/ml in men, > 20 ng/ml in women) were recorded in 27% of the men and in 28% of the women. The mean basal GH concentration was 37.3 ± 43.1 ng/ml in 93 normo- and 38.3 ± 33.5 ng/ml in 36 hyperprolactinemic patients; there was no correlation between GH and PRL levels (r = -0.025).

Hypothalamic vs. Tumoral Origin of Hyperprolactinemia

The study of PRL secretion in basal conditions and in response to stimulatory or inhibitory agents does not help in distinguishing if PRL hypersecretion originates from tumor cells or from hypothalamic disconnection. Mildly elevated basal levels of PRL and similar responses to dynamic testing may be found in patients with hypothalamic disconnection and in those with mixed (GH/PRL) adenoma. Moreover, contrary to patients with prolactinomas, in hyperprolactinemic acromegalic patients with mixed tumor serum, PRL may rise after thyrotropin-releasing hormone (TRH) administration in more than 50% of cases (56% in our series), while it may show blunted or absent responses also in normoprolactinemic patients (44% in our series). Unfortunately, testing with dopamine antagonists does not help in distinguishing between tumoral and hypothalamic hyperprolactinemia (34,35).

Therefore, this distinction can be achieved only by immunohisto- chemical studies on excised tumors. Kanie et al. (19) utilizing the immunoperoxidase technique, observed that 6 of 21 tumors from acromegalic patients with prolactin excess did not show immunoreactive PRL cells. We have observed similar findings (3 of 8 cases) in our studies.

Mixed GH/PRL Adenomas

It has been reported that GH responsiveness to TRH and suppressibil- ity by dopamine agonists is more frequent in hyper- than in normoprolac- tinemic acromegalic patients, and that a homogeneity of response is present in about 70% of cases (15,36). This PRL-like behavior of GH has been assumed to be indirect evidence for the presence of mammosomatotropic adenomatous cells. However, the frequency of mammosomatotropic cells reported in the large series by Horvath et al. (37) was only 5.8%.

These conflicting findings prompted us to reexamine this intriguing problem by reevaluating our own hormonal data and by carrying out immuno- cytochemical studies. In our series, no difference in the frequency of positive GH responses to TRH and suppressibility to dopamine (DA) between normo- and hyperprolactinemic patients has been found. In fact, GH increase after TRH occurred in 43 of 93 (46%) normoprolactinemic and in 17 of 36 (47%) hyperprolactinemic patients while GH suppression by DA infu- sion occurred in the 51% and 54% of cases, respectively. In 80 acro- megalics investigated with both agents, we observed concordant responses in 61% of the cases without any difference between the 60 normo- (61%) and the 20 hyperprolactinemic patients (60%). Moreover, 12 of 32 (37%) patients who responded to TRH were DA-unresponsive, and 19 of 39 (49%) DA-responsive patients were TRH-unresponsive. No clear-cut difference in GH secretory pattern was found either in patients subdivided according to their degree of hyperprolactinemia (i.e., less than or greater than 30 ng/ml), or in patients tested with bromocriptine instead of DA. On the whole, our data do not confirm that acromegalic patients with high PRL levels show a greater sensitivity to TRH and dopaminergic agents than those with normal PRL levels as previously suggested (15,36).

We carried out immunocytochemistry by a double-labeling method utilizing the protein A-gold electron microscopic technique. With this method it was possible not only to identify the presence of hormones by the reaction between the specific antibody and protein A conjugated with gold particles of definite sizes, but also to investigate ultrastructural details such as the mono- or bihormonal nature of the secretory granules.

Twenty GH-secreting adenomas, surgically removed from 8 hyper- and 12 normoprolactinemic patients, were studied. Five adenomas from hyperprolactinemic patients (PRL: 26–453 ng/ml) were positive for both GH and PRL. All the GH/PRL adenomas showed a large number of cells positive for both GH and PRL, generally localized in the same secretory granule (Fig. 2 and 3). In these 5 patients, GH responses to TRH, DA, growth hormone-releasing factor (GRF)·, and somatostatin (SRIF) paralleled those of PRL (Fig. 2 and 3, and Table 1), but the pattern of response was different from patient to patient. Two cases were unresponsive to TRH, and one was unresponsive to DA while the hormonal behavior considered "typical" for mammosomatotropic cell (GH and PRL increase in response to TRH and inhibition to DA) was recorded in only 2 cases. These data are in contrast with the results obtained with traditional morphologic methods by which mixed GH- and PRL-producing cells were identified in a small number of adenomas (31,37). However, this discrepancy can be attributable, at least in part, to the use of light microscopic methods which cannot resolve immunoreactive product when present in small amounts. In fact, of the five GH/PRL-secreting adenomas described above, immunofluorescence studies at the light microscopic level allowed us to clearly identify mammosomatotropes in only two cases (38).

In 3 other hyperprolactinemic patients (PRL: 33–52 ng/ml), no cells positive for PRL were observed, suggesting a hypothalamic lesion. Surprisingly, in 2 of these patients no PRL response to TRH was observed and only one showed GH and PRL increase after TRH administration, thus confirming the inability to differentiate the origin of the hyperprolactinemia by clinical tests, and to attribute any value to the GH responsivity to TRH as a diagnostic criteria in identifying the existence of mammosomatotropic tumors.

In 12 adenomas from normoprolactinemic patients the great majority of cells were positive only for GH. Furthermore, the GH and PRL responses to

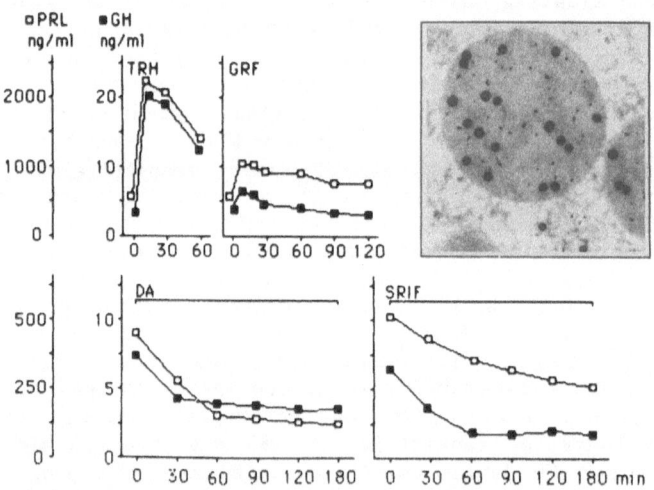

Fig. 2. Typical mixed GH- and PRL-secreting pituitary adenoma. The responses of both hormones to TRH (200 µg IV), GRF (1 µg/Kg IV), dopamine infusion (2 µg/kg/min over 180 min), SRIF (3.3 µg/min over 180 min) were parallel. Protein A-gold double immunolabeling showed that GH (small particles) and PRL (large particles) coexisted in the same secretory granules; 80% of adenoma cells were positive for both GH and PRL.

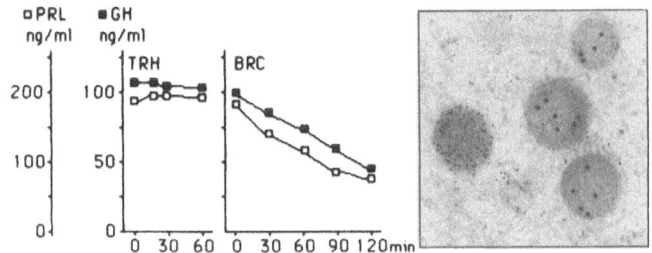

Fig. 3. Mixed GH- and PRL-secreting pituitary adenoma. The responses of both hormones to TRH and bromocriptine (2.5 mg p.o.) were parallel. However, neither hormone responded to TRH although they were inhibited by bromocriptine. Protein A-gold double immunolabeling showed that GH (small particles, left) and PRL (large particles, right) coexisted in the same cell but in different secretory granules; 70% of adenoma cells were positive for both GH and PRL.

provocative stimuli were not parallel (Fig. 4 and 5). As shown in Table 1, GH secretion was stimulated by TRH and inhibited by DA in 9 and 11 patients, respectively, whose adenomas did not show PRL positive cells. The finding that the pattern of GH secretion shows a PRL-like behavior in acromegalic patients when either a pure GH-secreting adenoma or a mixed GH/PRL- secreting adenoma is present seems to weaken the hypothesis that these abnormal GH responses reflect the presence of mammosomatotropic cells. By contrast, PRL responses to releasing and inhibiting factors specific for GH were only observed in mixed GH/PRL adenomas (Fig. 2), which is in agreement with previous observations (33).

Table 1. Immunohistochemical findings in comparison with basal levels of serum GH and PRL and their responses to stimulatory or inhibitory agents in 20 acromegalic patients.

| | | Pure GH Adenomas (80-100% of cells positive for GH only) (n=15) | | Mixed Adenomas (30-100% of cells positive for both GH and PRL) (n=5) | |
		GH	PRL	GH	PRL
Basal levels (ng/ml ± SD)		37 ± 31	16 ± 15	47 ± 52	137 ± 141
	↑[a]	15/15[b]	3/15[b]	5/5[b]	5/5[b]
TRH	↑	9/15[c]	11/15[c]	3/5[c]	3/5[c]
DA	↓	11/14[c]	14/14[c]	4/5[c]	5/5[c]
GRF	↑	6/11[c]	0/11[c]	1/1[c]	1/1[c]
SRIF	↓	5/5[c]	0/5[c]	1/1[c]	1/1[c]

[a] Arrows indicate high basal hormone levels or responsiveness to tests.
[b] Patients with high basal hormone levels/total number of patients.
[c] Patients with positive response/number of tested patients.

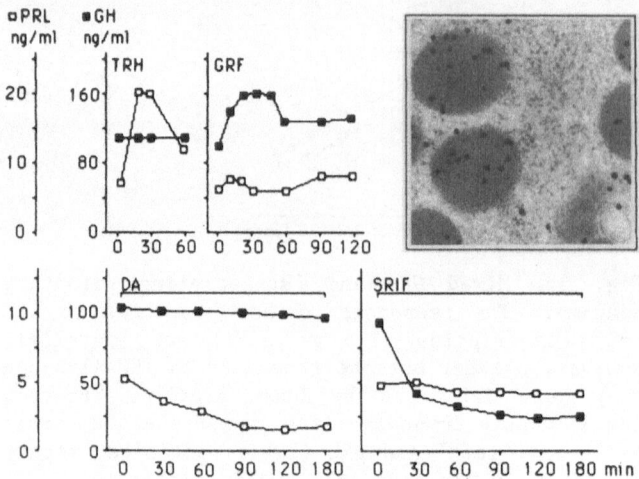

Fig. 4. Typical pure GH-secreting pituitary adenoma. The patient was normoprolactinemic. GH, but not PRL, increased after GRF and was inhibited by SRIF. PRL, but not GH, increased after TRH and was inhibited by dopamine infusion. Protein A-gold double immunolabeling showed GH only (large particles) secretory granules; 100% of adenoma cells were positive for GH only.

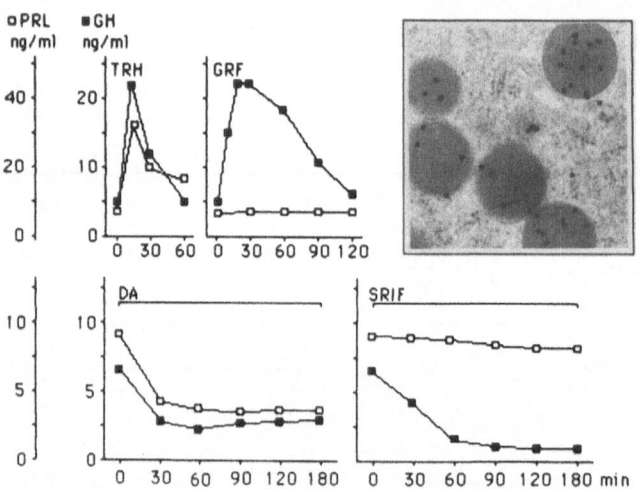

Fig. 5. Pure GH-secreting pituitary adenoma. The patient was normoprolactinemic. GH, but not PRL, increased after GRF and was inhibited by SRIF. However, both PRL and GH increased after TRH and were inhibited by dopamine infusion. Protein A-gold double immunolabeling showed GH only (large particles) secretory granules; 100% of adenoma cells were positive for GH only.

ASSOCIATED HYPERSECRETION OF GROWTH HORMONE AND THYROTROPIN

Thyrotropin hypersecretion has been documented to be a possible cause of hyperthyroidism in acromegaly (24). Beck-Peccoz et al. have described 19 patients with associated hypersecretion of GH and TSH (44). Dynamic hormone secretion studies, although carried out in a small number of patients, have revealed variable patterns of response (44).

Three out of 129 (2.3%) acromegalic patients in our series had associated TSH-induced hyperthyroidism. In these 3 patients, serum TSH concentrations, measured by the new ultrasensitive immunoradiometric assay which is able to clearly distinguish suppressed from unsuppressed TSH levels (40), were detectable in spite of high levels of circulating free thyroid hormones. In addition, serum-free alpha-sub levels were high, resulting in alpha-sub/TSH molar ratios > 1. In one patient, the immuno-reactive TSH had (apparent) decreased molecular weight and enhanced biological activity (41). In this patient, alpha-sub response to dynamic tests paralleled that of GH rather than that of TSH. In fact, after TRH administration, TSH did not show any significant increase while GH and alpha-sub showed a marked increment. The same pattern of response was observed when TRH was injected during SRIF infusion, or when sulpiride (100 mg) was administered during DA infusion (Fig. 6). After successful selective adenomectomy, GH and alpha-sub levels fell into the normal range and did not respond to further provocative stimuli. The patient became euthyroid and the (apparent) molecular weight of TSH was normalized (41). Morphological studies showed that the tumor was composed of a single type of cells. A few small secretory granules were seen, mainly aligned under the plasma membrane. Double gold immunolabeling (Fig. 6) showed that the large majority of the cells were positive for GH and alpha-sub, while only a very few cells were positive for GH and TSH-β. These few cells were also positive for alpha-sub, thus indicating that complete TSH originated from a minority of tumor cells. No increase in serum TSH, alpha-sub, or GH was observed after administration of the three above-mentioned tests to the 2 other patients.

Due to the rarity of this association, there are only a few studies on in vitro hormone release from GH/TSH-secreting adenomas. Lamberts et al. (42) reported that TSH and GH secretion by cultured cells from one mixed tumor was stimulated by TRH and gonadotropin-releasing hormone (GnRH), but unaffected by bromocriptine, and that TSH release was inhibited by triiodothyronine and dexamethasone.

We studied the in vitro hormone secretion from two GH/TSH-secreting adenomas. In short-term incubation of tissue fragments, the tumor re-leased large amounts of TSH, TSH-β, alpha-sub and GH which were inhibited by DA and SRIF in one case, and unaffected in the other one (Table 2). It is noteworthy that a good correlation between in vivo and in vitro respon-siveness to DA and SRIF was observed.

ASSOCIATED HYPERSECRETION OF GROWTH HORMONE AND GLYCOPROTEIN HORMONE ALPHA-SUBUNIT

Glycoprotein hormones (TSH, LH, FSH, and chorionic gonadotropin) are composed of two noncovalently bound subunits, alpha and beta, the former being virtually identical for all glycoprotein hormones, the latter conferring the specificity of action.

Although alpha-sub levels are usually high in blood of subjects with increased concentration of the complete hormone (43), elevated levels of circulating free alpha-sub may also be found in patients with pituitary

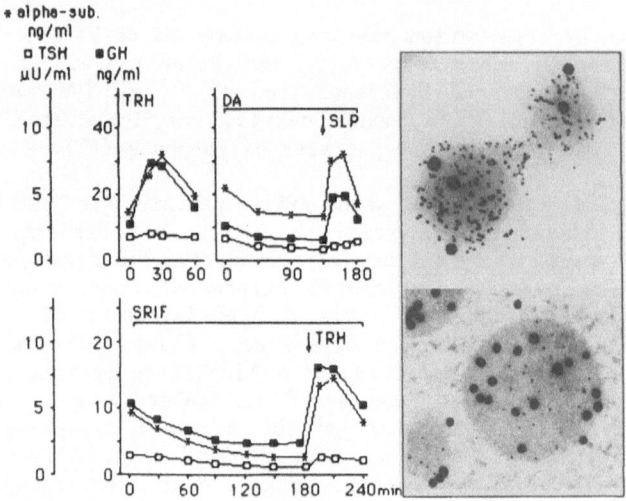

Fig. 6. GH- and TSH-secreting pituitary adenoma.
The patient was acromegalic and hyperthyroid with
unsuppressed TSH. GH and alpha-subunit showed
parallel responses to TRH, dopamine, sulpiride
(100 mg IV administered at 120 min during dopamine
infusion), SRIF (250 μg IV bolus followed by an
infusion of 5 μg/min), and TRH administered during
SRIF infusion. Serum TSH did not show significant
changes during the above dynamic tests. Protein
A-gold double immunostaining showed that GH (small
particles) and alpha-sub (large particles) were
co-localized in the same secretory granules in the
large majority of cells (upper right panel). Only
a minority of cells showed the coexistence of both
TSH-β (large particles) and GH (lower right
panel).

Table 2. Effects of SRIF and DA on hormone release from 2
cultured TSH/GH-secreting pituitary adenomas.

| | | Hormone release (per mg prot. x 30 min) | | |
		Baseline	SRIF 10^{-7}M	DA 10^{-7}M
Case 1	TSH (μU)	19.3 ± 3.1	7.2 ± 1.0*	7.0 ± 1.2*
	alpha-sub.(ng)	66.3 ± 5.0	40.1 ± 3.0*	45.0 ± 2.8*
	GH (ng)	4.1 ± 0.9	1.8 ± 0.3*	2.0 ± 0.5*
Case 2	TSH (μU)	5.0 ± 1.0	5.0 ± 1.5	4.9 ± 1.0
	alpha-sub.(ng)	28.2 ± 6.2	29.2 ± 2.0	30.2 ± 5.0
	GH (ng)	10.4 ± 1.2	9.8 ± 2.0	10.1 ± 1.5

*P < 0.01

adenomas irrespective of complete hormone hypersecretion (22,43). MacFarlane et al. (22,23) reported that 13 out of 46 (28%) acromegalic patients showed high levels of serum alpha-sub, and of 8 acromegalics examined, 6 showed increased alpha-sub levels after TRH and 3 after GnRH administration. In 2 of these patients bromocriptine was effective in lowering alpha-subunit levels. Unfortunately, the authors did not report whether alpha-sub secretion was parallel to that of GH.

We investigated basal and dynamic secretion of alpha-sub in 75 acromegalic patients, some of whom have already been reported (44). Thirteen patients (17%) had serum alpha-sub above the upper limit of normal (calculated as mean ± 3 SD of appropriate control groups). GH and alpha-sub showed a superimposable pattern of response to several stimuli. A parallel increase in GH and alpha-sub levels was recorded in 1 of 3 patients with elevated basal alpha-sub levels after GnRH, in 2 of 4 after TRH, in 4 of 6 after sulpiride administered during DA infusion, in 1 of 2 after insulin-induced hypoglycemia, and 4 of 4 after GRF injection (Fig. 7), compared to patients with normal alpha-sub levels. Seven patients with elevated alpha-sub levels who were successfully operated upon showed normalization of both GH and alpha-sub levels. In 2 of them alpha-sub response after GRF disappeared, though a definite GH elevation was still present. Alpha-subunit was released in large amounts from in vitro cultured adenoma fragments of these 2 patients, both in basal conditions and after GRF (10^{-7}M) stimulation, while neither spontaneous nor GRF-stimulated release of alpha-sub was seen from adenomas of patients with normal alpha-sub levels (Table 3).

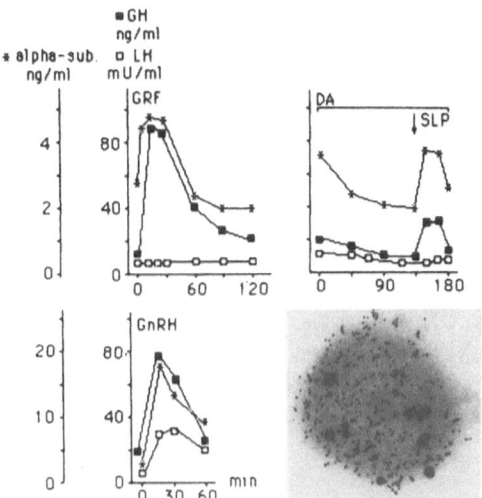

Fig. 7. GH and alpha-sub mixed pituitary adenoma. Both GH and alpha-sub showed parallel responses to GRF, GnRH (100 μg IV), dopamine, and sulpiride administered during dopamine infusion. A slight increase in LH secretion was observed in response to GnRH, but not to GRF or dopamine. Protein A-gold double immunolabeling showed that GH (large particles) and alpha-subunit (small particles) were co-localized in the same secretory granules in the large majority of cells.

Table 3. Effect of GRF on in vivo and in vitro GH and alpha-subunit release in acromegalic patients with (cases 1 or 2) or without (cases 11, 16, 20) alpha-sub hypersecretion.

Case	In vivo levels (ng/ml)				In vitro release (ng/mg prot. x 30 min)			
	Basal		Peak after GRF		Basal		10^{-7}M GRF	
	GH	α-sub	GH	α-sub	GH	α-sub	GH	α-sub
1	11	2.8	96	5.8	3,470	534	9,430	976
2	7	1.2	26	2.4	2,985	388	7,143	875
11	7	0.8	22	1.0	1,000	12	1,178	11
16	43	0.7	98	0.7	11,950	6	10,344	5
20	57	0.8	69	0.7	4,970	16	10,930	16

Protein A-gold double immunolabeling showed that the great majority of cells contained secretory granules positive for both GH and alpha-sub (Fig. 7), whereas alpha-sub, nonsecreting tumors showed only GH immunoreactivity.

CONCLUSIONS

The hypersecretion of anterior pituitary hormones other than GH frequently occurs in acromegaly. Hormonal dynamic tests are unable to discriminate if hormonal hypersecretion originates from the tumor or from a hypothalamic disorder. However, in mixed tumors, the concordance of GH and associate hormone response to specific releasing or inhibiting factors and immunocytochemical studies, carried out by a highly sensitive technique, suggest that bihormonal hypersecretion results from a unique tumoral cell rather than from distinct cell populations. Thus, it is conceivable that the adenomatous cell originates from a common multipotential stem cell or, alternatively, that multiple hormone production may be ascribed to derepression of the genetic code when cells undergo neoplastic transformation. However, the reason why so frequently in acromegaly, but not in other hypersecreting pituitary tumors, one cell type is capable of producing two hormones even markedly different in molecular structure (i.e., GH/alpha-subunit, GH/TSH) remains to be elucidated.

ACKNOWLEDGMENTS

This work was partially supported by Italian National Research Council (CNR), Special Project Oncology.

REFERENCES

1. Verga A. Caso singolare di prosopectasia. Reale Istituto Lombardo di Scienze e Lettere, Classe Scienze Matematiche e Naturali 1864; R.cl.1,1:111.
2. Davidoff LM. Studies in acromegaly. II. Historical note. Endocrinology 1926; 10:453.
3. Marie P. Sur deux cas d'acromegalie. Hypertrophie singuliere non congenitale des extremites superieures, inferieures et cephaliques. Rev Med 1886; 6:297.

4. Fraenkel A, Stadelmann E, Benda C. Klinische und anatomische Beitraege zur Lehre von der Akromegalie. Dtsch Med Wochenschr 1901; 27:513, 536, 564.

5. Roth O. Auftreten von Milchsekretion bei enem an Akromegalie leidenden patienten. Berl Klin Wchnschr 1918; 53:305.

6. Frantz AG, Kleinberg DL. Prolactin: evidence that it is separate from growth hormone in human blood. Science 1970; 170:745.

7. Hwang P, Guyda H, Friesen H. A radioimmunoassay for human prolactin. Proc Natl Acad Sci USA 1971; 68:1902.

8. Turkington RW. Secretion of prolactin by patients with pituitary and hypothalamic tumors. J Clin Endocrinol Metab 1972; 34:159.

9. Jacobs LS, Daughaday WH. Pathophysiology and control of prolactin secretion in patients with pituitary and hypothalamic disease. In: Pasteels JL, Robyns C, eds. Human prolactin. Amsterdam: Excerpta Medica, 1973.

10. Franks S, Jacobs HS, Nabarro JDN. Prolactin concentrations in patients with acromegaly: clinical significance and response to surgery. Clin Endocrinol (Oxf) 1976; 5:63.

11. Wass JAH, Thorner MO, Morris DV, et al. Long-term treatment of acromegaly with bromocriptine. Br Med J 1977; i:875.

12. Tucker HS, Grubb SR, Wigand JP, Watlington CO, Blackard WG, Becker DP. The treatment of acromegaly by transsphenoidal surgery. Arch Intern Med 1980; 140:795.

13. Arafah BM, Brodkey JS, Kaufman B, Velasco B, Manni M, Pearson OH. Transsphenoidal microsurgery in the treatment of acromegaly and gigantism. J Clin Endocrinol Metab 1980; 50:578.

14. De Pablo F, Eastman RC, Roth J, Gorden P. Plasma prolactin in acromegaly before and after treatment. J Clin Endocrinol Metab 1981; 53:344.

15. Lamberts SWJ, Liuzzi A, Chiodini PG, Verde S, Klijn JGM, Birkenhager JC. The value of plasma prolactin levels in the prediction of the responsiveness of growth hormone secretion to bromocriptine and TRH in acromegaly. Eur J Clin Invest 1982; 12:151.

16. Hulting A-L, Werner S, Wersaell J, Tribukait B, Anniko M. Normal growth hormone secretion is rare after microsurgical normalization of growth hormone levels in acromegaly. Acta Med Scand 1982; 212:401.

17. Quabbe HJ. Treatment of acromegaly by trans-sphenoidal operation 90-Yttrium implantation and bromocriptine: results in 230 patients. Clin Endocrinol (Oxf) 1982; 16:107.

18. Nieuwenhuijzen Kruseman AC, Bots GThAM, Roelfsema F, Froelich M, Van Dulken H. Immunocytochemical growth hormone and prolactin in pituitary adenomas causing acromegaly and their relationship to basal serum hormone. Clin Endocrinol (Oxf) 1983; 19:1.

19. Kanie N, Kageyama N, Kuwayama A, Nakane T, Watanabe M, Kwaoi A. Pituitary adenomas in acromegalic patients: an immunohistochemical study with special reference to prolactin-secreting adenoma. J Clin Endocrinol Metab 1982; 57:1093.

20. Teasdale G. Surgical management of pituitary adenoma. Clin Endocrinol Metab 1983; 121:789.

21. Lamberg B-A, Ripatti S, Gordin A, Juustila H, Sivula A, Bjorkesten G. Chromophobe pituitary adenoma with acromegaly and TSH-induced hyperthyroidism associated with parathyroid adenoma. Acta Endocrinol (Copenh) 1969; 60:157.

22. MacFarlane IA, Beardwell CG, Shalet SM, Darbyshire PJ, Hayward E, Sutton ML. Glycoprotein hormone alpha-subunit secretion by pituitary adenomas: influence of external irradiation. Clin Endocrinol (Oxf) 1980; 13:215.

23. MacFarlane IA, Beardwell CG, Shalet SM, Ainsle G, Rankin E. Glycoprotein hormone alpha-subunit secretion by pituitary adenomas: influence of TRH, LHRH and bromocriptine. Acta Endocrinol (Copenh) 1982; 99:847.

24. Heitz PU. Multihormonal pituitary adenomas. Horm Res 1979; 10:1.
25. Melmed S, Braunstein GD, Horvath E, Ezrin C, Kovacs K. Pathophysiology of acromegaly. Endocr Rev 1983; 4:271.
26. Schatz H, Daun M, Leicht R, Stracke H, Saeger W, Zierski J. Immunohistochemical examination of pituitary adenomas. Comparison to clinical and endocrinological findings. Horm Res 1985; 21:246.
27. Tournaire J, Trouillas J, Chalender D, Bonneton-Emptoz A, Goutelle A, Girod C. Somatotropic adenoma manifested by galactorrhea without acromegaly. J Clin Endocrinol Metab 1985; 61:451.
28. Badawy SZA, Anderson GH, Shende MC, Marshall L. Development of acromegaly in a patient with prolactinemia: a case study. Fertil Steril 1984; 42:926.
29. Tolis G, Bertrand G, Carpenter S, McKenzie JM. Acromegaly and galactorrhea-amenorrhea with two pituitary adenomas secreting growth hormone and prolactin. Ann Intern Med 1978; 89:343.
30. Lamberts SWJ, Klijn JGM, Kwa GH, Birkenhaeger JC. The dynamics of growth hormone and prolactin secretion in acromegalic patients with mixed tumors. Acta Endocrinol (Copenh) 1979; 90:198.
31. Lamberts SWJ, Klijn JGM, van Vroonhoven CCJ, Stefanko SZ. Different responses of growth hormone secretion to guanfacine, bromocriptine, and thyrotropin-releasing hormone in acromegalic patients with pure growth hormone (GH)-containing and mixed GH/prolactin-containing pituitary adenomas. J Clin Endocrinol Metab 1985; 60:1148.
32. Zimmerman EA, Defendini R, Frantz AG. Prolactin and growth hormone in patients with pituitary adenomas. A correlative study of hormone in tumor and plasma by immunoperoxidase technique and radioimmunoassay. J Clin Endocrinol Metab 1974; 38:577.
33. Ishibashi M, Yamaji T. Effects of hypophysiotropic factors on growth hormone and prolactin secretion from somatotroph adenomas in culture. J Clin Endocrinol Metab 1985; 60:985.
34. Camanni F, Massara JF, Santia M, Molinatti GM, Mantegazza P, Muller EE. Impaired prolactin responsiveness to dopamine antagonists in acromegaly. Metabolism 1982; 31:1090.
35. Prescott RWG, Weightman DR, Kendall-Taylor P, Johnston DG. Different and PRL responses to dopamine receptor blockade in acromegaly. Clin Endocrinol (Oxf) 1984; 21:369.
36. Liuzzi A, Chiodini PG, Botalla L, Silvestrini F, Muller EE. Growth hormone-releasing activity of TRH and GH lowering effect of dopaminergic drugs in acromegaly: homogeneity of the two responses. J Clin Endocrinol Metab 1974; 39:871.
37. Horvath E, Kovacs K, Killinger DW, Smyth HS, Weiss MH, Ezrin C. Mammosomatotroph cell adenoma of the human pituitary: a morphologic entity. Virchows Arch [A] 1983; 398:277.
38. Bassetti M, Spada A, Arosio M, Vallar L, Brina M, Giannattasio G. Morphological studies on mixed growth hormone (GH)- and prolactin-(PRL) human pituitary adenomas. Coexistence of GH and PRL in the same secretory nodule. J Clin Endocrinol Metab 1986; 62:1093.
39. Faglia G, Beck-Peccoz P, Piscitelli G, Medri G. Pituitary inappropriate secretion of thyrotropin. Horm Res (in press).
40. Beck-Peccoz P, Piscitelli G, Medri G, Ballabio M, Faglia G. Thyroid test strategy. Lancet 1985; 1:1456.
41. Beck-Peccoz P, Piscitelli G, Amr S, et al. Endocrine, biochemical, and morphological studies of a pituitary adenoma secreting growth hormone, thyrotropin (TSH), and alpha-subunit: evidence for secretion of THS with increased bioactivity. J Clin Endocrinol Metab 1986; 62:704.
42. Lamberts SWJ, Oosterom R, Verleun T, Krenning EP, Assies JH. Regulation of hormone release by cultured cells from a thyrotropin-growth hormone secreting tumor. Direct inhibiting effects of 3,5,3'-triiodothyronine and dexamethasone on thyrotropin secretion. J Endocrinol Invest 1984; 7:313.

43. Kourides IA, Weintraub BD, Ridgway EC, Maloof F. Secretion of alpha-subunit of glycoprotein hormones by pituitary adenomas. J Clin Endocrinol Metab 1976; 43:97.
44. Beck-Peccoz P, Bassetti M, Spada A, et al. Glycoprotein hormone alpha-subunit response to growth hormone (GH)-releasing hormone in patients with active acromegaly. Evidence for alpha-subunit and GH coexistence in the same tumoral cell. J Clin Endocrinol Metab 1985; 61:541.

18

EFFECT OF GROWTH HORMONE ON CARBOHYDRATE AND LIPID METABOLISM: AN OVERVIEW

Mayer B. Davidson, M.D.

Department of Medicine
Cedars-Sinai Medical Center
Los Angeles, California 90048

Approximately 60 years ago, Houssay and his colleagues described hypersensitivity to insulin in hypophysectomized (hypox) animals (1). Further work documented a primary effect of growth hormone (GH) in this phenomenon (1). Over the ensuing years, numerous investigators have sought to define the role of GH in carbohydrate and lipid metabolism. Unfortunately, no unified picture has emerged. Both "insulin-like" and "anti-insulin-like" effects have been documented although the physiological significance of the former is uncertain. Major controversies surround the relationship between structure and function of the GH molecule. Indeed, some believe that most of the reported effects of GH are due to contaminants in the hormone preparation. With two exceptions (2,3), reviews in this area (4-10) have focused mainly on the author's own work in a circumscribed field, e.g., in vivo effects after GH administration (6,7,9), tissue effects in vitro (5,7), or effects on lipolysis (4,8,10). Furthermore, these reviews were published more than 10 years ago.

I have reviewed the current information regarding the effect of GH on carbohydrate and lipid metabolism. Since the last general review of this was published in 1965 (3), a literature search (English language) from 1966 through 1985 was conducted. All told, nearly 400 papers were surveyed. The information was separated into the following categories: (a) individual tissue effects when the tissue is either initially exposed to GH in vitro or removed from GH-injected animals; (b) in vivo effects of exogenous GH administration; (c) in vivo effects of physiological or pathological (i.e., tumor) GH secretion; (d) lipolytic (both in vitro and in-vivo) effects of GH; (e) structure-function relationships of the GH molecule evaluated by using hormones synthesized by recombinant DNA technology; and (f) possible mechanism(s) of the effect of GH on carbohydrate and lipid metabolism.

Data describing the effects of GH on carbohydrate and lipid metabolism are conflicting. The following conclusions seem reasonable although all investigators in this field may not agree entirely.

CONCLUSIONS

The "insulin-like" effects of GH involve enhanced glucose utilization (probably at the glucose transport step) and anti-lipolysis. They can be demonstrated both in vitro and in vivo but they are clearly easier to show if the tissue has had little or no recent prior exposure to GH. For this reason, the "insulin-like" effects of GH are not important physiologically because of frequent bursts of endogenous secretion of the hormone.

The "anti-insulin-like" effects of GH involve impaired glucose utilization, inducing a refractory state to the "insulin-like" effects of the hormone and stimulating lipolysis. The first two can be demonstrated in vitro but only inferred to occur in vivo. Increased lipolysis can easily be shown to occur both in vitro and in vivo but only after a definite lag period of several hours.

GH definitely antagonizes the action of insulin. This effect of GH is much easier to demonstrate in vivo. This implies that GH does not cause insulin antagonism directly but may do so secondarily.

The mechanism of GH effects on carbohydrate and lipid metabolism remains unclear and may not be due to GH itself. Studies with inhibitors of RNA and protein synthesis suggest that many of the effects of GH may involve a protein whose synthesis is stimulated by GH. Several studies suggest that the insulin antagonistic (but not the "anti-insulin-like") effects of GH may be secondary to the increased lipolysis via the glucose-fatty acid cycle. It is disappointing to note that this was the conclusion of the last general review of this subject over 20 years ago (3) and we have made little progress in substantiating or refuting this hypothesis. On a subcellular level, the adenyl cyclase-c-AMP-protein kinase system may be involved; however, the data are extremely confusing. There may be different biochemical mechanisms for the different effects of GH but there are little data directed specifically at this speculation.

Data concerning the structure-function relationships of GH are also very confusing. Several aspects of the existing dilemma have been considered. For example, are the diabetogenic and lipolytic effects of GH intrinsic to the molecule, or are they due to another factor(s) carried along in the pituitary extraction and purification of GH? The data from studies with DNA-synthesized hormones would suggest that GH itself is diabetogenic and probably lipolytic. Another important question involves the naturally occurring 20K variant of the peptide. Does this form of the hormone have effects similar to those of the 22K isomer? Although the 20K preparations isolated from pituitary glands were inactive, the DNA-derived molecule was active suggesting an intrinsic activity to this isomer.

Only limited progress has been made in understanding the fundamental mechanisms of GH effects on carbohydrate and lipid metabolism since the last general review on this subject over 20 years ago (3). With the newer technologies available today and an expanding knowledge of hormone action in general, we can expect to see many of the unanswered questions posed in this overview resolved in the next 20 years.

REFERENCES

1. Houssay BA. The hypophysis and metabolism. N Engl J Med 1936; 214:961.
2. De Bodo RC, Altszuler N. Insulin hypersensitivity and physiological insulin antagonists. Physiol Rev 1958; 38:389.
3. Weil R. Pituitary growth hormone and intermediary metabolism. I. The hormonal effect on the metabolism of fat and carbohydrate. Acta Endocrinol (Copenh) 1965; 49(suppl):98.
4. Fain JN. Studies on the role of RNA and protein synthesis in the lipolytic action of growth hormone in isolated fat cells. In: Weber

      G, ed. Adv in enzyme regulation. Oxford: Pergamon Press, 1967.

5. Goodman HM. Growth hormone and the metabolism of carbohydrate and lipid in adipose tissue. Ann NY Acad Sci 1968; 148:419.

6. Steele R. The effects of growth hormone on carbohydrate and lipid metabolism in the dog. Ann NY Acad Sci 1968; 148:441.

7. Mahler RJ, Szabo O. A postulated mechanism for the insulin synergistic and insulin antagonistic action of growth hormone. Adv Metab Disord 1970; 1(suppl 1):147.

8. Fain JN, Saperstein R. The involvement of RNA synthesis and cyclic AMP in the activation of fat cell lipolysis by growth hormone and glucocorticoids. Horm Metab Res 1970; 2:20.

9. Altszuler N. Action of growth hormone and carbohydrate metabolism. In: Knobil E, Sawyer WH, eds. Handbook of physiology. Washington, DC: American Physiological Society, 1974.

10. Rao AJ, Ramachandran J. Growth hormone and the regulation of lipolysis. In: Li CH, ed. Hormonal proteins and peptides. New York: Academic Press, 1977.

19

THE DIAGNOSIS OF ACROMEGALY

Harold E. Carlson, M.D.

Northport VA Hospital, Northport, NY 11768, and
Department of Medicine, State University of New York at
Stony Brook, Stony Brook, NY 11794

As one would expect, there have been many advances in the diagnosis of acromegaly in the last one hundred years. Although the diagnosis is now firmly established on the basis of laboratory measurements of serum growth hormone (GH), there is, in nearly all cases, an initial clinical diagnosis which leads to the appropriate biochemical testing.

Thus, the original description of acromegaly and the diagnosis of subsequent cases were made primarily on clinical grounds by Marie and other early investigators. It was, of course, the striking physical appearance of acromegalic patients that called attention to their condition. Even today, enlargement of the hands, feet and facial features are the usual findings which lead us to suspect the diagnosis. Many of the early cases were undoubtedly long-standing and most involved large pituitary tumors. Thus, Marie and others frequently noted hypogonadism as a presenting symptom of the disorder, probably due to compromise of normal pituitary function by the tumor. Polyuria was commonly observed, and was due to either diabetes mellitus (secondary to insulin antagonism by GH) or diabetes insipidus (reflecting damage to the hypothalamus and posterior pituitary by the sellar mass lesion). Visual field defects were commonly found as a consequence of optic chiasmal compression (1).

Clinical findings in acromegaly are not limited to the above symptoms; many other signs and symptoms may be present (2-7) (Table 1). Some of these, such as hypertension and degenerative arthritis, are so common in the general population as to be of little diagnostic value, whereas others, such as carpal tunnel syndrome and galactorrhea, are unusual enough to make one consider the diagnosis of acromegaly as an explanation for their occurrence.

Pituitary and sellar enlargement were noted in autopsied cases by Marie and his collaborator, Souza-Leite, but these findings were used in diagnosis only when skull roentgenography became widespread in the first decade of the twentieth century (8). Modern series have noted sellar enlargement on plain skull X-rays in 75-95% of patients. Using the more sensitive technique of computed tomography, a pituitary tumor can be demonstrated in nearly all patients (9) (Fig. 1).

Apart from glucose measurements, the first laboratory test to be applied to the diagnosis of acromegaly was the measurement of serum

Table 1. Clinical features of acromegaly.

	% occurrence
Acral enlargement	98
Increased sweating	75
Fatigue/lethargy	60
Headache	60
Paresthesias	50
Hypertension	25
Goiter	30
Osteoarthritis	55
Visual problems	15
Menstrual abnormality	60
Decreased libido/impotence	35
Galactorrhea	6
Skin tags	50
Acanthosis nigricans	50
Diabetes mellitus/impaired glucose tolerance	40
Hypercalcinuria	60
Nephrolithiasis	7

inorganic phosphorus. Elevated serum phosphorus levels in acromegaly were first described by Reifenstein, Kinsell and Albright in 1946 (10). This elevation reflects the effect of GH in promoting renal phosphate reabsorption. Subsequent series have noted the variability of serum phosphorus measurements; only about 50% of acromegalic patients have an elevated value (that is, greater than 4.5 mg/dl) (Fig. 2) and there may be significant day-to-day variation in any single subject (3-5,11,12). Thus, serum phosphorus measurements have not found great favor as a diagnostic test.

In the 1950s and 1960s, considerable attention was given to radiographic findings in acromegaly (13). Of these, quantitation of soft

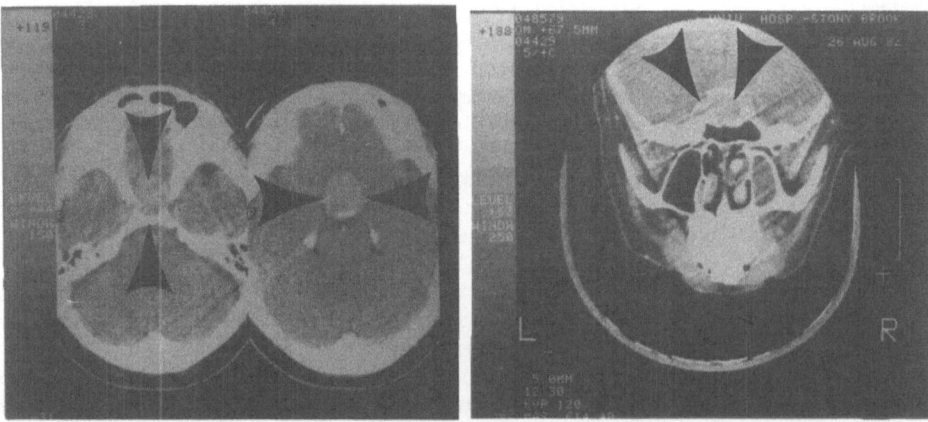

Fig. 1. Cranial computed tomography demonstrating a large pituitary macroadenoma (arrows) on axial (left) and coronal (right) sections. (Scans courtesy of Department of Radiology, State University of New York at Stony Brook.)

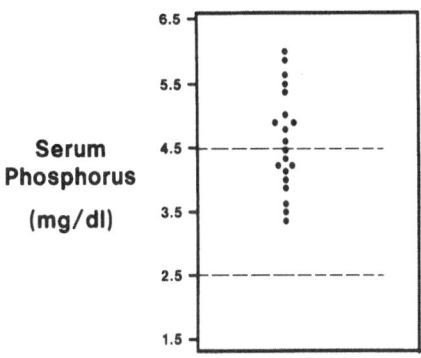

Fig. 2. Serum phosphorus levels in untreated acromegalics. About 50% of untreated patients have elevated phosphorus levels. (Data plotted from references 11,12,44.)

tissue enlargement by measurement of heel pad thickness was found to be one of the most useful measurements and was proposed as a diagnostic test (14-18). Lack of a uniform method led to considerable confusion regarding upper limits of normal values. Subsequently, however, the method of Kho et al. (18) standardized the procedure (Fig. 3) which allowed comparison of data between institutions. Even with this technique, however, there is overlap of normal values with those obtained in acromegalics (Fig. 4). Some of the higher values obtained in normals may be due to obesity, or to

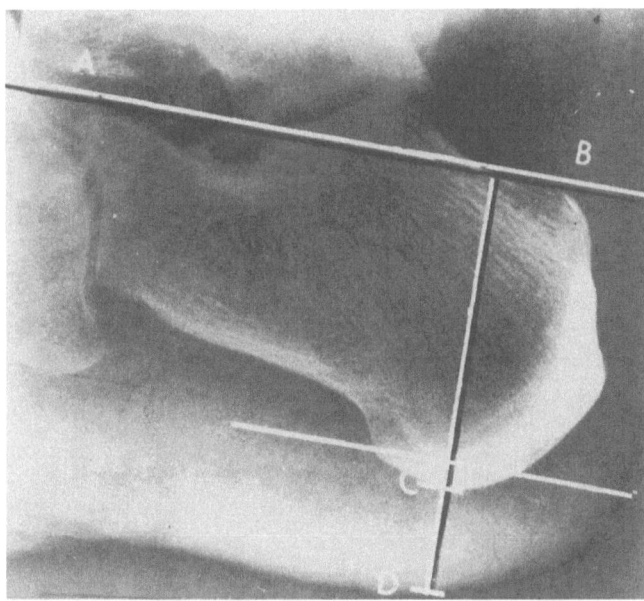

Fig. 3. Assessment of heel-pad thickness according to Kho et al. (18). Measurement is made from the skin surface to the lowest point on the calcaneus (C-D) perpendicular to a line connecting its anterior and posterior angles (A-B). (Reprinted by permission of K. R. Kattan, Thickening of the heel pad associated with long-term Dilantin therapy, Am J Roentgenol 1975; 124:52. Copyright, American Roentgen Ray Society.)

phenytoin therapy, both of which are associated with heel pad thickening (18-20). Although values greater than 22 mm are suggestive of acromegaly, the test is not specific enough to be used in diagnosis; however, heel pad measurements, along with measurements of skin thickness (21), hand volume and ring size, have found their greatest utility in following the effects of therapy in acromegaly.

In the early 1960s a truly revolutionary advance in the diagnosis of acromegaly was brought about by the development of sensitive and specific radioimmunoassays for the measurement of serum GH. Measurement of GH in random or fasting serum specimens soon demonstrated that although some patients with acromegaly have grossly elevated values (e.g., > 100 ng/ml), many have only slightly elevated serum GH levels (e.g., 5-20 ng/ml). Such minor elevations may also be found in normal subjects, presumably reflecting physiologic GH elevations secondary to various types of stress (22) (Fig. 5). Thus, the observation of Roth et al. (23) in 1963 that glucose administration suppressed serum GH in normals, but not acromegalics, led to the use of this maneuver in diagnosis. Assessment of the GH response to an oral glucose load of 75-100 gm remains the single most useful and most definitive diagnostic test for acromegaly. Nearly all normal subjects will suppress serum GH to values less than 5 ng/ml one hour after glucose ingestion, and values fall to less than 2 ng/ml in most individuals. In contrast, nearly all patients with acromegaly show serum GH values greater than 5 ng/ml postglucose, and some show a "paradoxical" stimulation of GH following glucose loading (24) (Fig. 6).

Ancillary tests of GH secretion which may be useful in the diagnosis of acromegaly include: (a) TRH administration (normals rarely show GH stimulation by TRH, but 70-90% of acromegalics have at least a 50% rise in serum GH after TRH [25-27] [Fig. 7]; unlike TSH, the GH response to TRH is not altered by thyroid hormones [28] so the test may be performed in patients receiving thyroid supplements); (b) L-dopa testing (most normals

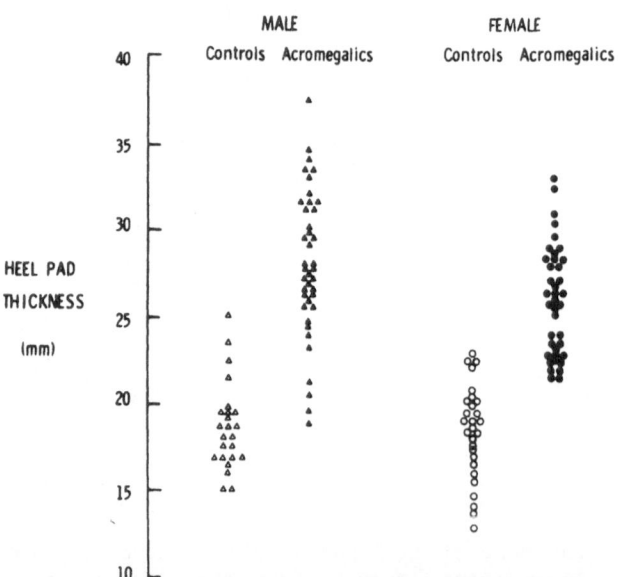

Fig. 4. Overlap of heel-pad thickness measurements in 52 normals and 79 untreated acromegalics. (Reprinted by permission of K. M. Kho et al., Heel pad thickness in acromegaly, Br J Radiol 1970; 43:119. Copyright, The British Institute of Radiology.)

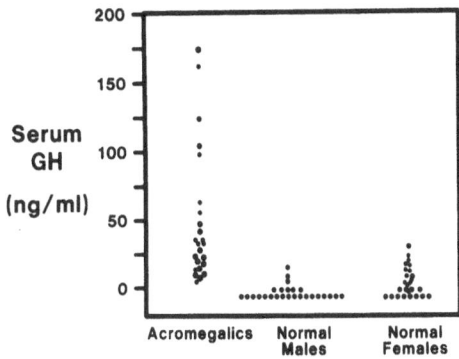

Fig. 5. Random serum GH measurements in normal subjects and in
patients with acromegaly. Small
circles indicate treated patients.

show GH stimulation following oral administration of 500 mg of L-dopa, but
50-100% of acromegalics show GH suppression following L-dopa [29-31]
[Fig. 8]); and, (c) the 24-hour GH profile, in which serum GH is measured
at 30-60 min intervals throughout the day and night (normals show very low
serum GH values [< 1-2 ng/ml] at some time during the period, while
acromegalics almost never achieve such low values [32-35] [Fig. 9]).
Although abnormal GH responses to each of these tests may be obtained in a
variety of illnesses (e.g., renal failure, protein-calorie malnutrition,
anorexia nervosa [36]), these states can usually be readily distinguished
from acromegaly on clinical grounds. GH responses to hypoglycemia,
arginine and GHRH are nondiscriminating and have generally not been useful
diagnostic criteria (32,34-39).

     Circulating serum GH is found in a variety of forms in humans.
Monomeric or "little" GH (MW = 22,000 daltons) is the most abundant
species with dimeric or "big" GH and larger ("big, big" GH) forms compris-
ing up to about 30% of the total serum immunoreactive GH (40). The
relative proportions of the various species are similar in acromegalic and

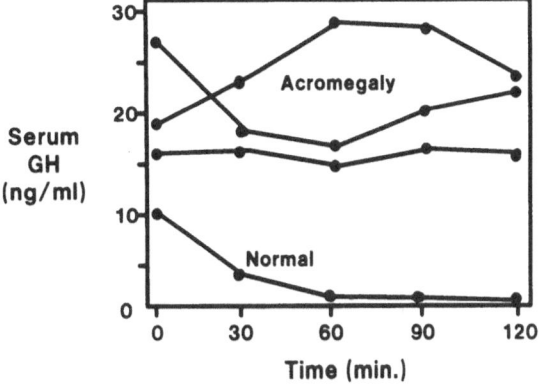

Fig. 6. Glucose ingestion (at time zero
min) suppresses serum GH to low levels
in normal subjects (bottom line), but
produces only partial suppression, no
change, or a rise in serum GH in
patients with acromegaly (top 3 lines).

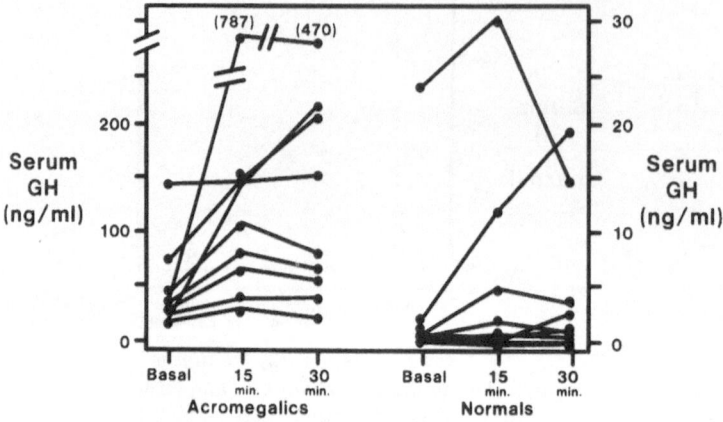

Fig. 7. Injection of TRH (IV) produces at least a 50%
rise in serum GH in the majority of acromegalics
(left); normal subjects generally show little change
in serum GH following TRH administration (right).

normal sera, however, and the quantitation of these forms has not proven
useful in diagnosis of the disorder (41-43).

Measurements of serum somatomedin activity using in vitro bioassays
developed by Daughaday and others showed that many, but not all, acromegalics have elevated values (44,45). More recently, somatomedin-C
(IGF-I) radioimmunoassays have demonstrated elevated values in nearly all
patients with acromegaly (46,47) (Fig. 10). Thus the measurement of serum
somatomedin-C can be a useful ancillary diagnostic test. Such assays are
now readily available through commercial laboratories and provide the
simplest objective index of the biologic effect of GH hypersecretion.

The role of growth hormone-releasing hormone (GHRH) in acromegaly
will be discussed in much greater detail by others at this symposium. As
a diagnostic test, however, the measurement of plasma GHRH has thus far
been useful only in the diagnosis of secondary acromegaly, in which plasma

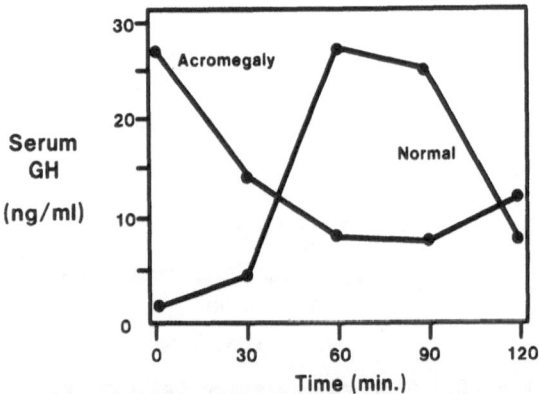

Fig. 8. Effects of L-dopa on GH secretion in normal and acromegalic patients.
Oral administration of L-dopa stimulates
GH secretion in normals but frequently
suppresses serum GH in acromegalics.

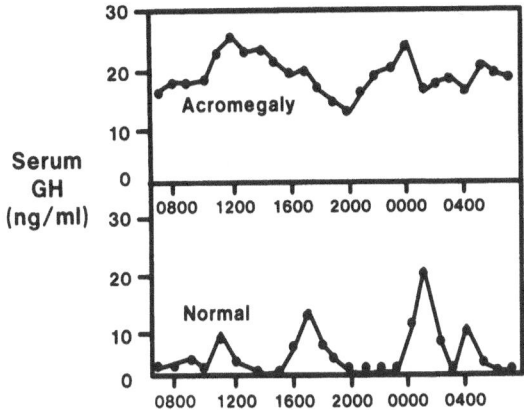

Fig. 9. Variations in GH levels in
normal and acromegalic patients over a
24-hour period. In normal individuals
(bottom panel), serum GH levels are low
(less than 1-2 ng/ml) at some time
during a 24-hour period; acromegalics
(top panel), rarely achieve such low
values.

GHRH is usually massively elevated due to its production by a neoplasm
(Fig. 11). Plasma GHRH concentrations have generally been normal in most
"ordinary" cases of the disorder (48,49), and assays for GHRH are currently available only in a few research laboratories.

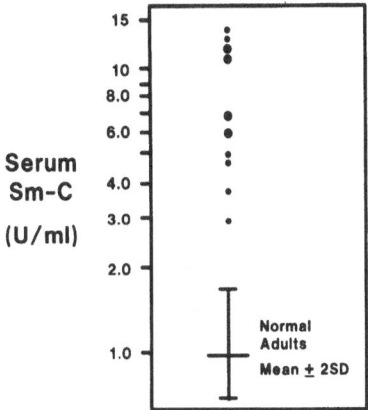

Fig. 10. Immunoreactive serum
somatomedin-C (IGF-I) levels
in acromegalics and in normal
subjects. Circulating levels
of SM-C are usually elevated
in acromegaly compared to normals; small circles indicate
treated patients. Note logarithmic scale. (Data adopted
from H. E. Carlson et al.,
Effect of bromocriptine on
serum hormones in acromegaly,
Horm Res 1984; 19:142.)

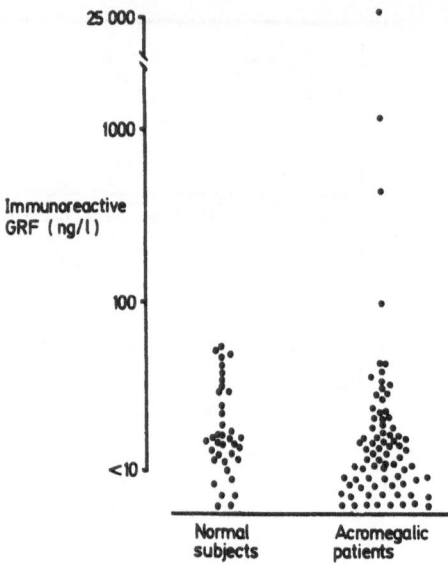

Fig. 11. Plasma immunoreactive GHRH in normal subjects and patients with acromegaly. In most patients with acromegaly, GHRH values are normal; however, grossly elevated values are found in patients with secondary acromegaly due to GHRH secretion by a neoplasm. Note logarithmic scale. (Reprinted by permission of E. S. Penny et al., Circulating growth hormone releasing factor concentrations in normal subjects and patients with acromegaly, Br Med J 1984; 289:453. Copyright, British Medical Association.)

In summary, then, the routine diagnosis of acromegaly can usually be accomplished by demonstrating elevated basal and postglucose serum GH levels in a patient with clinical findings of the disorder. In cases of borderline GH suppression by glucose, assessment of serum somatomedin-C and the GH response to TRH are simple and useful confirmatory tests (46,50). L-dopa tests are less often diagnostic and the 24-hour GH profile may be too cumbersome for routine use.

Some patients with the clinical findings of acromegaly but normal GH secretion have been given a diagnosis of "acromegaloidism" (51,52). Somatomedin levels are normal in these subjects but they may have excessive circulating concentrations of other growth factors (52) (Fig. 12). The origin, nature and role of these factors remain unknown and there is no effective treatment for the disorder.

Finally, the spectrum of clinical findings in acromegaly has been enlarged over the years. Clinicians still need a high index of suspicion to make the diagnosis of acromegaly early in the course of the disease. Recent reports have emphasized the occurrence of acromegaly as a component of multiple endocrine neoplasia, Type I (53) and a new, as yet unnamed familial syndrome of spotty mucocutaneous pigmentation, cardiac and cutaneous myxomas and endocrine overactivity (54,55).

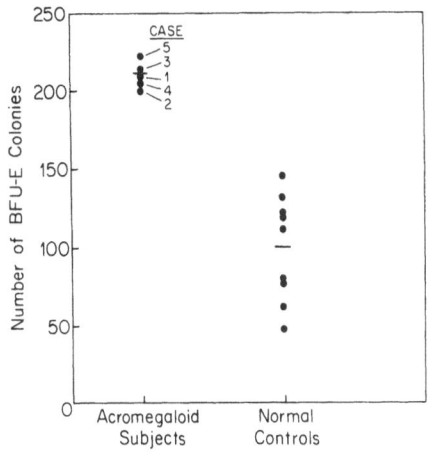

Fig. 12. Erythroid precursor stimulation (burst-forming units; BFU-E) in normal subjects and in patients with acromegaloidism. Some patients with "acromegaloidism" have elevated serum levels of a growth factor which can be measured by assessing stimulation of primitive erythroid precursors in culture. (Reprinted by permission of M. W. Ashcraft et al., A unique growth factor in patients with acromegaloidism, J Clin Endocrinol Metab 1983; 57:272. Copyright, The Endocrine Society.)

Additional associations with sleep apnea (which may be seen in up to 40% of patients) (56) and colonic neoplasia (which may occur in as many as 45% of acromegalics) (57-59) may provide new clues to the diagnosis. The presence of multiple skin tags may serve as a marker for colon polyps or cancer in acromegaly as well as in normal subjects (57,58,60). Thus, like Marie, we must remain keenly attuned to the clinical findings in our patients in order to make optimal use of the sophisticated and sensitive laboratory tools now available for the diagnosis of the disorder which he named acromegaly.

REFERENCES

1. Medvei VC. A history of endocrinology. Lancaster: MTP Press, Ltd., 1982.
2. Davidoff LM. Studies in acromegaly. III. The anamnesis and symptomatology in one hundred cases. Endocrinology 1926; 10:461.
3. Hamwi GJ, Skillman TG, Tufts KC Jr. Acromegaly. Am J Med 1960; 29:690.
4. Gordon DA, Hill FM, Ezrin C. Acromegaly: a review of 100 cases. Can Med Assoc J 1962; 87:1106.
5. Lawrence JH, Tobias CA, Linfoot JA, et al. Successful treatment of acromegaly; metabolic and clinical studies in 145 patients. J Clin Endocrinol Metab 1970; 31:180.
6. Levin SR. Manifestations and treatment of acromegaly. Calif Med 1972; 116:57.
7. Jadresic A, Banks LM, Child DF, et al. The acromegaly syndrome. Q J

Med 1982; 51:189.

8. Cushing H. The pituitary body and its disorders. Philadelphia: JB Lippincott, 1912.

9. Kendall B. Current approaches to hypothalamic-pituitary radiology. Clin Endocrinol Metab 1983; 12:535.

10. Reifenstein EC, Kinsell LW, Albright F. Observations on the use of the serum phosphorus level as an index of pituitary growth hormone activity; the effect of estrogen therapy in acromegaly [Abstract]. J Clin Endocrinol 1946; 6:470.

11. Beck P, Schalch DS, Parker ML, Kipnis DM, Daughaday WH. Correlative studies of growth hormone and insulin plasma concentrations with metabolic abnormalities in acromegaly. J Lab Clin Med 1965; 66:366.

12. Ikkos D, Ljunggren H, Luft R. Basal metabolic rate in relation to body size and cell mass in acromegaly. Acta Endocrinol (Copenh) 1956; 21:237.

13. Steinbach HL, Feldman R, Goldberg MB. Acromegaly. Radiology 1959; 72:535.

14. Steinbach HL, Russell W. Measurement of the heel-pad as an aid to diagnosis of acromegaly. Radiology 1964; 82:418.

15. Fields ML, Greenberg BE, Burkett LL. Roentgenographic measurement of skin and heel-pad thickness in the diagnosis of acromegaly. Am J Med Sci 1967; 254:528.

16. Puckette SE Jr, Seymour EQ. Fallibility of the heel-pad thickness in the diagnosis of acromegaly. Radiology 1967; 88:982.

17. Gonticas SK, Ikkos DG, Stergiou LH. Evaluation of the diagnostic value of heel-pad thickness in acromegaly. Radiology 1969; 94:304.

18. Kho KM, Wright AD, Doyle FH. Heel pad thickness in acromegaly. Br J Radiol 1970; 43:119.

19. Jackson DM. Heel pad thickness in obese persons. Radiology 1968; 90:129.

20. Kattan KR. Thickening of the heel-pad associated with long-term Dilantin therapy. Am J Roentgenol 1975; 124:52.

21. Meema HE, Sheppard RH, Rapoport A. Roentgenographic visualization and measurement of skin thickness and its diagnostic application in acromegaly. Radiology 1964; 82:411.

22. Utiger RD, Parker ML, Daughaday WH. Studies in human growth hormone. I. A radioimmunoassay for human growth hormone. J Clin Invest 1962; 41:254.

23. Roth J, Glick SM, Yalow RS, Berson SA. Secretion of human growth hormone: physiologic and experimental modification. Metabolism 1963; 12:577.

24. Earll JM, Sparks LL, Forsham PH. Glucose suppression of serum growth hormone in the diagnosis of acromegaly. JAMA 1967; 201:134.

25. Irie M, Tsushima T. Increase of serum growth hormone concentration following thyrotropin-releasing hormone injection in patients with acromegaly or gigantism. J Clin Endocrinol Metab 1972; 35:97.

26. Faglia G, Beck-Peccoz P, Ferrari C, Travaglini P, Ambrosi B, Spada A. Plasma growth hormone response to thyrotropin-releasing hormone in patients with active acromegaly. J Clin Endocrinol Metab 1973; 36:1259.

27. Schalch DS, Gonzalez-Barcena D, Kastin AJ, Schally AV, Lee LA. Abnormalities in the release of TSH in response to thyrotropin-releasing hormone in patients with disorders of the pituitary, hypothalamus and basal ganglia. J Clin Endocrinol Metab 1972; 35:609.

28. Carlson HE, Sowers JR, Rand RW. Lack of effect of thyroid hormones on the growth hormone response to thyrotropin-releasing hormone in acromegaly. Metabolism 1977; 26:801.

29. Liuzzi A, Chiodini PG, Botalla L, Cremascoli G, Silvestrini F. Inhibitory effect of L-DOPA on GH release in acromegalic patients. J Clin Endocrinol Metab 1972; 35:941.

30. Mims RB, Stein RB, Bethune JE. The effect of a single dose of L-DOPA on pituitary hormones in acromegaly, obesity and in normal subjects. J Clin Endocrinol Metab 1973; 37:34.

31. Delitala G, Masala A, Alagna S, Devilla L, Lotti G. Growth hormone and prolactin release in acromegalic patients following metergoline administration. J Clin Endocrinol Metab 1976; 43:1382.

32. Cryer PE, Daughaday WH. Regulation of growth hormone secretion in acromegaly. J Clin Endocrinol Metab 1969; 29:386.

33. Carlson HE, Gillin JC, Gorden PE, Snyder F. Absence of sleep-related growth hormone peaks in aged normal subjects and in acromegaly. J Clin Endocrinol Metab 1972; 34:1102.

34. Cryer PE, Jacobs LS, Daughaday WH. Regulation of growth hormone and prolactin secretion in patients with acromegaly and/or excessive prolactin secretion. Mt Sinai J Med (NY) 1973; 40:402.

35. Mims RB, Bethune JE. Acromegaly with normal fasting growth hormone concentrations but abnormal growth hormone regulation. Ann Intern Med 1974; 81:781.

36. Ho KY, Evans SS, Thorner MO. Disorders of prolactin and growth hormone secretion. Clin Endocrinol Metab 1985; 14:1.

37. Lawrence AM, Goldfine ID, Kirsteins L. Growth hormone dynamics in acromegaly. J Clin Endocrinol Metab 1970; 31:239.

38. Losa M, Schopohl J, Stalla GK, Muller OA, Von Werder K. Growth hormone releasing factor-test in acromegaly: comparison with other dynamic tests. Clin Endocrinol (Oxf) 1985; 23:99.

39. Gelato ME, Merriam GR, Vance ML, et al. Effects of growth hormone-releasing factor on growth hormone secretion in acromegaly. J Clin Endocrinol Metab 1985; 60:251.

40. Chawla RK, Parks JS, Rudman D. Structural variants of human growth hormone: biochemical, genetic and clinical aspects. Annu Rev Med 1983; 34:519.

41. Goodman AD, Tanenbaum R, Rabinowitz D. Existence of two forms of immunoreactive growth hormone in human plasma. J Clin Endocrinol Metab 1972; 35:868.

42. Gorden P, Hendricks CM, Roth J. Evidence for "big" and "little" components of human plasma and pituitary growth hormone. J Clin Endocrinol Metab 1973; 36:178.

43. Dimond RC, Wartofsky L, Rosen SW. Heterogeneity of circulating growth hormone in acromegaly. J Clin Endocrinol Metab 1974; 39:1133.

44. Daughaday WH, Salmon WD Jr, Alexander F. Sulfation factor activity of sera from patients with pituitary disorders. J Clin Endocrinol Metab 1959; 19:743.

45. Grant DB. Sulfation factor. Clin Endocrinol (Oxf) 1972; 1:387.

46. Clemmons DR, Van Wyk JJ, Ridgway EC, Kliman B, Kjellberg RN, Underwood LE. Evaluation of acromegaly by radioimmunoassay of somatomedin-C. N Engl J Med 1979; 301:1138.

47. Rieu M, Girard F, Bricaire H, Binoux M. The importance of insulin-like growth factor (Somatomedin) measurements in the diagnosis and surveillance of acromegaly. J Clin Endocrinol Metab 1982; 55:147.

48. Penny ES, Penman E, Price J, et al. Circulating growth hormone releasing factor concentrations in normal subjects and patients with acromegaly. Br Med J 1984; 289:453.

49. Frohman LA. Growth hormone-releasing factor: a neuroendocrine perspective. J Lab Clin Med 1984; 103:819.

50. Feingold KR, Lorenz TJ. Acromegaly with "normal" growth hormone levels. West J Med 1985; 142:95.

51. Mims RB. Pituitary function and growth hormone dynamics in acromegaloidism. J Natl Med Assoc 1978; 70:919.

52. Ashcraft MW, Hartzband PI, Van Herle AJ, Bersch N, Golde DW. A unique growth factor in patients with acromegaloidism. J Clin Endocrinol Metab 1983; 57:272.

53. Yamaguchi K, Kameya T, Abe K. Multiple endocrine neoplasia type I.

Clin Endocrinol Metab 1980; 9:261.

54. Carney JA, Gordon H, Carpenter PC, Shenoy BV, Go VLW. The complex of myxomas, spotty pigmentation, and endocrine overactivity. Medicine (Baltimore) 1985; 64:270.

55. Carney JA, Hruska LS, Beauchamp GD, Gordon H. Dominant inheritance of the complex of myxomas, spotty pigmentation, and endocrine over-activity. Mayo Clin Proc 1986; 61:165.

56. Hart TB, Radow SK, Blackard WG, Tucker HS, Cooper KR. Sleep apnea in acromegaly. Arch Intern Med 1985; 145:865.

57. Klein I, Parveen G, Gavaler JS, Van Thiel DH. Colonic polyps in patients with acromegaly. Ann Intern Med 1982; 97:27.

58. Ituarte EA, Petrini J, Hershman JM. Acromegaly and colon cancer. Ann Intern Med 1984; 101:627.

59. Pines A, Rozen P, Ron E, Gilat T. Gastrointestinal tumors in acrome-galic patients. Am J Gastroenterol 1985; 80:266.

60. Chobanian SJ, Van Ness MM, Winters C, Cattau EL. Skin tags as a marker for adenomatous polyps of the colon. Ann Intern Med 1985; 103:892.

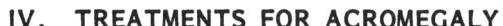

IV. TREATMENTS FOR ACROMEGALY

20

CONVENTIONAL SUPERVOLTAGE RADIATION IN THE TREATMENT OF ACROMEGALY

Phillip Gorden,* Eli Glatstein,[2] Edward Oldfield,[3] and Jesse Roth*

*Diabetes Branch, NIDDK; [2]Radiation Oncology Branch, NCI; [3]Surgical Neurology Branch, NINCDS; NIH, Bethesda, MD 20892

INTRODUCTION

In the present work, we will review our previous studies on the use of conventional supervoltage radiation in the treatment of acromegaly (1-5), present more extended data on the total group of patients that we have treated and followed over the past 22 years (1964-1986), and present data on patients who were irradiated following unsuccessful surgical therapy.

HISTORICAL PERSPECTIVE

Acromegaly is due to growth hormone (GH) hypersecretion predominantly from benign tumors of the pituitary gland. Thus, it was logical that when megavoltage X-ray sources became available approximately 30 years ago that this modality of therapy would be used to treat growth hormone secreting pituitary tumors. When pituitary irradiation was first used, however, methods were not available to measure GH in plasma and there was no other clinical or laboratory method that provided a sensitive measure of efficacy. When RIA for GH was developed in the early 1960s it was found that patients treated by pituitary irradiation may have persistent elevation of GH in plasma and the efficacy of irradiation therapy was unclear.

More recently it has become clear that conventional megavoltage irradiation does reduce GH concentration in the plasma of acromegalics but that this effect occurs over a period of years (1). Since over the last 20 years many other modalities of therapy have been introduced, the role of conventional megavoltage irradiation must continue to be defined. Certainly no surgical, X-ray, or pharmacologic treatment has emerged as definitive for all patients and attempts should be made to see if specific clinical situations are best treated by specific therapies, individually or in combination.

The Development of Radiotherapeutic Technique

The earliest experience of physicians with radiation therapy was limited; they had little or no understanding of the physical nature or the biological effects of the mysterious rays with which they worked. There were no reliable dose measurements, and no agreed-upon dose units.

Equipment was primitive and too limited in energy to permit treatment of anything other than the most superficial tumors. Early in this century radiation therapists utilized techniques that involved massive exposures which were intended to eradicate tumors in a single treatment. Thus, it is not surprising that the extensive morbidity from such massive exposure was often comparable to that of major ablative surgery of the same era.

The major developments in the first half of this century reflected a progressive understanding of the biological principles of radiation therapy on the basis of fractionation. Beginning in 1919, a classic series of experiments was carried out by Regaud and his co-workers in which they convincingly demonstrated that spermatogenesis in the testes of experimental animals could be completely eradicated by the administration of successive small daily doses of fractionated irradiation. Regaud and his colleague, Henri Coutard, applied the principles of protracted fractionated irradiation therapy to the treatment of patients with cancers, especially in the head, neck, and breast. Within a few years, physicians from the Fondation Curie reported surprisingly good 5-year survival data for a variety of cancers of the oral cavity, pharynx, and larynx. Daily small doses of radiation made treatment more tolerable and more effective. This is the heart of what radiotherapists call "fractionation" and, indeed, the principles of today's treatment are not different from what Regaud and Coutard pioneered in the 1920s.

The second important development in radiation therapy was the evolution at mid-century of megavoltage radiation beams, utilizing either Cobalt 60 or electronic devices such as the linear accelerator. The development of high energy beams generated by such devices liberated the radiation therapist from the physical limitations imposed by the kilovoltage units of the first half of the century. A beam of megavoltage energy has the capability of producing its maximum ionization at a significant depth below the skin surface, obviating the radiation tolerance of the skin as the dose-limiting factor. Moreover, these beams generally have relatively sharply defined lateral edges that greatly diminish lateral scatter and enable these beams to be used in a much more refined and sophisticated fashion than the kilovoltage beams of the first half of this century. Because of the enormous increase in energy that such beams have, compared to the old-fashioned kilovoltage X-rays, their penetration is enormously greater and more effective for deeply located tumors.

An important technological development in pituitary radiation was the marked improvement in tumor localization afforded by computerized axial tomography (CAT) scanning. Prior to the CAT scanning, definition of tumor volume was largely defined on the basis of skull films, tomograms through the sella, arteriogram to rule out an aneurysm, and a pneumoencephalogram to see if the ventricles had been displaced. It is now clear that gross underestimation of appropriate tumor volume was common prior to CAT scanning. This must be taken into account when the results of radiation therapy of the pituitary gland include patients treated from the prior era. Thus, modern CAT scanning has had a tremendous influence not only on the surgical approach to such patients, but also on their radiotherapeutic management, by defining the target volume of interest with unprecedented precision.

Method of Supervoltage Irradiation Used at the Clinical Center of the NIH

Acromegaly tends to be associated with relatively modest-sized pituitary neoplasms; tumor volumes of 5 to 6 cm are typically adequate to encompass the involved area. However, in those patients who have CAT evidence of significant suprasellar extension, or who have radiographic evidence of extension into the sphenoid sinus, more generous fields may be

212

required. Confidence in tumor localization will permit the construction of relatively small tumor volumes, since histologically benign tumors, such as most pituitary adenomas, do not require the same generous margins to account for infiltration that are generally necessary in the radiation treatment of malignant tumors.

Technically, the equipment required for modern treatment of the pituitary region includes a simulator and a megavoltage radiotherapy unit with rotational isocentric capability. Since radiation is both attenuating and diverging as it transverses tissue, special care with respect to the eyes must be taken before radiation is actually delivered. The simulator is essential to set up the radiotherapy portals in such a way that the tumor volume is consistently within all treatment portals but the eyes are excluded from the radiation beams.

An essential element in establishing the radiation portals is absolute immobilization of the patient's head during treatment. This will usually require a headboard when the patient is recumbent, or a bite block that has been customized to fit the patient's teeth, or both.

Beam direction and field size are established by simulation. This process refers to a mock procedure that duplicates everything to be done in treatment, except that a diagnostic X-ray beam is used rather than a megavoltage beam. Because of the preferential absorption according to atomic number, with a diagnostic low-energy X-ray beam, radiologic detail can be seen in arranging the portals with a simulator film. Inasmuch as a megavoltage beam does not absorb according to atomic number, anatomic detail cannot be identified well by examining megavoltage films.

A headboard elevates the neck and head at an angle of approximately 30° with respect to the top of the treatment couch. This elevation effectively moves the eyes out of the plane of axis of the rotating gantry and thus allows the orbits to be excluded from the tumor volume of interest, not only for the entering photon beam, but also for the exiting photon beam. Fluoroscopy and image intensifiers permit visualization of the field during simulation. When the patient is comfortably positioned on the headboard, we prefer to mark three separate points on the skin which serve to define the critical plane for rotational arcing of the gantry. These three points are obtained by laser light markings that correspond to the isocenter from three separate directions, based on simulator imaging. This type of laser light system is available both in the simulation room and in the treatment room. We generally use a 220° arcing or rotational field treatment. For very large lesions, we may resort to a three-field isocentric arrangement, utilizing two large wedged lateral fields and one anterior field.

Although any megavoltage beam is adequate to treat pituitary tumors, higher energies have more skin sparing and result in a more homogeneous radiation dosage across the central tumor volume than does ^{60}Co equipment. Accordingly, 6 to 15 MeV X-ray beams from a linear accelerator are probably optimal conventional energies for the treatment of pituitary lesions.

Because the pituitary region is central within the skull, a wedge of approximately 45° is commonly employed in the treatment of pituitary tumors to compensate for the sloping contours of the skull. We prefer a 220° arcing rotational field in the coronal plane, above the level of the orbits, as advocated by Kramer and colleagues. We utilize a 45° wedge starting counterclockwise at the lowest edge of the treatment field (from an approximate 200° angle), with the thick edge of the wedge pointed upward toward the top of the skull; as the gantry rotates to the vertex (90°), the treatment is stopped and the wedge is rotated 180° so that the thick edge of the wedge will ultimately point downward as the arc resumes. The treatment is then continued to complete a 220° arc (to -20°). If a three-field isocentric treatment plan is used, wedges are used on the two lateral fields to optimize their integration with the anterior field by eliminating any hot spot. We do not recommend the use of opposing lateral fields as the sole means of treatment of the pituitary, inasmuch as they deliver higher doses to the temporal lobes of the brain than will be received by the pituitary region, and thus predispose them to neurologic injury.

The dose that is recommended is 4500-5000 rads over 5 to 6 weeks. Treatment delivery is 5 days a week at the rate of 180 rads a day. The total tumor dose to the volume in question does not exceed 5000 rads over 6 weeks, thereby eliminating most of the major complications of radiation therapy resulting from the pituitary treatment. It is important to realize that most of the radiation injury reported from the treatment of pituitary tumors is seen either following doses in excess of 5000 rads or when similar doses of radiation have been delivered in very short periods of time, rather than at the rate of 180 rads per day. If the treatment has been properly planned and well administered, the major complications should occur rarely, since the major areas of risk (other than the pituitary region itself) should be outside the high-dose tumor volume.

Results of Conventional Supervoltage Irradiation
in Previously Untreated Patients

Sixty-two previously untreated patients have undergone irradiation therapy and have been followed from 2 to 15 years. Patients 1-47 (Fig. 1) have been previously reported (1) and are here updated with respect to follow-up time. Specific variations in the radiation technique from that described (see above) are given in reference 1. The additional patients shown in Figure 1 are previously unreported and more recently treated. To the extent that they can be compared, the response to therapy in the more recently treated group is about the same as in the previously reported group. Patients range in age from 13-63 years and mean pretreatment GH for the group is 52 ng/ml (range of 8-275 ng/ml). Most of our patients have enlargement of the sella on plain or tomographic skull X-ray (4). All have abnormalities on computerized axial tomograms of the sella. By 2 years following irradiation mean percent fall in GH = 50%, and by 5 years = 75% (Fig. 2). Although after 5 years the rate of fall of GH decreases, there is a slow persistent fall between 5 and 15 years. This same trend is evident when mean GH concentration is followed (Fig. 3). Again, there is a rapid fall for up to 5 years, with a slower but persistent decrease extending up to 15 years. Thus, by 10 years after therapy, 79% of patients have GH $\leq$10 ng/ml and 59% have values $\leq$5 ng/ml.

Though there is a positive correlation between the size of the pituitary tumor and plasma GH, the percent fall in plasma GH is independent of size, or of invasive or bone erosive properties of the tumor (4). This is an important consideration when making therapeutic decisions about surgery vs. irradiation in patients with large tumors who have relatively low plasma GH.

Though we have no systematic data on the gel filtration pattern or radioreceptor activity of plasma GH following irradiation, we have noted no qualitative changes in GH in the small group of patients whom we have studied. Further, we have no systematic data on IGF-I/somatomedin-C. However, the correlation coefficient between plasma GH and somatomedin-C in a representative group of irradiated patients (r = 0.7). We, therefore, believe that the immunoreactive GH concentration is an adequate measure of therapeutic efficacy.

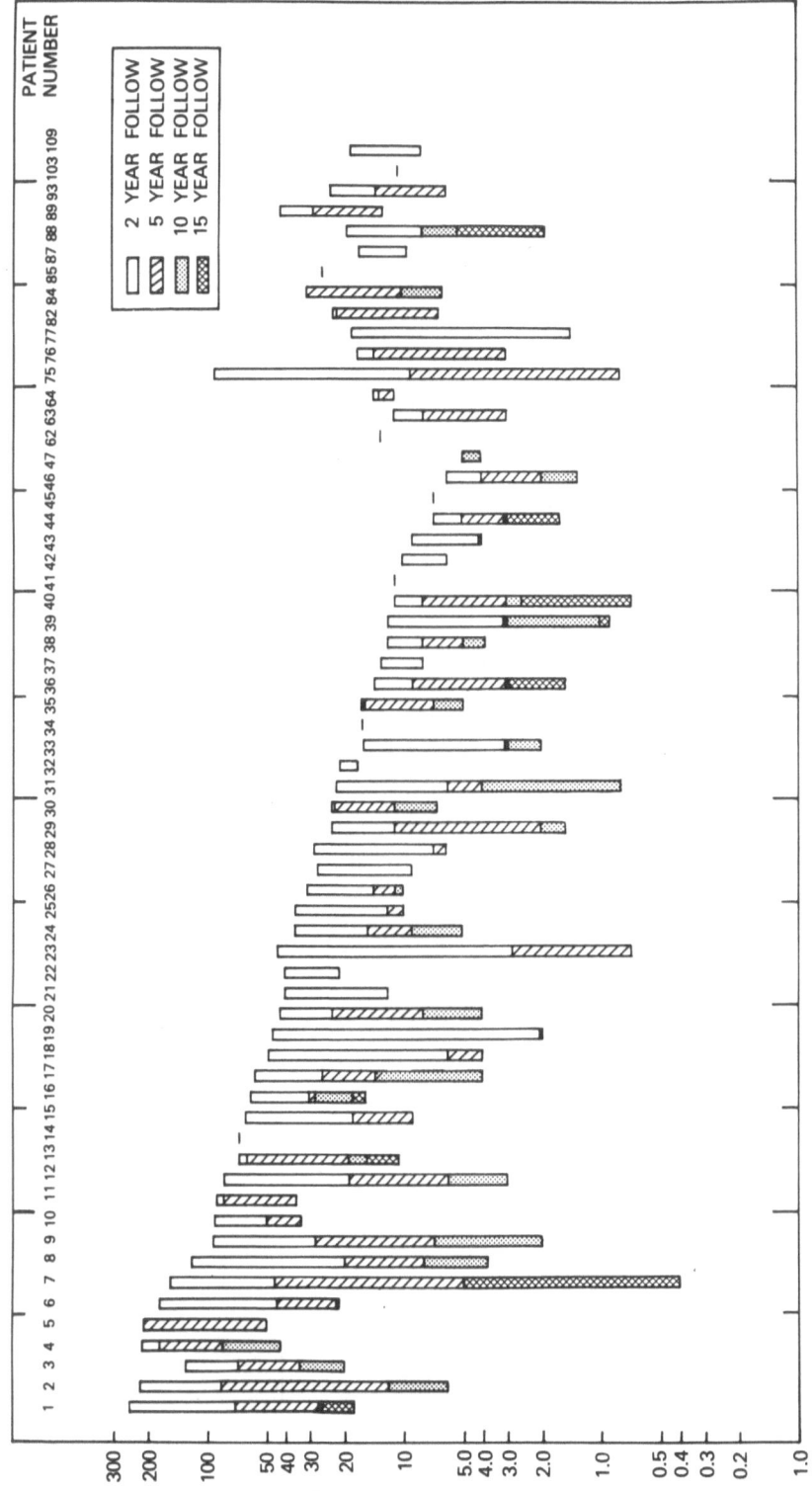

Fig. 1. Plasma growth hormone values of 62 acromegalic patients followed from 2 to 15 years following megavoltage radiation to the pituitary. These patients were untreated prior to irradiation therapy. The top of each bar represents the mean of 3 or more GH values of bloods collected in the morning from fasted inpatients. The different bar designations represent the mean GH at different follow-up times after radiation as shown in the key. Numbers 1-47 represent previously reported patients that are now updated (see Figure 1 of reference 1). The remaining patients are more recently treated.

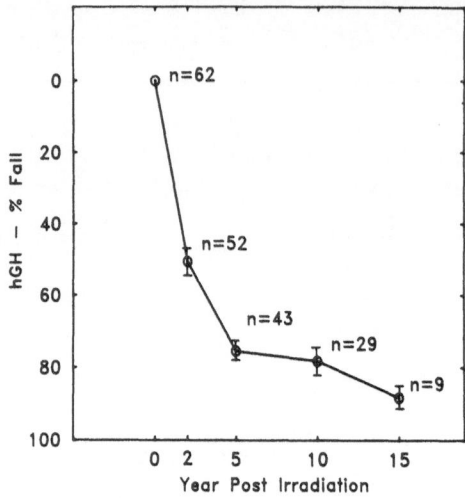

Fig. 2. Mean percent fall in GH plotted as a function of time following radiation therapy. These are the mean data from individual patients shown in Figure 1. N = number of patients followed at each time period.

Results of Pituitary Irradiation in Patients Previously Treated by Surgery

Sixteen patients treated by pituitary surgery, but who continued to have persistent elevation of plasma GH, were further treated by pituitary irradiation (Fig. 4). In the 12 patients who have been followed for 2 years or longer, the response to irradiation was similar to the group which received irradiation only. Thus, at 2 years following irradiation therapy, there was a mean decrease in GH = 65% (n=12) and at 5 years or more a mean percent decrease in GH = 85% (n=7).

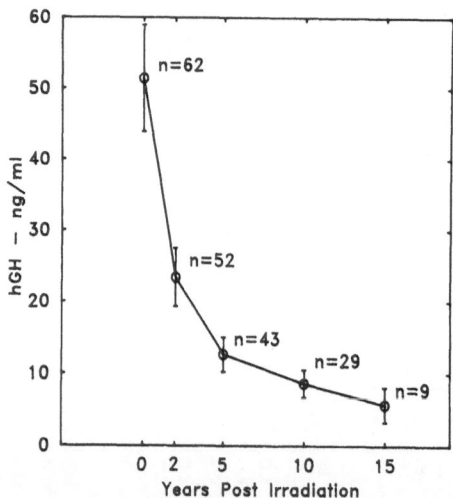

Fig. 3. Mean GH concentration plotted as a function of time following irradiation therapy. Same patients as Figures 1 and 2.

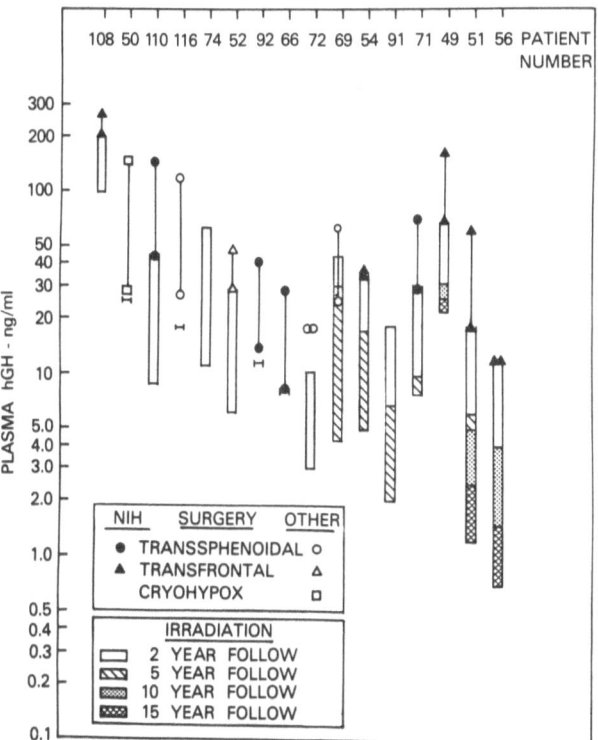

Fig. 4. GH values of patients previously
treated by surgery. Form of surgery and
whether surgery was performed at the NIH is
shown by symbol in the key. The bar designation is exactly as shown in Figure 1 and the
key above. When no bar is shown, no follow-up
data are yet available.

Clinical Response to Irradiation Therapy

If acromegaly is present for a significant period prior to therapy,
many features of the disease are not reversible. Changes in skeletal
features are difficult to document objectively, but as best we can determine, they remain stable or are moderately improved in our patients.

None of the patients developed clinical signs or symptoms of extrasellar extension after irradiation. It is also important to note that
none of the 78 patients reported here (i.e., 62 treated by irradiation
alone and 16 treated by surgery + irradiation) required any further
therapy for tumor growth. In approximately 75% of patients with headaches
prior to therapy, there was symptomatic improvement; but in about 10% of
patients without headaches prior to treatment, headaches developed. After
treatment there is a significant decrease in serum phosphorus and in both
basal glucose values and in glucose values after glucose administration.
(For a more complete description of clinical features, see reference 1.)

Untoward Effects of Radiation

One patient who had received 5000 rads in 5 weeks developed a visual
field defect 3 months after radiation; this defect cleared spontaneously
after one week and there was no further occurrence. The only permanent

complication in the 78 treated patients occurred 15 years ago in a patient with pulmonary, cutaneous, and uveal sarcoidosis. Because this patient required steroid therapy, she received 5600 rads in 6 weeks. Eighteen months after radiation she developed constitutional symptoms, which were thought to represent an exacerbation of her sarcoidosis, and she received prednisone, 80 mg per day. Over the subsequent year she developed progressively severe dementia and visual field loss associated with retinal lesions characteristic of uveal sarcoidosis. Pneumoencephalography revealed an empty sella, and fundus examination showed bilateral optic atrophy. CAT scans were unavailable at that time. However, radioisotope brain scanning was normal and CSF protein was 52 mg%. Though we have no clear explanation of her problem, we cannot exclude that this is a complication of radiation therapy and, since then, we have never delivered greater than 5000 rads over 5-6 weeks. Thus, over the past 15 years we have had no detectable complication of irradiation therapy.

Effect of Irradiation Therapy on Other Pituitary Hormones

With respect to pituitary dysfunction after treatment, there is a progressively increased incidence of hypopituitarism. By 10 years after therapy, approximately 19% of patients are hypothyroid, 38% hypoadrenal, and up to 50% hypogonadal. These figures include those patients with hypopituitarism prior to treatment as well as those who acquired hypopituitarism as a function of time after therapy. Therefore, these figures include both the effect of the natural history of the pituitary tumor as well as the possible additive effect of irradiation on the induction of pituitary insufficiency (1).

An additional endocrinologic feature of acromegaly is that about one-third of patients have elevations of serum prolactin concentration. In our experience, GH has a prolactin-like biologic potency equivalent to prolactin; therefore, we can assume that the sum of prolactin + GH = total prolactin activity. Under these circumstances the total prolactin-like activity of plasma is elevated in the majority of acromegalic patients. Thus, apparent hypogonadotropic hypogonadism can result from destruction of gonadotropin-producing cells or from inhibition of gonadotropin secretion secondary to elevation of total prolactin activity. After pituitary irradiation, serum prolactin concentration tends to fall in those patients in whom it was initially elevated and to rise modestly over the first 2 years following therapy in those patients in whom it was normal or low (6).

THERAPEUTIC CHOICES

Situations in Which the Pituitary Tumor is Dominant

In patients with visual impairment or other manifestations of extrasellar extension of the tumor, therapeutic decisions must be made in collaboration with a neurosurgeon. The unique combination of clinical, endocrinologic and anatomic features of each patient should be considered. Usually surgery, and in some instances surgery plus irradiation, is required.

Situations in Which the Elevated Concentration of GH is Dominant

These patients can be classified into at least two groups. First are patients in whom it is necessary to reduce the GH concentration rapidly. This includes patients with congestive heart failure. While the relationship of acromegaly to the pathogenesis of a specific cardiomyopathy is uncertain, it is clear that in patients with acromegaly and coexistent heart disease, regardless of cause, the prognosis is generally poor. Thus, management of coexistent heart disease, and possibly of severe hypertension, is facilitated by successful treatment of acromegaly. Patients requiring similar considerations are those with arthritis and joint fixation. This is relatively common in acromegaly, and it is not clear whether, once the arthritic process is established, treatment of the acromegaly ameliorates the arthritis. In some patients there may be urgency because of the severity of symptoms, e.g., sweating, loss of stamina, renal stones and hypercalcinuria. In instances in which it is necessary to decrease GH concentration rapidly, transsphenoidal microsurgery is the treatment of choice. If it is not curative, irradiation should follow.

In the second group, the typical acromegalic patient is one who is middle-aged, has had the disease for 10 years or longer at the time of diagnosis, and is only moderately symptomatic. At present, therapeutic choices for this type of patient are made by regional preference and expertise. There is no available information to tell us whether one therapy or another is more beneficial with respect to longevity; we cannot even be certain whether rapid reduction in GH is beneficial with respect to morbidity. The therapeutic dilemma is that those patients who will respond completely and/or rapidly to either irradiation or surgery cannot be predicted in advance. Conventional supervoltage irradiation produces a consistent, but slow, reduction in GH; this is independent of the size of the pituitary tumor or its bone-erosive or invasive properties. In most instances following irradiation, pituitary tumor growth is stabilized, and within 5 to 10 years the growth hormone concentrations return to normal in about 75% of patients (7-10). Patients with large pituitary tumors and a high GH concentration (i.e., 50 ng/ml or greater) are unlikely to achieve a normal growth hormone concentration following surgery alone. There is less morbidity with irradiation than with surgery for pituitary macroadenomas.

In summary, there are two clear options for therapy. Decisions must be made on an individual basis. If one elects surgery, then irradiation can be used if surgery is not successful. The decision can also be for irradiation first and surgical intervention at a later date, if necessary. At present, medical management with bromocriptine or long-acting somatostatin therapy should be used only for those patients in whom irradiation, surgery, or both has been unsuccessful. In selected cases these agents may be used as an adjunct to irradiation to achieve a more rapid reduction in GH. The patient should be monitored closely, however, and the drug therapy discontinued if its efficacy cannot be shown by reduction in plasma GH concentration.

REFERENCES

1. Eastman RC, Gorden P, Roth J. Conventional supervoltage irradiation is an effective treatment for acromegaly. J Clin Endocrinol Metab 1979; 48:931.
2. Roth J, Gorden P, Brace K. Efficacy of conventional pituitary irradiation in acromegaly. N Engl J Med 1970; 282:1385.
3. Gorden P, Roth J. The treatment of acromegaly by conventional pituitary irradiation. In: Kohler PO, Ross GT, eds. Diagnosis and treatment of pituitary tumors. New York: American Elsevier Pub Co, 1973:230.
4. Dons RF, Rieth KG, Gorden P, Roth J. Size and erosive features of the sella turcica in acromegaly as predictors of therapeutic response to supervoltage irradiation. Am J Med 1983; 74:69.
5. Gorden P, Glatstein E, Roth J. Acromegaly. In: Krieger DT, Bardin

CW, eds. Current therapy in endocrinology 1983–1984. St. Louis: CV Mosby, 1983:43.

6. DePablo F, Eastman RC, Roth J, Gorden P. Plasma prolactin in acromegaly before and after treatment. J Clin Endocrinol Metab 1981; 53:344.

7. Bloom B, Kramer S. Conventional radiation therapy in the management of acromegaly. In: Black P McL, Zervas NT, Ridgeway EC, Martin JB, eds. Secretory tumors of the pituitary gland. (Progress in endocrine research, vol 1.) New York: Raven Press, 1984:179.

8. Sheline GE, Wara WM. Radiation therapy of acromegaly and nonsecretory chromophobe adenomas of the pituitary. In: Seydel HG, ed. Tumors of the nervous system. New York: Wiley, 1975:117.

9. Lawrence AM, Pinsky SM, Goldfine ID. Conventional radiation therapy in acromegaly. Arch Intern Med 1971; 128:369.

10. Feek CM, McLelland J, Seth J, et al. How effective is external pituitary irradiation for growth hormone-secreting pituitary tumours? Clin Endocrinol (Oxf) 1984; 20:401.

21

LONG-TERM EFFECTS OF PROTON BEAM THERAPY FOR ACROMEGALY

Bernard Kliman, M.D., Raymond N. Kjellberg, M.D.,
Billie Swisher, R.N., and William Butler

Medical and Neurosurgical Services, Massachusetts
General Hospital, Boston, Massachusetts 02114

INTRODUCTION

The first heavy particle treatment program for patients with acromegaly was developed at the Berkeley Cyclotron by Dr. John H. Lawrence and his associates who used alpha particles in a fractionated dose schedule (1). Starting 25 years ago, Dr. Raymond N. Kjellberg proposed a single dose approach by utilizing the Bragg peak of the proton beam at the Harvard Cyclotron (2). The success of this program is indicated by the achievement of a treatment group which now numbers 562 acromegaly patients, the largest group treated by a single therapist with a single modality. The need for lifetime patient follow-up was anticipated in order to assess the benefits and risks of proton beam therapy in the long term. The assistance of referring physicians, the patients themselves and a computer-generated inquiry schedule has provided data on 435 patients followed for one to 20 years after initial treatment. The major findings have been reported elsewhere (3) and are now supplemented by new evaluations of the rate of incidence and nature of hypopituitarism, an analysis of proton dosage and changes in anterior pituitary function and the probability of a favorable outcome in relation to tumor size and treatment dose. These assessments provide a unique capability for prediction of the future clinical course and the prospects for retained pituitary function. The almost complete absence of relapse after achievement of a normal fasting growth hormone (GH) level, 5 ng/ml or less, distinguishes proton beam therapy from open surgical methods and approaches the goal of lifetime effectiveness in the treatment of acromegaly. Since no medical therapy has yet emerged for convenient long-term treatment, the Bragg peak method is a major resource for the treatment of newly diagnosed patients and for patients who have failed to obtain a cure by surgical means. Proton beam therapy deserves consideration when choices of treatment are being selected. The ability to provide a therapy with no mortality and minimal morbidity is a modern advance in the care of patients with active acromegaly.

PATIENT ASSESSMENT

The typical patient with acromegaly is recognized after the insidious development of physical changes described as acral overgrowth. At the stage of recognition, the rate of progression of the disease is determined retrospectively and may not follow a predictable course. Other cases are detected after medical complications lead to diagnostic studies. In two unusual cases in our series, the presence of known acromegaly in a family member led to early examination and diagnosis of the disease. Exceptional cases with a history of abnormal growth are found to be in a remission when first examined, presumably due to spontaneous necrosis of the pituitary tumor. Our own experience consists of three such cases and includes one with mild residual acromegaly, a large 3 cm diameter tumor mass with a large central defect shown by cisternography and elevated serum prolactin. Accordingly, an initial clinical diagnosis of acromegaly is almost invariably proved to be active and will merit consideration for treatment. One study has revealed progression of the disease in untreated cases (4). The reduced longevity of acromegaly patients prior to modern means of therapy provides another indication for prophylactic treatment as opposed to expectant observation for signs of progression (5).

Activity of acromegaly is currently defined as the presence of GH levels which are unresponsive to normal control mechanisms. Since GH is subject to normal physiologic stimuli such as exercise, especially in women (6), and after ingestion of food, the assay of a "basal" sample, fasting and at rest for one or more hours, is compatible with active disease when the level exceeds 5 ng/ml. Confirmation of elevated GH requires a suppression test with oral glucose in which normal subjects have GH levels at or below 2 ng/ml within 1 to 2 hours. The glucose values also provide an indication of the degree of glucose intolerance as a measure of one of the clinical manifestations of acromegaly. In recent years, it has been established that active acromegaly is associated with elevation of plasma unbound somatomedin-C concentration (7). The somatomedin-C (SM-C) level is not altered by exercise or glucose and is lowered rather than increased by estrogen (8). We found this test to be convenient for follow-up of ambulatory outpatients, as a means of confirmation of activity in cases with borderline GH levels, and as a better correlate to clinical changes than the fasting or postglucose GH values (7).

The severity of acromegaly is difficult to define in quantitative terms because of the complex interaction of the duration of the disease, the absolute levels of GH and SM-C and the variables of host response. Each of these factors can be assessed for individual patients in comparison to pretreatment test results and clinical assessments. It is also possible to compare laboratory and clinical findings in groups of patients provided that a large population sample is studied. In this respect, the longitudinal study of proton beam treated patients affords an opportunity to make valid group comparisons at varying time intervals after initial therapy.

GOALS OF PROTON BEAM THERAPY

The purpose of proton beam therapy of acromegaly is to obtain the greatest possible degree of improvement with the least possible risks and complications. The actual goals for individual patients are defined in terms of the existing disease process and the presence of adverse factors such as large tumor size or established complications of osteoarthritis, hypertension, diabetes mellitus or hypopituitarism. It has also become evident that remodeling of bone is not observed with any form of treatment in current use. Nevertheless, surgical correction of skeletal or superficial deformities becomes possible when the disease process is arrested. Correction of prognathism by oral surgery has been attempted in advanced cases. Sleep apnea due to voluminous nasopharyngeal tissues is also amenable to surgical repair. In most cases, carpal tunnel syndrome subsides without surgical intervention.

The management of the medical complications is often simplified as GH levels decrease, except for hypopituitarism which is usually permanent. Hypogonadism alone in either sex may improve if coexistent hyperprolactinemia is the cause of gonadotropin deficiency and responds to the treatment provided for acromegaly. In a unique case in this series, one patient also had ACTH-dependent Cushing's disease which resolved in advance of the remission of acromegaly. Associated disorders of the MEN-I (multiple endocrine neoplasia Type I) syndrome, do not improve with cure of the acromegaly and require specific therapy, most commonly surgical parathyroidectomy for primary hyperparathyroidism. Although difficult to assess, the patient with active disease is subject to psychological disorders involving a change in body image or concerns about disease complications and expectations for cure. Three of our cases developed apoplexy-like signs and symptoms: fever, nuchal rigidity, headache, prostration and a dramatic fall in GH and other pituitary hormones within 48 hours after proton beam therapy. The symptoms resolved rapidly with high dose steroid therapy. This type of response is unexpected and is attributed to central necrosis and hemorrhagic infarction of tumor.

Although we have accepted several patients with prior X-ray therapy of less than 4000 rads given at 180 rads per day, the limitations of a supplemental proton beam dose and the risks of side effects make such patients unsuitable candidates. In general, we now avoid using heavy particle therapy after X-ray has been given.

METHOD OF TREATMENT

The initial evaluation of a prospective candidate for proton beam therapy is based on review of medical records and a recent CAT scan. Patients with more than 2 mm of suprasellar extension or with parasellar extension are normally excluded at this stage. Evidence of tumor activity is confirmed by GH and SM-C levels, results of glucose suppression tests or abnormal GH release with TRH. Patients with other medical disabilities can usually be treated. For example, one young patient was receiving dialysis treatments while awaiting a renal transplant. Angina pectoris in several patients did not interfere with treatment or preparative testing. Advanced age is not a limitation unless major mental or physical disabilities are present which would not be corrected by remission of acromegaly. Potential problems are discussed with the referring physician prior to scheduling patients for hospital admission. No patient has died during or soon after therapy.

The first stage of treatment consists of an in-hospital evaluation. Endocrine studies are obtained as a pretreatment baseline and include fasting GH levels, SM-C, FBS, calcium, phosphorus, alkaline phosphatase, 8 a.m. cortisol, thyroxine, T3 resin uptake, free T4 index, total T3, TSH, prolactin, FSH, LH, and plasma testosterone or estradiol. A TRH test is performed for TSH and prolactin response, or for prolactin alone if the patient is taking thyroid hormone replacement. A one-hour Cortrosyn test is combined with TRH testing. Overnight metyrapone tests are performed with a midnight dose of 2.5 to 3.0 grams taken with milk or antacid and followed by 8 a.m. 11-deoxy-cortisol and cortisol assays. Neuroophthalmologic consultation includes visual fields, visual acuity, and a general eye examination. Radiographic procedures are required to define the treatment target zone, to accurately measure the dimensions of intrasellar contents and to localize adjacent anatomic structures. A contrast-enhanced CAT scan is obtained with axial sections which are processed to multiplanar reconstructions in sagittal and coronal planes. Tumor enhancement, effects of prior surgery if present, and the path of the cavernous sinus vessels are noted. Marker skull films are prepared by means of headbands containing lead spheres of known diameter which will provide magnification factors for the films made during cisternography with a hyperbaric, water-soluble contrast medium such as metrizamide or iopamidol. This procedure is performed by a neurologist member of the team to assure constant technique. Phenobarbital is given before and immediately after instillation of contrast into the spinal fluid as prophylaxis against seizures. Analgesic or antiemetic agents may be needed within the first few hours after the study while on a mandatory 8-hour bedrest schedule. No complications have been experienced except for uncommon spinal headache which responds well to rest, fluids and pain medication. The cisternogram consists of sella polytomes and a subsequent CAT scan of the contrast shown in the cerebrospinal fluid. With this method, the location of each optic nerve is determined and used to guide the placement of the beam field. The third radiographic procedure is a digital subtraction angiogram performed by venous catheterization of an antecubital or femoral vein. The cavernous portions of both internal carotid arteries are visualized and the intercavernous distance is measured to define the degree to which opposed beam portals will be overlapped within the sella. A treatment plan is developed to provide a customized pattern for each patient.

It has been customary to treat patients in-hospital; however, some insurers have requested outpatient care whenever possible. If otherwise well, the patient can be discharged to the local area and will return for final instructions and informed consent on the day prior to treatment, proton therapy the next day, and a postoperative visit on the day after treatment. This option has been successful in reducing hospital days to 4 instead of 7 with expected savings of about $1,000 for the insurer, and the cost of treatment has remained below that required for transsphenoidal surgery.

On the treatment day, each patient is transported to the Cyclotron where stereotactic fixation is done using local anesthesia and the proton beam therapy is performed in a single visit lasting about 90 minutes. Patients are ambulatory after the procedure and return the next morning for examination of the four stereotactic fixation sites which are protected by Band-Aids and to inspect the ear canals and eardrums since the halo headframe is temporarily positioned using blunt rods within the external ear canals. Cerumen impaction is removed if present, and the patient is instructed to apply cortisporin ear drops for two days after treatment. It is usual to plan a return to full-time activities immediately afterwards. The schedule for follow-up with their attending physicians is discussed and consists at minimum of 6 monthly visits in the first year, then annually. A computerized mailing program is used to confirm follow-up.

RESULTS OF TREATMENT WITH BRAGG PEAK PROTON BEAM THERAPY

The follow-up of 435 patients one to 20 years after proton beam therapy has been analyzed and was reported at the first international conference on the therapy of pituitary tumors (3). Growth hormone fell progressively to 10 ng/ml or less in 97.5%, and to 5 ng/ml or less in 87.5% of patients who received no subsequent surgery or radiotherapy. Results were similar when all cases were considered (Table 1). The median fall in GH was 80% from baseline in the first 24 months. Clinical improvement was frequently correlated with a favorable decrease in GH levels to 10 ng/ml or less. (Only one case experienced recurrence of activity of acromegaly after an initial GH fall to below 5 ng/ml.) For comparison to transsphenoidal surgery, Laws et al. (9) reported an 82% normalization of basal GH to less than 5 ng/ml in 17 acromegaly patients with microadenomas and 54% in 75 patients with macroadenomas. Ten of the patients with macroadenomas received postoperative radiation therapy. Five of the remaining 65 patients had recurrence of acromegaly within 18 to 36 months after achieving a postoperative GH of 5 ng or less, a 7.7% recurrence rate in three years, or an annualized recurrence rate of 2.6% per year.

SIDE EFFECTS OF TREATMENT

There is rarely any immediate morbidity associated with proton beam therapy and only 3 patients have experienced a course consistent with early apoplexy leading to rapid onset of hypopituitarism including cure of the tumor. Within the first year, a small percentage of cases, 1.74% or 8 cases, experienced diplopia which was transient in 6 cases and episodic over a longer interval (4 to 10 years) in only 2 cases. An additional 8 cases (1.74%) experienced partial visual impairment of which 2 lost vision in both eyes. This type of complication appears to have been eliminated by the advent of modern radiological preparation and by exclusion of patients with more than a total of 4000 rads of X-ray or a greater than 180 rads per day X-ray dosage schedule. A mortality rate of 11.7% observed during follow-up was analyzed and found to be unrelated to treatment except for one case of sarcoma without prior X-ray therapy and one case of sarcoma with prior X-ray therapy. This compares favorably to the rate seen after conventional radiation alone (10).

Hypopituitarism is a major complication of surgery, conventional X-ray, or proton beam therapy. In this proton beam treated group, thyroid, adrenal, or gonadal deficiencies developed in 9.7%, 9.0% and 6.7%, respectively. These changes are considerably less than those reported by two groups utilizing conventional radiotherapy (11,12) as compared in Table 2. Replacement therapy is sufficient to resolve symptoms and gonadotropin therapy has been used to restore fertility in some patients. Laws et al. (13) reported a need for pituitary hormone replacement in 5 of 133 acromegaly patients after transsphenoidal surgery, a rate of 3.8%. Wilson found that 5% of 102 patients developed partial hypopituitarism after transsphenoidal surgery when no postoperative radiotherapy was provided (14). The relative preservation of pituitary function afforded by proton beam therapy is attributed to a low dosimetry, 100-500 rads, in the zone

Table 1. Life table analysis of 435 cases of acromegaly followed for 1 to 20 years after proton beam therapy.

Time (years)	All cases	No other therapy
GH = 10 ng/ml or less		
2	47.5%	47.5%
5	68.6	70.0
10	87.5	90.0
20	97.5	97.5
GH = 5 ng/ml or less		
2	27.5%	30.0%
5	56.2	49.6
10	75.0	77.5
20	92.5	87.5

of the hypothalamus and the ability of a pituitary remnant to respond to hypothalamic releasing factors.

The onset of anterior pituitary hormone deficiencies was detected between one day to 9.3 years after proton beam therapy. The median time of appearance of function loss was 2.8 years, and 90.2% of these cases were noted within the first 5 years. Diabetes insipidus was exceptional in 2 cases, one of whom required treatment with antidiuretic hormone preparations prior to eventual return of normal serum and urine osmolality off treatment. The second such case has recently been observed to have a partial impairment of urine concentrating ability and has not required medication. Both patients had a partially empty sella by CAT scan. Since the anterior supraoptic nuclei receive a comparatively small dosage of under 500 rads, a mechanical process involving the pituitary stalk may explain this finding.

To date, we are aware of only 3 cases of temporal lobe seizures after proton beam therapy, a lower frequency than has been noted in untreated acromegaly (15). The low proton beam dosimetry outside the sella turcica should serve to avoid this possible complication.

CURRENT AND FUTURE DEVELOPMENT OF TREATMENT

An analysis of probability of achieving a curative level of growth hormone and probability of experiencing loss of anterior pituitary hormones has been applied to the data base of this treatment program. The individual doses were compared to the beam diameter and to development of hypopituitarism. In our experience, there is an association between higher dosage and an inverse correlation to beam portal diameters in relation to remission rate. Pituitary function loss could also be related to the treatment dose. Optimal therapy is related to maximum cure rate and minimum incidence of pituitary hormone deficiency. These factors may ultimately be used to optimize selection of dosage and beam portal sizes.

The early recognition and diagnosis of active acromegaly has potential for the improvement of treatment outcome. Somatomedin-C assay appears to be useful for this purpose and has provided an early warning in

Table 2. Risk of new pituitary hormone deficiencies following proton beam or conventional X-ray therapy for acromegaly.

Reference	Method	Dose	Cases	Years	Thyroid	Adrenal	Gonadal
Kliman, Kjellberg et al., 1984	Proton beam	10-12 Krads	435	2-20	9.7%	9.0%	6.7%
Eastman, Gordon, Roth, 1979	X-ray	4.0-5.6 Krads	47	10	10%	32%	39%
Feek et al., 1984	X-ray	3.8 Krads	36	10	16%	30%	47%

two familial and two random cases (16). The waiting period for diagnosis would have been reduced if we had relied on the SM-C value as the basis for a treatment plan. Follow-up is convenient with this test since it does not require fasting, rest or oral glucose suppression to collect blood for analysis.

The ability to reduce hospitalization time and costs has only recently been possible because of the acceptance by insurance carriers of an outpatient approach to the treatment procedure. Further efficiency may be achieved by expected developments in magnetic resonance imaging to reduce the need for multiple contrast procedures which include a CAT scan, a cisternogram and a digital subtraction angiogram. The new technology will need to demonstrate the paths of the optic nerves, tumor location and exact dimensions of the intrasellar lesion.

HISTORICAL PERSPECTIVE AND CONCLUSIONS

Heavy particle therapy for acromegaly has undergone an evolution during the past 25 years. Alpha particle therapy was introduced at the Berkeley Cyclotron, required multiple treatments and the Bragg peak was not utilized. The development of a stereotactic method allowed the use of the desirable features of the Bragg peak of the proton beam at the Harvard Cyclotron. Cumulative experience has shown that favorable long-term benefits are achieved with few disadvantages and a low rate of hypopituitarism. Since many patients receive initial transsphenoidal surgery, it is important to note that residual or recurrent tumor can be treated effectively with the proton beam. Removal of suprasellar extension by open surgery prepares the patient for proton beam therapy. Macroadenomas without suprasellar or parasellar extension allow the option of initial treatment with proton beam which facilitates avoidance of secondary treatment should failure or recurrence occur after open surgery. We conclude that Bragg peak proton beam therapy is an established and effective method for selected patients with active acromegaly.

ACKNOWLEDGMENTS

The clinical investigation of selected patients was carried out under the auspices of the Clinical Research Center, Massachusetts General Hospital, with the assistance of grant No. MO1-RR01066 from the U.S. Department of Health and Human Services. Computer services were rendered by the Harvard School of Public Health under the supervision of Raymond Neff, Ph.D., and Elizabeth Allred, who contributed to the design of the data processing and statistical programs. The research analyst services of Vicky Martin and Judith Priestley are greatly appreciated.

REFERENCES

1. Lawrence JH, Tobias CA, Linfoot JA. Successful treatment of acromegaly: metabolic and clinical studies in 145 patients. J Clin Endocrinol Metab 1970; 31:180.
2. Kjellberg RN, Shintani A, Frantz AG, Kliman B. Proton beam therapy in acromegaly. N Engl J Med 1968; 278:689.
3. Kliman B, Kjellberg RN, Swisher B, Butler W. Proton beam therapy of acromegaly: a 20 year experience. In: Black PMcL, et al., eds. Secretory tumors of the pituitary gland. New York: Raven Press, 1984.
4. Roth J, Gorden P, Brace K. Efficacy of conventional pituitary irradiation in acromegaly. N Engl J Med 1970; 282:1385.

5. Wright AD, Hill DM, Lowy C, Fraser TR. Mortality in acromegaly. Q J Med 1970; 39:1.
6. Frantz AG, Rabkin MT. Effects of estrogen and sex difference on secretion of human growth hormone. J Clin Endocrinol Metab 1965; 25:1470.
7. Clemmons DR, Van Wyk JJ, Ridgway EC, Kliman B, Kjellberg RN, Underwood LE. Evaluation of acromegaly by radioimmunoassay of somatomedin-C. N Engl J Med 1979; 301:1138.
8. Clemmons DR, Underwood LE, Ridgway EC, Kliman B, Kjellberg RN, Van Wyk JJ. Estradiol treatment of acromegaly: reduction of immunoreactive somatomedin-C and improvement in metabolic status. Am J Med 1980; 69:571.
9. Laws ER Jr, Scheithauer BW, Carpenter S, Randall RV, Abboud CF. The pathogenesis of acromegaly. J Neurosurg 1985; 63:35.
10. Waltz TA, Brownell B. Sarcoma: a possible late result of effective radiation therapy for pituitary adenoma. J Neurosurg 1966; 24:901.
11. Eastman RC, Gorden P, Roth J. Conventional super-voltage is an effective treatment for acromegaly. J Clin Endocrinol Metab 1979; 48:931.
12. Feek CM, McLelland J, Seth J, et al. How effective is external pituitary irradiation for growth hormone-secreting pituitary tumors? Clin Endocrinol (Oxf) 1984; 20:401.
13. Laws ER Jr, Randall RV, Abboud CF. Surgical treatment of acromegaly: results in 140 patients. In: Givens JR, ed. Hormone-secreting pituitary tumors. Chicago: Year Book Medical Publishers, 1982: 225-8.
14. Wilson CB. A decade of pituitary microsurgery. J Neurosurg 1984; 61:814.
15. Davidoff LM. Studies in acromegaly. III. the anamnesis and symptomatology in one hundred cases. Endocrinology 1926; 10:461.
16. Kliman B, MacLaughlin RA, Kjellberg RN. Somatomedin-C radioimmunoassay for early detection of active acromegaly. Baltimore: Program of the 67th annual meeting of the Endocrine Society, 1985.

22

RESULTS OF TRANSSPHENOIDAL RESECTION OF GROWTH HORMONE-SECRETING PITUITARY ADENOMAS

Donald A. Ross, M.D., and Charles B. Wilson, M.D.

Department of Neurological Surgery, School of Medicine
University of California, San Francisco
San Francisco, California

INTRODUCTION

There is still controversy regarding which of the therapeutic modalities available for the management of growth hormone-secreting pituitary adenomas is safest and most effective (1-5). With a view toward resolving aspects of the question, we summarize the results of a long-term follow-up review of a large series of patients managed by transsphenoidal microsurgical resection, providing data for comparison with other surgical series and with the documented results of irradiation (6-12) and medical therapies (12-15).

CLINICAL MATERIAL AND METHODS

From 1970 to 1984, 221 patients with acromegaly were seen at our institution, of whom 214 underwent transsphenoidal microsurgical resection of a pituitary adenoma (16). Historical, neurologic, endocrine, radiographic, operative, and pathologic data were gathered from the patients medical records. After these data were correlated, the adenomas were classified by amount of sellar destruction (grade) and suprasellar extension (stage) according to a system described elsewhere (17-20). Each procedure was tailored to the size, shape, location, and consistency of the individual tumor (3); preoperative preparations and the surgical technique have been described (17,18,20-23). The tumor's size and the extent of resection were ascertained at surgery. Alternative procedures and their indications are detailed elsewhere (24). Preoperative and postoperative endocrine evaluations were performed by the referring endocrinologist. Follow-up reviews were obtained through the patients and/or their physicians between October 1985 and February 1986.

RESULTS

The mean age of the 221 patients in the series was 41.6 years; 132 patients (59.7%) were male and 89 (40.3%), female. Nearly two-thirds of the tumors were Grade II adenomas (Table 1), and there were only 16 (13.8%) true microadenomas (<1 cm in diameter). Median tumor size was in the range of 1.6 to 2.0 cm; 78.5% of the adenomas were confined to the sella or suprasellar cisterns. Seventeen patients (8.3%) had fasting morning growth hormone (GH) levels <10 ng/ml, whereas 69 (33.8%) had levels >50 ng/ml. One patient had suffered pituitary apoplexy. Sixty-one patients (27.6%) had undergone radiation therapy, surgery, and/or medical therapy before their referral to our institution.

Results of the complete preoperative endocrinologic evaluation were available for 77 patients: 45 (58.4%) had at least one abnormal axis, gonadotropin levels being low in 37, adrenal responsiveness was inadequate in 20, and thyroid function in 15 patients. Seventeen (22%) of the 77 patients had hyperprolactinemia.

A total of 224 transsphenoidal operations were performed on 214 patients. During 221 procedures, an adenoma was found. There were 202 cases of gross total resection, but the surgeon was confident of cure in only 158 of these cases (78.2% of total resections or 70.9% overall).

Immediately postoperative fasting morning GH levels were in the records of 204 patients; 117 patients (57.4%) had levels <5 ng/ml and 160 (78.4%) had levels <10 ng/ml. Postoperative GH levels were <5 ng/ml in 62% of the patients who had had no previous therapy, but were <5 ng/ml in only 47% of those who had prior treatment (P < 0.05 by Chi square test). Only 1 patient with a postoperative GH level <10 ng/ml did not have clinical remission. Fifty-two patients were referred for postoperative radiation therapy, 40 because of persistently elevated GH levels, 10 prophylactically for invasive tumor, and 2 for recurrence of tumor.

All complications occurring perioperatively and throughout the period of follow-up were compiled. Of the 224 operations evaluated, 47 (21.0%) resulted in one or more complications (Table 2). There were no serious permanent sequelae: no deaths, persistent neurologic deficits, or permanent diabetes insipidus. Cerebrospinal fluid (CSF) leaks, occurring in 11 patients, were controlled, although two patients (of whom 1 had previously been operated on elsewhere and the other had undergone preoperative irradiation) required a craniotomy to correct the leak. Among the more serious surgical complications, 4 of 5 CSF leaks requiring surgical repair, 4 of 6 simple CSF leaks, and 1 of 4 cases of meningitis occurred in previously treated patients.

Long-Term Follow-Up Review

Follow-up review ranging from 12 to 157 months (mean, 76 months) was obtained for 174 patients, none of whom at that time had clinically active acromegaly; some of these patients, however, continued to be hypertensive

Table 1. Grade and stage of adenomas in 224 transsphenoidal operations.*

Tumor grade	Number of patients (%)		Tumor stage	Number of patients (%)	
I	19	(8.7)	0	110	(50.5)
II	131	(60.1)	A	61	(28.0)
III	37	(17.0)	B	9	(4.1)
IV	31	(14.2)	C	10	(4.6)
			D	2	(0.9)
			E	26	(11.9)

*No tumor found in 3 cases; in 3 others, data not known.

Table 2. Postoperative complications.

Complication	Number of patients (%)[a]	Complication	Number of patients
Death/stroke	0	Negative exploration	3
CSF leak requiring surgical repair	5 (2.2)	Carotid injury	2
		Operative hemorrhage	3
CSF leak responding to simple measures	6	Medical illness[b]	13
		Minor oronasal	17
Meningitis	4 (1.8)	Graft site	2[c]
Cranial nerve palsy	3		

CSF = cerebrospinal fluid.
[a] Percentages facilitate comparison with other published data.
[b] Chest pain, gastrointestinal hemorrhage, hyponatremia, pneumonia.
[c] One an infection, the other a hematoma.

or to suffer from progressive osteoarthritis. Of the 165 patients for whom most recent morning fasting GH levels were available, 131 (79.1%) had levels <5 ng/ml and 153 (92.7%), <10 ng/ml. Nine other patients had been in clinical remission for a mean period of 69 months but had not had recent GH determinations. There was no difference in long-term outcome between previously treated and primarily operated patients, with 7.3% of either group having most recent GH levels >10 ng/ml, and 80% having levels <5 ng/ml.

Follow-up evaluations were obtained for 44 of the 52 patients who had postoperative radiation therapy. Thirty of these had postoperative GH levels >5 ng/ml, of whom 21 (70.0%) now have levels <5 ng/ml and 24 (80%) have levels <10 ng/ml. The 10 patients irradiated prophylactically continue to be in remission. Two patients irradiated for recurrent tumor presently have GH levels <5 ng/ml. Two of these 44 patients (4.5%) suffered serious complications of irradiation; 1 developed radiation necrosis of the temporal lobes and the other suffered progressive visual loss. Panhypopituitarism had developed in 23 of 42 (54.8%) of the irradiated patients, whereas 8 (19.0%) were still eupituitary an average of 44 months after the completion of radiation therapy.

Five patients (2.3%) were considered therapeutic failures because their GH levels remain >10 ng/ml despite surgery, irradiation, and bromocriptine therapy. All had preoperative GH levels >100 ng/ml and tumors >15 mm in diameter that produced sellar destruction. All have shown a slow, steady decline in their GH levels since completing radiation therapy from 1 to 6 years earlier.

Nine patients underwent a second transsphenoidal procedure because they had persistently or recurrently elevated GH values; one of these required a third exploration. Residual tumor was resected in 7 cases. Postoperative GH levels were <5 ng/ml in 3 of these 7 patients; 2 have required no additional therapy, and 5 underwent radiation therapy. In 3 cases, no tumor was found: in 1, an error in GH determinations performed at a referring institution was the basis for an unnecessary reexploration; in another, an intracavernous tumor was detected by selective venous sampling; in the third case, the cause of the disease was not identified but the patient responded to sellar irradiation. Of the 8 patients reoperated because of verified GH elevations, 6 have most recent GH levels <5 ng/ml, and 2 (only 1 of whom had postoperative radiation therapy) have levels between 5 and 12 ng/ml.

Nine patients (4.0%) who did not undergo postoperative irradiation had a new onset of hypofunction in one or more anterior pituitary axis postoperatively. Four patients currently require thyroid replacement and 1, testosterone injections. Only 4 patients (1.9%) were rendered panhypopituitary by their operation; 1 had previously undergone a cryohypophysectomy and 2 had been irradiated. Three of the 4 had preoperative dysfunction in at least one axis, a factor linked to an increased likelihood of further dysfunction postoperatively (25). Thus, only 1 of the 107 patients who received no therapy other than surgery was rendered panhypopituitary by the operation (0.9%), and this was also the only patient who had normal function preoperatively and diminished function in more than a single axis after surgery.

Eighty-nine patients who had no therapy other than transsphenoidal surgery were available for follow-up evaluation. Only 5 (5.6%) had new anterior pituitary hypofunction postoperatively, 1 of whom had pituitary apoplexy. Only 14 of the 89 (15.7%) have any diminution in anterior pituitary function after a mean period of 69 months postoperatively.

Of the 117 patients with immediately postoperative GH levels <5 ng/ml, 5 (4.3%) had resumption of biochemical and/or clinical signs of active acromegaly after a period of time with normal GH levels. There was no pattern of characteristics among these patients predictive of a high likelihood of recurrence. One apparent recurrence resolved after a short course of bromocriptine therapy, casting doubt on its validity (13,15,26,27). One patient was apparently cured by reoperation and 2 are in remission after undergoing radiation therapy. Recurrence could not be confirmed in 1 case, as the patient has died.

Postoperative testing of GH dynamics has been advocated in assessing the adequacy of resection and the need for adjunctive irradiation (28-37). Seventy-one patients available for follow-up review underwent such tests. Of these, 36 (51%) either failed to suppress with glucose (37-40) or stimulated with thyrotropin-releasing hormone (TRH) (28,30,31,36,37,41-43); 14 of these 36 had immediately postoperative GH levels <5 ng/ml. Fifteen of the 36 patients for whom GH dynamics predicted therapeutic failure have had no clinically or biochemically evident recurrence of their disease over a mean follow-up period of 101 months, despite their having no postoperative therapy of any kind. Of the other 21 patients predicted to have therapeutic failure, 16 had radiation therapy; 15 of these had most recent fasting morning GH levels <10 ng/ml, and 1 had a level of 11.9 ng/ml. Four have had no further treatment and have levels between 5 and 10 ng/ml. One underwent sellar exenteration and, 13 years later, had a level <1 ng/ml. Of 35 patients for whom dynamic testing predicted a good outcome or was equivocal, 3 had a recurrence.

DISCUSSION

Published reports on the transsphenoidal microsurgical approach to GH-secreting adenomas include 31 series (3,30-33,35,37,39,40,44-65). The immediately postoperative GH levels in these series correspond closely with those in our own. The rate of new hypopituitarism among our patients was slightly lower than that generally reported for surgical therapy (15-20%) (3,25,62,63,66,67) and much lower than that reported for primary radiation therapy (20-65%) (6-8,68-72). The overall complication rates are difficult to compare, however, because most reports cite only the most serious complications, such as CSF leak or meningitis. Laws et al. (73), in a thorough review, detailed complications of 810 transsphenoidal procedures for all indications. The case mortality rate was 0.5%; CSF rhinorrhea occurred in 1.5%, stroke in 0.5%, meningitis in 0.3%, and permanent diabetes insipidus in 1.2% of cases. The higher overall rate in our series is accounted for by our inclusion of all complications, including the minor ones, accruing over the entire period of follow-up review. CSF rhinorrhea was more common in our patients, perhaps due to acromegalic changes in the sinuses and mucosa.

The recurrence rate in our series is only 4.3%. The cause of these recurrences may have been incomplete resection (46), but the possibility that they resulted from abnormal hypothalamic-pituitary interaction (28,74-77) or multifocal adenomas (78-80) cannot be excluded. Three of these 5 patients underwent testing of GH dynamics postoperatively. Two had normal glucose suppression tests (with serum GH levels going from 3.4 to 1.2 ng/ml and from 1.4 to 2.0 ng/ml with oral glucose loading); the third underwent TRH stimulation with a baseline value of 5.3 rising to 6.9 ng/ml.

Our results indicate that patients treated initially with transsphenoidal microsurgery fared better than those who had undergone prior therapy. This difference persisted when controls for confounding factors, such as preoperative GH level and tumor size, grade, and stage, were applied. Subgroup analysis showed that patients who had had prior surgery were the largest subgroup with poorer results among the previously treated patients, while those who had received radiation or bromocriptine therapy preoperatively suffered no loss of benefit from surgery. These findings confirm those in other series (3,19,48,66,78). This discrepancy did not persist over the course of long-term follow-up, however; only 7% of previously treated or primarily operated patients have most recent GH values that remain clearly abnormal. This convergence of outcome may be attributable to a delayed reduction in GH levels in the previously treated patients who underwent irradiation before (31 of 61) or after (21 of 61) their operation (11,81). The deleterious effects of as much as 6 additional years of excessive GH levels in some of these patients have not been documented, but the claim that such effects are negligible (1) must be viewed with caution (82).

Eight patients underwent reoperation for persistently or recurrently elevated GH levels, 3 of whom have not required radiation therapy. The potential benefit of reoperation has been debated, and several authors counsel against repeated operation (62,63). The higher complication rate for previously operated patients implies that only experienced pituitary surgeons should perform the second operation. We presently adhere to the following indications for consideration of reoperation: (1) recurrence after what was considered to a curative total resection; (2) radiologic evidence of a recurrent intrasellar mass; (3) cases in which irradiation is undesirable or contraindicated.

Several factors other than previous treatment had prognostic significance. Patients who had Grade IV tumors fared considerably worse than those with lower grade lesions (18,67); there was no significant difference in the immediate outcome for patients with tumors of Grades I through III. Patients with extrasellar extension (Stages C, D, E) were also less likely to be in remission postoperatively. Tumor size correlated only weakly with outcome, a rather surprising result (66). Outcome correlated with preoperative GH level, there being a linear decline in remission rate with respect to increasing preoperative GH level. Similar results have been reported for other series (19,26,28,32,44,45,54), but they varied in the threshold GH level used, and at least one series does not show such a correlation (30). All 6 therapeutic failures in our series were in patients with preoperative GH levels >100 ng/ml (3,18).

The surgeon's assessment of the curative potential of the operation, based on the appearance of the sella, the consistency of the tumor, and evidence of tumor invasion of bone or dura, had predictive value as well. Among the 174 patients who had long-term follow-up evaluations, the surgeon had been confident of cure in 122 cases; 94 of 115 patients (81.7%) who have recently had GH determinations performed have GH levels <5 ng/ml. Among 50 patients for whom cure was not predicted, 34 of 47 (72.3%) have GH levels <5 ng/ml. However, only 18 (14.8%) of the group for which cure was predicted underwent postoperative irradiation, whereas 25 (50%) of those in whom cure was not expected have been irradiated. This finding may be useful in evaluating patients who have had total surgical resections for subsequent radiation therapy.

We do not consider histologic signs of invasiveness useful in planning treatment (83,84). Rates of microscopic dural invasion as high as 85% have been reported for pituitary adenomas in general (83), and the presence of a true plane of dissection between adenoma and gland has been questioned (84). The presence of persistent tumor at autopsy, despite clinical and biochemical evidence of cure during life, has been reported (85). These findings are cited as a basis for the use of such topical agents as absolute alcohol or Zenker's solution (84), for the routine use of postoperative irradiation (83-85), and for total hypophysectomy (32). As our recurrence rate does not approach the incidence of disturbing histologic findings, the validity and significance of these data require further interpretation.

Precise biochemical criteria for cure or remission are difficult to define (26,28,31-37,40,86-90), and methods for doing so include GH levels, a variety of dynamic tests, measurement of the circadian rhythm of GH secretion, and determination of somatomedin levels. As more than 40% of the patients in this series who had persistently abnormal dynamic test results postoperatively have shown no sign of recurrence an average of nearly 9 years later, we cannot advocate these tests as the sole determinant of the need for adjunctive therapy (26). In evaluating the usefulness of the postoperative fasting morning GH level, we noted that, among 117 patients with levels <5 ng/ml, only 5 (4.3%) have had a recurrence. Only 10.6% of our patients with postoperative GH levels <5 ng/ml have required any additional therapy for acromegaly, whereas 21.2% of patients with levels of between 5 and 10 ng/ml and 82.4% of those with levels >10 ng/ml have required subsequent therapy. Among the 174 patients who had long-term follow-up evaluation are 89 patients for whom their operation was the only form of therapy administered; 69 of these (84.1%) have most recent GH levels <5 ng/ml, and all have levels <11 ng/ml. The recommendation that postoperative irradiation be given to all patients (84,85), or to those with persistent abnormal GH dynamics (32), must be reconsidered in the light of these findings.

It is evident that there is a group of patients who will have long-lasting remission postoperatively with no further therapy. What is needed is a method for determining which patients, among those who show clinical improvement and have postoperative GH values <10 ng/ml, will require prophylactic irradiation in order to ensure permanent arrest of their disease. This determination must be made immediately postoperatively, when the patients' tumor burden is at its minimum and when they are most likely to benefit from radiation therapy (91).

Transsphenoidal microsurgery, with adjunctive radiation therapy when indicated, offers the acromegalic patient an excellent chance for a durable remission with a high likelihood of preservation of anterior pituitary function and a low risk of permanent complications. Earlier detection of the disorder, and consequently earlier operation, would reduce the number of patients having poor prognostic factors and would contribute to an improvement in operative results. Further data are needed to assess the effects of persistently abnormal GH dynamics on longevity and of histologic signs of invasiveness on recurrence rates, but the classification of acromegaly as a "more or less intractable [disorder]" (1) would no longer seem justified.

REFERENCES

1. Christy NP. Choosing the best treatment for acromegaly. JAMA 1982; 247:1320.
2. Eastman RC, Roth J. Treatment of acromegaly [Abstract]. Syllabus of the 32nd Annual Postgraduate Assembly of the Endocrine Society. New York, October 27-31, 1980:118.
3. Hardy J, Somma M, Vezina JL. Treatment of acromegaly: radiation or surgery? In: Morley TP, ed. Current controversies in neurosurgery. Philadelphia: WB Saunders, 1976:377.
4. Nusynowitz ML. Skinning the cat. JAMA 1975; 233:1302.
5. Spark RF, Baker R, Bienfong DC, Bergland R. Bromocryptine reduces pituitary tumor size and hypersecretion. Requiem for pituitary surgery? JAMA 1982; 247:311.
6. Eastman RC, Gorden P, Roth J. Conventional supervoltage irradiation is an effective treatment for acromegaly. J Clin Endocrinol Metab 1979; 48:931.
7. Linfoot JA. Alpha particle pituitary irradiation in the primary and postsurgical management of pituitary microadenomas. In: Faglia G, Giovanelli MA, MacLeod RM, eds. Pituitary microadenomas. Proceedings of the Serono Symposia, vol 29. New York: Academic Press, 1980:515.
8. Kjellberg RN, Shintani A, Frantz AG, Kliman B. Proton-beam therapy in acromegaly. N Engl J Med 1968; 278:689.
9. Dawson DM, Dingman JF. Hazards of proton-beam pituitary irradiation (Letter). N Engl J Med 1970; 282:1434.
10. Lawrence JH. Metabolic and therapeutic studies on 246 patients with acromegaly treated with heavy particles. In: Pecile A, Muller EE, eds. Growth hormone and related peptides. Proceedings of the Third International Symposium on Growth Hormone. International Congress Series 381. New York: American Elsevier, 1976:312.
11. Lawrence AM, Pinsky SM, Goldfine ID. Conventional radiation therapy in acromegaly: a review and reassessment. Arch Intern Med 1971; 128:369.
12. Ross DA, Wilson CB. Primary therapy for acromegaly: a comparison of surgery, radiation therapy, and medical management. [Unpublished observations, 1986.]
13. Corenblum B. The medical treatment of the hypersecreting pituitary gland. Can J Neurol Sci 1985; 12:243.
14. Baskin DS, Wilson CB. Bromocriptine treatment of pituitary adenomas. Neurosurgery 1981; 8:741.
15. Liuzzi A, Chiodini PG, Cozzi R, et al. The medical treatment of acromegaly. In: Derome PJ, Jedynak CP, Peillon F, eds. Pituitary adenomas: biology, physiopathology, and treatment. Paris: Asclepios, 1980:269.
16. Ross DA, Wilson CB. Results of transsphenoidal microsurgery for growth hormone-secreting pituitary adenoma in a series of 214 patients. [Unpublished observations, 1986.]
17. Hardy J. Transsphenoidal surgery of hypersecreting pituitary tumors. In: Kohler PO, Ross GT, eds. Diagnosis and treatment of pituitary

tumors. New York: American Elsevier, 1973:179.

18. Hardy J, Robert F, Somma M, Vezina JL. Acromegalie-gigantisme: traitement chirurgicale par exerese transsphenoidale de l'adenome hypophysaire. Neurochirurgie 1973; 19(suppl 2):2.

19. Baskin DS, Boggan JE, Wilson CB. Transsphenoidal microsurgical removal of growth hormone-secreting pituitary adenomas: a review of 137 cases. J Neurosurg 1982; 56:634.

20. Wilson CB. A decade of pituitary microsurgery [The Herbert Olivecrona lecture]. J Neurosurg 1984; 61:814.

21. Hardy J. Transsphenoidal microsurgery of the normal and pathological pituitary. Clin Neurosurg 1969; 16:185.

22. Hardy J. Transsphenoidal hypophysectomy. J Neurosurg 1971; 34:582.

23. Wilson CB, Dempsey LC. Transsphenoidal microsurgical removal of 250 pituitary adenomas. J Neurosurg 1978; 48:13.

24. Landolt AM, Wilson CB. Tumors of the sellar and parasellar area in adults. In: Youmans JR, ed. Neurological surgery. 2nd ed, vol 5. Philadelphia: WB Saunders, 1982:3107.

25. McLanahan CS, Christy JH, Tindall GT. Anterior pituitary function before and after transsphenoidal microsurgical resection of pituitary tumors. Neurosurgery 1978; 3:142.

26. Watanabe M, Kuwayama A, Nakane T, et al. Long-term growth hormone responses to nonspecific hypothalamic hormones in acromegalic patients. Surg Neurol 1985; 24:449.

27. Roelfsema F, Goslings BM, Frohlich M, Moolenaar AJ, Van Seters AP, Van Slooten H. The influence of bromocryptine on serum levels of growth hormone and other pituitary hormones and its metabolic effects in active acromegaly. Clin Endocrinol (Oxf) 1979; 11:235.

28. Faglia G, Paracchi A, Ferrari C, Beck-Peccoz P. Evaluation of the results of transsphenoidal surgery in acromegaly by assessment of the growth hormone response to thyrotrophin-releasing hormone. Clin Endocrinol (Oxf) 1978; 8:373.

29. Abboud CF, Laws ER Jr. Clinical endocrinological approach to hypo-thalamic-pituitary disease. J Neurosurg 1979; 51:271.

30. Arafah BM, Brodkey JS, Kaufman B, Velasco M, Manni A, Pearson OH. Transsphenoidal microsurgery in the treatment of acromegaly and gigantism. Neurosurgery 1980; 50:578.

31. Arosio M, Giovanelli MA, Riva E, Nava C, Ambrosi B, Faglia G. Clinical use of pre- and postsurgical evaluation of abnormal GH responses in acromegaly. J Neurosurg 1983; 59:402.

32. Giovanelli MA, Motti EDF, Paraccha A, Beck-Peccoz P, Ambrosi B, Faglia G. Treatment of acromegaly by transsphenoidal microsurgery. J Neurosurg 1976; 44:677.

33. Hoyte KM, Martin JB. Recovery from paradoxical growth hormone responses in acromegaly after transsphenoidal selective adenomectomy. J Clin Endocrinol Metab 1975; 41:656.

34. Jaquet P, Guibout M, Jaquet C, et al. Circadian regulation of growth hormone secretion after treatment of acromegaly. J Clin Endocrinol Metab 1980; 50:322.

35. Leavens ME, Samaan NA, Jesse RH, Byers RM. Clinical and endocrinological evaluation of 16 acromegalic patients treated by transsphenoidal surgery. J Neurosurg 1977; 47:853.

36. Samaan NA, Leavens ME, Jesse RH Jr. Serum growth hormone and prolactin response to thyrotropin-releasing hormone in patients with acromegaly before and after surgery. J Clin Endocrinol Metab 1974; 38:957.

37. Schaison G, Couzinet B, Moatti N, Pertuiset B. Critical study of the growth hormone response to dynamic tests and the insulin growth factor assay in acromegaly after microsurgery. Clin Endocrinol (Oxf) 1983; 18:541.

38. Beck P, Parker ML, Daughaday WH. Paradoxical hypersecretion of growth hormone in response to glucose. J Clin Endocrinol Metab 1966;

26:463.

39. Quabbe H-J. Treatment of acromegaly by transsphenoidal operation, 90-yttrium implantation and bromocriptine: results in 230 patients. Clin Endocrinol (Oxf) 1982; 16:107.

40. Schuster LD, Bantle JP, Oppenheimer JH, Seljeskog EL. Acromegaly: reassessment of the long-term therapeutic efficacy of transsphenoidal pituitary surgery. Ann Intern Med 1981; 95:172.

41. Faglia G, Beck-Peccoz P, Ferrari C, Travaglini P, Ambrosi B, Spada A. Plasma growth hormone response to thyrotropin releasing hormone in patients with active acromegaly. J Clin Endocrinol Metab 1973; 36:1259.

42. Irie M, Tsushima T. Increase of serum growth hormone concentration following thyrotropin-releasing hormone injection in patients with acromegaly or gigantism. J Clin Endocrinol Metab 1972; 35:97.

43. Schalch DS, Gonzales-Barcena D, Kastin AJ, Schally AV, Lee LA. Abnormalities in the release of TSH in response to thyrotropin-releasing hormone in patients with disorders of the pituitary, hypothalamus, and basal ganglia. J Clin Endocrinol Metab 1972; 35:609.

44. Balagura S, Derome P, Guiot G. Acromegaly: analysis of 132 cases treated surgically. Neurosurgery 1981; 8:413.

45. Laws ER Jr, Randall RV, Abboud CF. Surgical treatment of acromegaly: results in 140 patients. In: Givens JR, ed. Hormone-secreting pituitary tumors. Chicago: Year Book Medical Publishers, 1982:225.

46. Ludecke D, Kautsky R, Saeger W, Schrader D. Selective removal of hypersecreting pituitary adenomas? An analysis of endocrine function, operative and microscopical findings in 101 cases. Acta Neurochir (Wien) 1976; 35:27.

47. Allen JP, Cook DM, Greer MA, Paxton H, Castro A. Serial plasma growth hormone concentration during selective removal of pituitary tumors in acromegaly. J Neurosurg 1974; 41:38.

48. Atkinson RL, Becker DP, Martins AD, et al. Acromegaly: treatment by transsphenoidal microsurgery. JAMA 1975; 233:1279.

49. Bøhmer T, Berdal P, Haugen HN. Transsphenoidal subtotal hypophysectomy in the treatment of acromegaly. Acta Endocrinol (Copenh) 1974; 77:477.

50. Bynke O, Karlberg BE, Kagedal B, Nilsson OR. Early post-operative growth hormone levels predict the result of transsphenoidal tumor removal in acromegaly. Acta Endocrinol (Copenh) 1983; 103:158.

51. Fletcher RF, Dalton GA. The treatment of acromegaly by transsphenoidal hypophysectomy. Acta Endocrinol [Suppl] (Copenh) 1973; 177:268.

52. Garcia-Uria J, del Pozo JM, Bravo G. Functional treatment of acromegaly by transsphenoidal microsurgery. J Neurosurg 1978; 49:36.

53. Guibout MP, Jaquet JC, Lissitzky JC, Grisoli F, Vincentelli F. Resultats de l'exerese transsphenoidale des adenomes hypophysaires secretants. Ann Endocrinol (Paris) 1978; 39:95.

54. Hulting A-L, Werner S, Wersall J, Tribukait B, Anniko M. Normal growth hormone secretion is rare after microsurgical normalization of growth hormone levels in acromegaly. Acta Med Scand 1982; 212:401.

55. Kinnman J. The prognosis in acromegaly treated by transanthrosphenoidal operation. Acta Otolaryngol (Stockh) 1976; 82:420.

56. Knappe G, Rohde W, Mennig H, Gerl H. 10-year follow-up of transsphenoidal pituitary surgery in acromegaly. Endocrinologie 1982; 79:423.

57. Kondo A, Handa H, Matsumura H, Makita Y. Operative treatments for acromegaly: comparison of transsphenoidal cryogenic and microsurgical hypophysectomy. Neurol Med Chir (Tokyo) 1979; 19:683.

58. Nabarro JDN. Management of acromegaly. J Clin Pathol 1976; 7(suppl 30):62.

59. Nowakowski H, Stahnke N, Espinoza A, Regler B. Selective removal of

pituitary adenomas in acromegaly and in Nelson's syndrome. Acta Endocrinol [Suppl] (Copenh) 1973; 177:267.

60. Richards SH, Thomas JP. Treatment of acromegaly by transethmoidal hypophysectomy. Q J Med 1980; 49:21.

61. Teasdale GM, Hay ID, Beastall GH, et al. Cryosurgery or microsurgery in the management of acromegaly. JAMA 1982; 247:1289.

62. Tindall GT, Tindall SC. Transsphenoidal surgery for acromegaly: long-term results in 50 patients. In: Black PMcL, Zervas NT, Ridgway EC, Martin JB, eds. Secretory tumors of the pituitary gland: progress in endocrine research and therapy, vol 1. New York: Raven Press, 1984:175.

63. Tucker HSG, Grubb SR, Wigand JP, Wathington CO, Blackard WG, Becker DP. The treatment of acromegaly by transsphenoidal surgery. Arch Intern Med 1980; 140:795.

64. Weiss MH. Medical and surgical management of functional pituitary tumors. Clin Neurosurg 1980; 28:374.

65. Zampieri P, Scanarini M, Sicolo N, Andrioli G, Mingrino S. The acromegaly-gigantism syndrome: report of four cases treated surgically. Surg Neurol 1983; 20:498.

66. Teasdale G. Surgical management of pituitary adenoma. Clin Endocrinol (Oxf) 1983; 12:789.

67. Weiss MH. Acromegaly: selection parameters and operative results. Clin Neurosurg 1979; 27:31.

68. Aloia JF, Archambeau JO. Hypopituitarism following pituitary irradiation for acromegaly. Horm Res 1978; 9:201.

69. Kjellberg RN, Kliman B, Swisher BJ. Radiosurgery for pituitary adenoma with Bragg peak proton beam. In: Derome PJ, Jedynak CP, Peillon F, eds. Pituitary adenomas: biology, physiopathology and treatment. 2nd European Workshop, La Pitie-Salpetriere. Paris: Ascelpios, 1980:209.

70. Lamberg B-A, Kivikangas V, Vartiainen J, Raitta C, Pelkonen R. Conventional pituitary irradiation in acromegaly. Effect on growth hormone and TSH secretion. Acta Endocrinol (Copenh) 1976; 82:267.

71. Lawrence JH, Chong CY, Lyman JT, et al. Treatment of pituitary tumors with heavy particles. In: Kohler PO, Ross GT, eds. Diagnosis and treatment of pituitary tumors. International Congress Series 303. New York: American Elsevier, 1973:253.

72. Sheline GE. Conventional radiation therapy in the treatment of pituitary tumors. In: Tindall GT, Collins WF, eds. Clinical management of pituitary disorders. New York: Raven Press, 1979:287.

73. Laws ER Jr. Complications of transsphenoidal microsurgery for pituitary adenoma. In: Brook M, ed. Modern neurosurgery. Berlin: Springer-Verlag, 1982:181.

74. Asa SL, Scheithauer BW, Bilbao JM, et al. A case for hypothalamic acromegaly: a clinicopathologic study of six patients with hypothalamic gangliocytomas producing growth hormone releasing factor. J Clin Endocrinol Metab 1984; 58:796.

75. Daughaday WH, Cryer PE, Jacobs LS. The role of the hypothalamus in the pathogenesis of pituitary tumors. In: Kohler PO, Ross GT, eds. Diagnosis and treatment of pituitary tumors. Amsterdam: Excerpta Medica, 1973:26.

76. Liuzzi A, Chiodini PG, Botella L, Cremascoli G, Silvestrini F. Inhibitory effect of L-dopa on GH release in acromegalic patients. J Clin Endocrinol Metab 1972; 35:941.

77. Scheithauer BW, Kovacs K, Randall RV, Horvath E, Okazaki H, Laws ER Jr. Hypothalamic neuronal hamartoma and adenohypophyseal choristoma: their association with growth hormone adenoma of the pituitary gland. J Neuropathol Exp Neurol 1983; 42:648.

78. Laws ER Jr, Fode NC, Redmond MJ. Transsphenoidal surgery following unsuccessful prior therapy. J Neurosurg 1985; 63:823.

79. Scheithauer BW. Surgical pathology of the pituitary: the adenomas.

Part 1. Pathol Annu 1984; 19:317.

80. Woosley RE. Multiple secreting microadenomas as a possible cause of selective adenectomy failure. Case report. J Neurosurg 1983; 58:267.

81. Gordon P, Roth J. The treatment of acromegaly by conventional pituitary irradiation. In: Kohler PO, Ross GT, eds. Proceedings of Conference on Diagnosis and Treatment of Pituitary Tumors, Bethesda, MD, Jan 15–17, 1973, International Congress Series 303. Amsterdam: Excerpta Medica, 1974:230.

82. Lawrence JH, Linfoot JA. Treatment of acromegaly, Cushing's disease, and Nelson's syndrome. West J Med 1980; 133:197.

83. Selman WR, Laws ER, Scheithauer BW, Carpenter S. The occurrence and significance of dural invasion in pituitary adenoma [Abstract]. Proceedings of the Annual Meeting of the American Association of Neurological Surgeons, Atlanta GA, April 21–25, 1985:66.

84. Wrightson P. Conservative removal of small pituitary tumors: is it justified by the pathological findings? J Neurol Neurosurg Psychiatry 1978; 41:2839.

85. Wrightson P, Holdaway I, Synek B. Criteria for cure in acromegaly: report of a case apparently cured in which persisting tumor was found at autopsy. Neurosurgery 1984; 14:750.

86. Clemmons DR, Van Wyk JJ, Ridgway EC, Kliman B, Kjellberg RN, Underwood LE. Evaluation of acromegaly by radioimmunoassay of somatomedin C. N Engl J Med 1979; 301:1138.

87. Daughaday WH. New criteria for evaluation of acromegaly. N Engl J Med 1979; 301:1175.

88. Faglia G, Arosio M, Ambrosi B, Moriondo P, Beck-Peccoz P, Travaglini P. Hypothalamic-pituitary function studies in the diagnosis and follow-up of acromegaly. In: Derome PJ, Jedynak CP, Peillon F, eds. Pituitary adenomas: biology, physiopathology, and treatment. Paris: Asclepios, 1980:131.

89. Kowarski A, Thompson RL, Blizzard RM. Integrated concentration of human growth hormone (ICGH) and true secretion rates (SR) in normal and abnormal states [Abstract]. In: Proceedings of the 52nd Annual Meeting of the Endocrine Society, St. Louis, MO, June 10–12, 1970:114.

90. Stonesifer LD, Jordan RM, Kohler PO. Somatomedin C in treated acromegaly: poor correlation with growth hormone and clinical response. J Clin Endocrinol Metab 1981; 53:931.

91. Wilson CB, Linfoot JA, Sheline GE. Role of transsphenoidal microsurgery in the primary and secondary management of pituitary tumors. In: Linfoot JA, ed. Recent advances in the diagnosis and treatment of pituitary tumors. New York: Raven Press, 1979:419.

23

LONG-TERM RESULTS OF TRANSSPHENOIDAL SURGERY FOR THE

MANAGEMENT OF ACROMEGALY

Edward R. Laws, Jr., M.D., Sandra M. Carpenter, R.N.,
Bernd W. Scheithauer, M.D., Raymond V. Randall, M.D.

Mayo Clinic
Rochester, MN

Although acromegaly as a medical entity was described as early as 1779, it was 100 years ago in 1886 that the French neurologist Pierre Marie (1) coined the term, acromegaly, and presented the clinical details of two cases. Considerable interest in acromegaly rapidly evolved, but the pathophysiology and etiology of the disorder was not at all clear to the initial investigators. Minkowski in 1887 and subsequently Marie and Marinesco (2) all noted that enlargement of the pituitary was a constant feature in autopsied cases of acromegaly, but this was thought by some to be merely part of a generalized process resulting in hypertrophy of various glands. By 1900 pathophysiologic correlations suggested an etiologic role for pituitary hypertrophy or neoplasia, and Dean Lewis in 1905 (3) propagated the concept among the surgical community.

The earliest reported attempt at the surgical management of acromegaly occurred in 1893, just 7 years after Marie's description of the disease. Acting upon the advice of Sir Victor Horsley, the British general surgeon F. T. Paul (4) performed a temporal decompression to relieve pain resulting from increased intracranial pressure in a patient with acromegaly. Paul had planned to remove the pituitary but was unable to reach it; the patient was relieved of his symptoms by the procedure. Horsley himself performed 10 operations for pituitary tumor between 1889 and 1906, initially using a subfrontal approach and subsequently a temporal approach; some (probably 3) of these patients were acromegalic.

In 1908-1909, three acromegalics were treated surgically using transsphenoidal approaches, by Hochenegg and Kocher in Vienna and by Harvey Cushing (5) in Baltimore. The fact that these surgeons reported "partial hypophysectomy" as the goal and result of their operative procedures indicates that the pathogenesis of acromegaly was still unclear to them.

In the winter of 1908, a 38-year-old farmer from Columbia, South Dakota, journeyed to Rochester, Minnesota, for medical care. He complained of headache, facial pain, and photophobia. He had enlargement of the tongue, jaw, hands, and feet, and general fatigue and loss of libido. The patient was examined by Dr. H. S. Plummer, who made the diagnosis of "acromegalia." Dr. C. H. Mayo was consulted and, obviously aware not only of the latest concepts of the pathogenesis of acromegaly but also of Dr. Harvey Cushing's particular expertise, he referred the patient to Cushing at the Johns Hopkins Hospital in Baltimore.

Cushing's operation on this patient, in March 1909, was his first surgical attempt to control acromegaly and his first operation using the transsphenoidal approach (5). The symptoms and signs of acromegaly rapidly improved, and there ensued a large series of patients operated on transsphenoidally for pituitary adenoma.

By 1912 Cushing had operated successfully upon 4 acromegalics and surgeons in other countries had also reported successes. The fact that the causative lesion was a neoplasm rather than hypertrophy of the gland was becoming generally accepted.

Ultimately, Cushing operated upon 67 patients with acromegaly, 60 transsphenoidally and 7 using a frontal craniotomy. These patients had large tumors and the mortality rates were 6.6% and 20%, respectively. Visual loss accompanied acromegaly in 18 of the 67 patients, and was improved postoperatively in 15 (83%).

Until the late 1920s, most acromegalics treated surgically were managed by one or another of the transsphenoidal approaches. As cranial surgery developed, however, this approach was also applied to pituitary adenomas of all types, including acromegaly. The success of such operations in the era before the development of steroid support and antibiotics is remarkable. The concept of the transsphenoidal approach was sustained and practiced in a few centers, notably by Norman Dott in Edinburgh, Oskar Hirsch in Boston, and Pierre Wertheimer in Lyon. This approach was popularized again by Guiot (6) and Hardy (7-9) in the early 1960s, with the selective microsurgical method ultimately becoming the current standard surgical technique.

MODES OF SURGICAL THERAPY

Approaches to the pituitary region have challenged surgeons for more than a century and have resulted in many innovative solutions. As mentioned, craniotomies of various kinds have been utilized, with approaches to the pituitary fossa subfrontally, temporally and along the sphenoid wing (10). As microsurgical techniques developed, most surgeons who selected a craniotomy for pituitary tumors used a so-called pterional approach (frontotemporal, along the sphenoid wing) which avoids the frontal sinus, so frequently enlarged in acromegaly.

Transsphenoidal approaches have included transpalatal, transantral and transethmoidal routes. However, most surgeons currently utilize a transrhinoseptal technique designed to maintain the anatomy and physiology of the nose and sinuses (11-17).

Stereotactic surgery was introduced in 1908, and this concept has been utilized to allow surgeons to reach the pituitary with needles and probes placed through the nose or through the cranium. Stereotactic implantation of radioactive isotopes and stereotactic ablation of the pituitary tumor in acromegaly by cold (cryotherapy) or by thermocoagulation with heat have been utilized in the past as part of our surgical armamentarium.

INDICATIONS FOR SURGERY AND PREOPERATIVE EVALUATION

Indications for surgical management of acromegaly are several, and vary somewhat with the clinical and laboratory assessment. Patients with clinical evidence of active acromegaly (including pathologically elevated levels of serum growth hormone, and radiographic [usually CT] evidence of a pituitary adenoma) make up the largest pool of patients. The vast majority of these cases can be managed successfully with transsphenoidal surgery designed to accomplish selective microsurgical ablation of the pituitary adenoma and preservation of normal pituitary function. Craniotomy is reserved for those rare patients with very large tumors extending into the anterior or middle fossae, or for those patients with sequestered suprasellar tumor nodules which are inaccessible from the transsphenoidal approach.

Surgery may be contraindicated in the occasional patient with severe debilitation, medical problems in other organ systems or active infection in the sinuses or elsewhere. Surgical management is inappropriate in those cases of acromegaly associated with somatotroph hyperplasia related to excess levels of GHRH (18-21). Such cases have accompanied hypothalamic hamartomas, empty sellas, neoplasms of the lung and pancreas, and may present idiopathically. Sellar enlargement secondary to hyperplasia may mimic neoplasm, and is potentially reversible if the basic problem is solved (e.g., excision of a GHRH secreting tumor).

Once a decision for surgical management has been reached, a standard preoperative assessment scheme is utilized (22). Each acromegalic has a careful general medical and neurologic evaluation with special attention to any disorders of the cardiovascular system. Some 30% of our patients are hypertensive and most are receiving medical therapy. Some degree of diabetes mellitus is also very common, and its therapy adds to the complexity of perioperative management. All patients have an ear, nose, throat and respiratory evaluation. Many acromegalics have partial upper airway obstruction and require evaluation and reassurance. Prior nasal surgery or injury influences the surgical approach as does prior sinus disease or surgery. Hypertrophy of the tongue and laryngeal structures can complicate anesthesia and endotracheal intubation, so that a preoperative anesthetic consultation is often advisable.

Pituitary endocrine assessment includes basal and dynamic assessment of GH, somatomedin-C and prolactin. Pituitary-adrenal, pituitary-thyroid and pituitary-gonadal axes are assessed appropriately for preoperative baseline function. Body weight is carefully measured and urinary concentrating ability documented in those patients where there is a suggestion clinically of posterior pituitary dysfunction. A neuro-ophthalmologic examination is carried out before and after surgery with measurement of visual acuity and visual fields using tangent screen and perimeter.

The ordinary preoperative radiographic assessment includes plain skull radiographs and a CT scan with contrast enhancement. Axial and coronal views both are recommended, but the latter are difficult to obtain in some patients because of restriction of neck motion. As technology advances, magnetic resonance imaging may complement or even replace CT scanning for some pituitary tumors. Angiography is performed when there is reason to suspect associated intracranial vascular disease, to determine details of vascular anatomy in large tumors with suprasellar or parasellar extensions, and whenever the added information may enhance the safety of the planned operative procedure.

SURGICAL TECHNIQUE AND RESULTS

The advantage of the surgical approach, and the goal, is the selective and, ideally, complete removal of pituitary tumor while preserving or even improving normal pituitary function. Postoperative assessment determines the measure of success and the need for adjunctive therapy, either medical or radiation or both.

The technique of transsphenoidal microsurgical excision of pituitary adenomas has evolved to a standard procedure which, in experienced hands, is remarkably safe and effective (23-38). The approach involves an endonasal or sublabial, transseptal exposure of the midline sphenoid sinus. There are no external scars, the cosmetic and functional aspects of the nose are preserved, and there is minimal pain or discomfort. Exposure involves removal of a portion of the bony nasal septum, the face of the sphenoid sinus and the anterior aspect of the sella turcica. Most of these structures are reconstructed during the closure. The incisions are repaired with dissolving sutures.

Surgery in the region of the sella is carried out under magnified vision and excellent illumination using the operating microscope. The position of the surgical instruments is monitored by a lateral X-ray image intensifier, offering further control and precision. In most cases, the goal is complete removal of the tumor which, usually, is soft in consistency and is readily separated from the sellar dura, the diaphragma sellae, and the residual normal pituitary gland. Some tumors (about 30%) invade dura and bone and may require more radical surgical techniques. Tumors with suprasellar or parasellar extension may require delicate dissection under radiographic control. In these cases the injection of air into the CSF via an indwelling lumbar needle or catheter can be a useful adjunct.

Following tumor removal, reconstruction is carried out within the sella as well. With small tumors, the tumor cavity is filled with hemostatic gelatin foam. In large tumors and those cases wherein an intraoperative CSF leak has occurred, the sella is filled with a graft of fat or muscle, taken from the abdomen or the thigh. The incidence of postoperative CSF rhinorrhea is very low (less than 1%) even in cases of large tumors with suprasellar extension and visual loss.

Following surgery, the nostrils are packed with gauze for 3 or 4 days. A postoperative endocrine evaluation is carried out during the recovery period and most patients are able to return home within one week of surgery and to resume work within two to four weeks.

It is probably not wise to consider independently the results of any one form of management of a disorder as complex as acromegaly. Neither is it prudent to place too much emphasis on early posttreatment assessment of endocrine results. Since each patient may present a particular therapeutic challenge with regard to the size, invasiveness, and endocrine activity of the pituitary adenoma, treatment should be individualized and long-term control of disease rather than short-term values of endocrine tests should be the goal.

Since November of 1972, initial therapy for nearly all acromegalics treated at the Mayo Clinic has been transsphenoidal microsurgery. A few patients who would not consider surgery were referred elsewhere for heavy particle radiation therapy, and one patient had acromegaly controlled by removal of a pulmonary carcinoid tumor which produced GHRH.

Transsphenoidal surgery has been followed by additional therapy as indicated to achieve more satisfactory long-term control. Patients with large or invasive tumors, and those who have abnormal postoperative GH levels, are given conventional radiation therapy (39,40). This is accomplished using multiple port or rotational technique with shielding of the eyes, using a linear accelerator and treating to a total dose of 4500-5500 rads in 180 rad daily fractions. Some patients in these categories are candidates for proton beam therapy and several have been treated with this modality postoperatively.

In order to assess the long-term efficacy of this therapeutic approach, the medical records of 100 patients treated for acromegaly and followed for the longest period of time were reviewed in a retrospective fashion.

These 100 patients were treated between November 1971 and February 1976. Postoperative follow-up is complete and ranges from 24 to 180 months with a mean follow-up of 96 months for those patients still alive. There were 62 men and 38 women treated. The age range was 17 to 75 years, with a mean age of 45 years.

The lesions found at surgery were classified as somatotrophic hyperplasia (2%), microadenoma ($\leq$10 mm in diameter—25%) and macroadenoma (73%). Invasion of bone or dura was observed macroscopically at surgery in 8 of the microadenomas and 17 of the macroadenomas. Studies of the pathologic specimens reveal a much higher incidence of microscopic invasion of pituitary dura, tending to increase with increasing size of the adenomas.

Long-term control of the clinical aspects of active acromegaly has been quite satisfactory. Gross signs and symptoms of acromegaly have remained quiescent in 93% of the patients. Recurrence clinically and hormonally developed in 7 patients and generally was controllable by radiation therapy (5 patients) or another transsphenoidal operation and radiation therapy (1 patient). One patient has not been treated for mild symptoms associated with recurrence. Detection of recurrence occurred between 6 and 60 months after surgery.

If loose criteria are used for the definition of satisfactory long-term control, this method of therapy is excellent. If the goal is arrest of active acromegaly and repeated follow-up fasting GH levels of 10 ng/ml or less, then success was achieved in both patients with hyperplasia, 96% of those with microadenomas and 79% of those with macroadenomas. It should be noted that 56% of the patients in this series have been managed by a combination of surgery and radiation therapy.

Although there was no treatment-related mortality, 8 of the 100 acromegalics have died during the follow-up period. The cause of death was myocardial infarction in 5 patients and unrelated malignancy in the other 3. Interestingly, 7 of these 8 patients had GH levels >10 ng/ml (12.4–74.3 ng/ml) at last follow-up before death. The significance, if any, of this latter finding is not known.

Complications of therapy have been relatively few, although hypopituitarism requiring replacement therapy is common in those patients treated by surgery and radiation therapy. Except for 2 patients with diabetes insipidus, long-term morbidity has not occurred.

The outcome of these 100 acromegalic patients treated initially with transsphenoidal microsurgery is given in Table 1. The fact that satisfactory long-term control, allowing fully active normal lives for these patients, has been achieved in 74% of these subjects is rewarding. Hopefully, these results will improve with time and experience. The advent of new forms of medical therapy can be anticipated (41), and the role of surgery may change, but it remains likely that a multiple modality approach will continue to provide the optimal results.

Table 1. Outcome in 100 acromegalics treated by
transsphenoidal surgery (10-year follow-up).

Status	Number of patients (%)
Living and well (no active acromegaly)	74
Living with disease (mild acromegaly)	11
Recurrent acromegaly	7
Expired	8

REFERENCES

1. Marie P. Sur deux cas d'acromegalie: hypertrophie singuliere non congenitale des extremites superieures, inferieures et cephalique. Rev Med Liege 1886; 6:297.
2. Marie P, Marinesco G. Sur l'anatomic pathologique de l'acromegalie. Arch de Med Exper et D'Anat Path (Paris) 1891; 3:539-65.
3. Lewis DD. Hyperplasia of the chromophile cells of the hypophysis as the cause of acromegaly, with report of a case. Johns Hopkins Med J 1905; 16:157-64.
4. Caton R, Paul FT. Notes on a case of acromegaly treated by operation. Br Med J 1893; 2:1421-3.
5. Cushing H. Partial hypophysectomy for acromegaly. Ann Surg 1909; 50:1002-17.
6. Guiot G. Considerations on the surgical treatment of pituitary adenomas. In: Fahlbusch R, von Werder KVM, eds. Treatment of pituitary adenomas. Stuttgart: Georg Thieme, 1978:202-18.
7. Hardy J, Robert F, Somma M, et al. Acromegalie-gigantisme: traitement chirurgical par exerese transsphenoidale de l'adenome hypophysaire. Neurochirurgie 1973; 19:1-184.
8. Hardy J, Somma M. Acromegaly: surgical treatment by transsphenoidal microsurgical removal of the pituitary adenoma. In: Tindall GT, Collins WF, eds. Clinical management of pituitary disorders. New York: Raven Press, 1979:209-17.
9. Hardy J, Somma M, Vezina JL. Treatment of acromegaly: radiation or surgery? In: Morley T, ed. Current controversies in neurosurgery. Philadelphia: Saunders Co., 1976:377-91.
10. Ray BS, Horwith M, Mautalen C. Surgical hypophysectomy as a treatment for acromegaly. In: Astwood EB, Cassidy CE, eds. Clinical endocrinology. New York: Grune & Stratton, 1968:93-102.
11. Collins WF. Pituitary tumor management: an overview. In: Tindall GT, Collins WF, eds. Clinical management of pituitary disorders. New York: Raven Press, 1979:179-86.
12. Fukushima T, Takakura K, Sano K. Sublabial rhinoseptoplastic microsurgery for functioning pituitary adenomas: a new technique. In: Sano K, Takakura K, Fukushima T, eds. Functioning pituitary adenoma. Proceedings of the first workshop on pituitary adenomas. Tokyo, 1980:61-76.
13. Giovanelli MA, Motti EDF, Paracchi A, et al. Treatment of acromegaly by transsphenoidal microsurgery. J Neurosurg 1976; 44:677-86.
14. Laws ER Jr. Transsphenoidal microsurgery in the management of acromegaly. In: Smith JL, ed. Neuro-ophthalmology focus. New York: Masson Publishing USA, Inc., 1980:289-93.

15. Laws ER Jr, Randall RV, Kern EB, Abboud CF, eds. Management of pituitary adenomas and related lesions with emphasis on transsphenoidal microsurgery. New York: Appleton-Century-Crofts, 1982.

16. Wilson CB. A decade of pituitary microsurgery. The Herbert Olivecrona lecture. J Neurosurg 1984; 61:814-33.

17. Zervas NT, Martin JB. Management of hormone-secreting pituitary adenomas. N Engl J Med 1980; 302:210-4.

18. Asa SL, Scheithauer BW, Bilbao JM, et al. A case for hypothalamic acromegaly: a clinicopathological study of six patients with hypothalamic gangliocytomas producing growth hormone-releasing factor. J Clin Endocrinol Metab 1984; 58:796-803.

19. Caplan RH, Koob L, Abellera RM, Pagliara AS, Kovacs K, Randall RV. Cure of acromegaly by operative removal of an islet cell tumor of the pancreas. Am J Med 1978; 64:874.

20. Scheithauer BW, Kovacs K, Randall RV, Horvath E, Okazaki H, Laws ER Jr. Hypothalamic neuronal hamartoma and adenohypophyseal neuronal choristoma: their association with growth hormone adenoma of the pituitary gland. J Neuropathol Exp Neurol 1983; 42:648.

21. Scheithauer BW, Carpenter PC, Block B, Brazeau P. Ectopic secretion of a growth hormone-releasing factor. Report of a case of acromegaly with bronchial carcinoid tumor. Am J Med 1984; 76:605-16.

22. Abboud CF, Laws ER Jr. Clinical endocrinological approach to hypothalamic-pituitary disease. J Neurosurg 1979; 51:271-91.

23. Balagura S, Derome P, Guiot G. Acromegaly: analysis of 132 cases treated surgically. Neurosurgery 1981; 8:413-6.

24. Baskin DS, Boggan JE, Wilson CB. Transsphenoidal microsurgical removal of growth hormone-secreting pituitary tumors: a review of 137 cases. J Neurosurg 1982; 56:634-41.

25. Ciric IS, Tarkington J. Transsphenoidal microsurgery. Surg Neurol 1974; 2:207-12.

26. Delalande G, Derome PJ, Jedynak CP, et al. Transsphenoidal surgery in acromegaly. Results in 102 patients according to the European enquiry. In: Derome PJ, Jedynak CP, Peillon F, eds. Pituitary adenomas. Biology, physiopathology and treatment. Paris: Asclepios, 1980; 320-1.

27. Fahlbusch R. Surgical treatment of pituitary adenomas. In: Beardwell C, Robertson GL, eds. Clinical endocrinology 1: the pituitary. London: Butterworths International Medical Reviews, 1981:76-105.

28. Garcia-Uria J, del Pozo JM, Bravo G. Functional treatment of acromegaly by transsphenoidal microsurgery. J Neurosurg 1978; 49:36-40.

29. Giovanelli MA, Fahlbusch R, Gaini SM, et al. Surgical treatment of growth hormone-secreting microadenomas. In: Faglia G, Giovanelli MA, MacLeod RM, eds. Pituitary microadenomas. New York: Academic Press, 1980:427-41.

30. Guibout M, Jaquet P, Lissitzky J-C, Grisoli F, Vincentelli F. Resultats de l'exerese trans-sphenoidale des adenomes hypophysaires secretants. Ann Endocrinol (Paris) 1978; 39:95-106.

31. Laws ER Jr, Piepgras DG, Randall RV, Abboud CF. Neurosurgical management of acromegaly: results in 82 patients treated between 1972 and 1977. J Neurosurg 1979; 50:454-61.

32. Laws ER Jr, Randall RV, Abboud CF. Surgical treatment of acromegaly: results in 140 patients. In: Givens J, ed. Hormone-secreting pituitary tumors. Chicago: Year Book Publishing Co., 1982:225-8.

33. Laws ER Jr, Fode NC, Redmond MJ. Transsphenoidal surgery following unsuccessful prior therapy. J Neurosurg 1985; 63:823-9.

34. Ludecke D, Kautzky R, Saeger W, et al. Selective removal of hypersecreting pituitary adenomas? An analysis of endocrine function, operative and microscopical findings in 101 cases. Acta Neurochir (Wien) 1976; 35:27-42.

35. Ludecke DK, Saeger W, William T. Effectiveness of microsurgery in

acromegaly. Study of 210 cases. Period Biol 1983; 85:59–66.

36. Teasdale G. Surgical management of pituitary adenoma. Clin Endocrinol Metab 1983; 12:789–823.

37. Sang H, Wilson CB, Tyrrell JB. Transsphenoidal microhypophysectomy
in acromegaly. J Neurosurg 1977; 47:840–52.

38. Williams RA, Jacobs HS, Kurtz AB, et al. The treatment of acromegaly
with special reference to transsphenoidal hypophysectomy. Q J Med
1975; 79–98.

39. Kramer S. Indications for, and results of, treatment of pituitary
tumors by external radiation. In: Kohler PO, Ross GT, eds. Diagnosis and treatment of pituitary tumors. New York: Excerpta Medica
American Elsevier, 1973:217–33.

40. Sheline GE, Goldberg MB, Feldman R. Pituitary irradiation for
acromegaly. Radiology 1961; 76:70–5.

41. Wass JAH, Thorner MO, Morris DV, et al. Long-term treatment of
acromegaly with bromocriptine. Br Med J 1977; 1:875–8.

24

THE USE OF SOMATOSTATIN ANALOGS IN THE TREATMENT OF

ACROMEGALY

Steven W. J. Lamberts

Department of Medicine
Erasmus University
Rotterdam, The Netherlands

INTRODUCTION

The hypothalamic hormones, somatostatin and growth hormone-releasing hormone (GHRH), play a central role in the regulation of normal growth hormone secretion. GH secretion by the cultured pituitary tumor cells of acromegalic patients has retained a high sensitivity to the inhibitory effect of somatostatin and the stimulatory effect of GHRH (1). Interestingly, on a molar base somatostatin inhibits GHRH-stimulated GH release by these tumor cells in a noncompetitive manner (1). Intravenous administration of natural somatostatin results in a marked inhibition of GH release in most acromegalic patients, but rebound hypersecretion occurs after discontinuation of the infusion (2,3,4). Chronic therapy with the native peptide was impractical because of its short half-life of about 3 min. For this reason, attempts have been made to synthesize analogs of somatostatin with a longer duration of action than the native form. Step by step modification of a conformationally stabilized analog of somatostatin, which was thought to be the essential active moiety, enabled Bauer et al. (5) to synthesize the analog termed SMS 201-995 (Sandostatin).

In vivo, SMS 201-995 was at least 45 times more potent than somatostatin in inhibiting GH secretion in monkeys. Its much longer duration of action is caused by resistance to proteolytic clearance. SMS 201-995 was also highly potent in inhibiting glucagon secretion, but much less so in the suppression of insulin secretion. Therefore, this analog was viewed as a promising agent for the treatment of acromegaly. In normal subjects, a single dose of 50 µg SMS 201-995 produced peak plasma SMS 201-995 levels of 2.0-3.0 ng/ml (1.6-2.5 pM) within 15-30 min after injection. Based on these observations, estimated half-life of SMS 201-995 was calculated to be 113 min (6).

THE ACUTE EFFECT OF SMS 201-995 ON GH RELEASE IN ACROMEGALY

A typical example of the effects of SMS 201-995 on circulating GH, glucose, and insulin levels is shown in Figure 1. In a 56-year-old untreated acromegalic male patient, basal GH levels over a 24-hour period were calculated at 36 ± 3 µg/l (mean ± SEM; n = 17). The subcutaneous administration of 25, 50 and 100 µg SMS 201-995 induced a rapid and pronounced inhibition of plasma GH levels, which was maximal 2 hours after the subcutaneous administration of the drug. The effect of these three doses of SMS 201-995 on GH secretion differed especially with regard to the duration of the inhibitory effect on GH release. In other more extensive studies in 7 acromegalic patients, we showed that 50 and 100 μg SMS 201-995 induced a similar reduction of GH levels by 85% and 86%, respectively, for 2-6 hours after administration. Administration of 100 μg SMS 201-995 caused a significantly longer inhibitory effect than 50 μg of the compound; for 2-10 hours after SMS 201-995 administration plasma GH levels were suppressed by 62% after 50 μg and by 81% after 100 μg (P < 0.01). The postprandial increment of glucose after breakfast increased in a dose-dependent manner after SMS 201-995 administration (Fig. 1, middle part). This was caused by a short-lived dose-dependent inhibition of insulin secretion for only about 2 hours. Of paramount importance for the potential further therapeutic use of this somatostatin analog was the absence of a rebound hypersecretion of GH (7).

The acute effect of the injection of 50 μg SMS 201-995 on plasma GH levels was measured in 22 acromegalic patients. Mean plasma GH levels were 44.0 ± 11.4 μg/l on the control day, and were inhibited to 8.6 ± 2.3 μg/l (-80 ± 5%) between 2 and 6 hours after SMS 201-995 administration. The plasma GH levels were suppressed to less than 5 μg/l in 14 of the 22 patients, and to less than 50% of the control levels in 16 subjects. These data point to a considerable variation in the sensitivity of GH secretion to SMS 201-995 in acromegalics, i.e., 6 of the 22 patients studied showed a rather low sensitivity to SMS 201-995. A further example of the powerful inhibitory effect of SMS 201-995 on GH release in some of these acromegalics is shown in Figure 2. Plasma GH levels were suppressed by 50 μg SMS 201-995 to below 5 μg/l for 9 hours, while the paradoxical increments of GH, in response to TRH, was significantly blunted (P < 0.01 vs. response to TRH on the placebo day).

CHRONIC THERAPY WITH SMS 201-995

We treated 8 acromegalic patients for 14-78 weeks with SMS 201-995 (200-300 μg/day in 2 or 3 subcutaneous injections). Part of these results have been published elsewhere (8). Chronic therapy with SMS 201-995 resulted in a rapid clinical improvement in all patients, varying from diminution to complete disappearance of the signs and symptoms of acromegaly within the first week of treatment: paresthesia, headache, backache, tender joints, excessive perspiration, tiredness and hypertension. A decrease in soft-tissue swelling was also evident in all patients, since wedding rings could be removed for the first time in many years and smaller shoe sizes were needed. Interestingly, a slight shrinkage of the pituitary tumors was observed at CT-scanning in 3 of the 6 patients in whom this could be evaluated.

The clinical improvement was accompanied by a "normalization" of GH levels (below 5 μg/l) for several hours after each injection of SMS 201-995 in all 8 patients. This powerful inhibitory effect of SMS 201-995 on GH secretion resolved rapidly, however, and was, in most instances, followed by a gradual increase toward the pre-injection levels of SMS 201-995 (Fig. 3). This tendency of the plasma GH levels to increase between injections of the analog was evident even after 78 weeks of therapy with SMS 201-995. Of great importance, however, is the observation that a slowly progressive further decrease in the profile of the plasma GH levels over 24 hours occurred even after 26 of 52 weeks of therapy with 200-300 μg SMS 201-995 daily.

Serum somatomedin-C (SM-C) and phosphate levels were increased in all patients before the start of therapy with SMS 201-995. During treatment

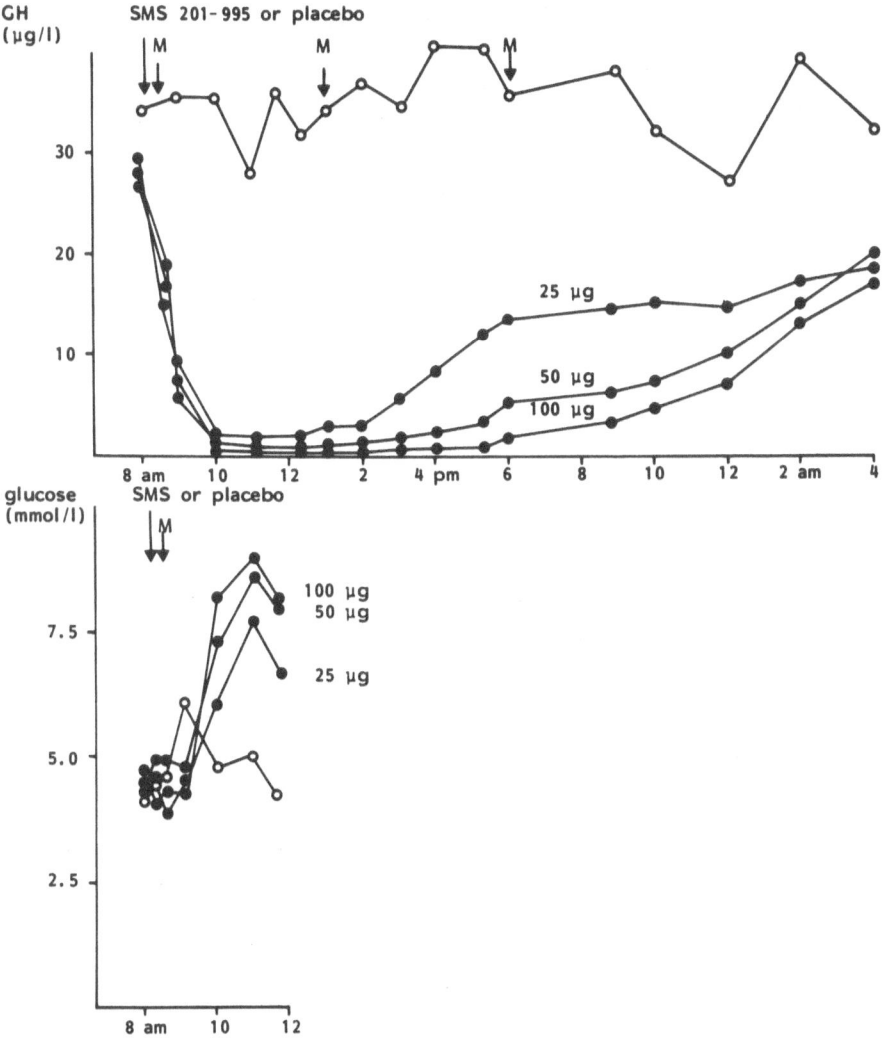

Fig. 1. A comparison between the effects of the subcutaneous administration of 25, 50 and 100 μg SMS 201-995 (●—●) and of placebo (○—○) on plasma GH, glucose and insulin levels of an untreated acromegalic patient.

there was a gradual decrease of SM-C and phosphate levels which was directly correlated with the decrease in the mean GH levels as measured over a 24-hour period (Fig. 4 and 5). Mean plasma GH and SM-C levels were suppressed by 60-90% in all patients and normalized in 5 of these 8 acromegalics.

All patients adapted well to self-administration of SMS 201-995. The injection sites on the anterior aspect of each thigh remained soft, without induration. No signs or symptoms that might be attributed to treatment were recorded, except the transient occurrence of steatorrhea in two patients. This was not accompanied, however, by a change in the number of bowel movements. Carbohydrate tolerance worsened slightly during the initial period of SMS 201-995 therapy, but normalized during chronic therapy in 6 patients. Blood glucose levels in 2 patients with

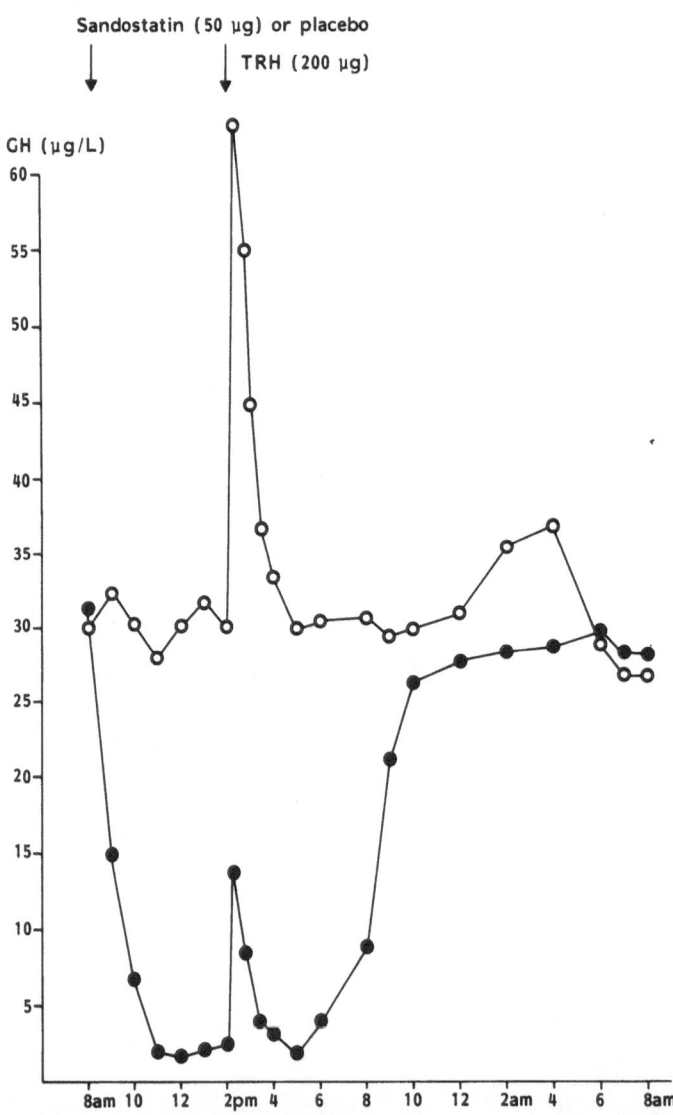

Fig. 2. The effect of TRH (200 μg intravenously) on GH levels of an acromegalic patient on a control day (o—o = placebo) and 6 hours after the subcutaneous administration of 50 μg SMS 201-995 (●—●).

type II diabetes mellitus at the start of SMS 201-995 therapy, diminished during the course of treatment. Sulfonylurea derivatives, however, completely overcame the SMS 201-995-induced inhibition of insulin release.

A COMPARISON BETWEEN THE EFFECTS OF SMS 201-995, BROMOCRIPTINE AND THEIR COMBINATION ON GH RELEASE IN ACROMEGALY

A number of studies have shown that chronic treatment with dopamine agonists like bromocriptine resulted in the normalization of plasma GH levels and disappearance of the clinical symptoms of acromegaly in about 30% of the patients (9–11). We have observed considerable variability in the sensitivity of GH release to bromocriptine. Interestingly, this variability appeared to be dependent on the presence of PRL within the GH-secreting tumors, thus making GH release from mixed GH/PRL-secreting adenomas more sensitive to bromocriptine (12–14). In an immunohisto-chemical study of pituitary tumors from 41 acromegalic patients, we observed that 25 tumors contained only GH, while PRL was also found in 16 of the adenomas. Hyperprolactinemia was present in only 10 of the 16 patients with mixed GH/PRL-containing tumors and in 1 of the 25 patients

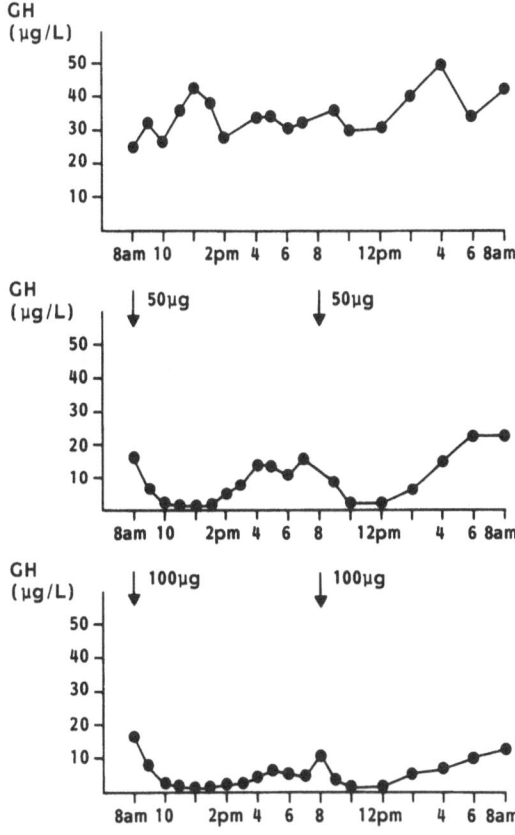

Fig. 3. Plasma GH response to various doses of SMS 201-995 over 24 hours in an acromegalic patient. Profiles are shown before treatment (top graph) and after 4 weeks of therapy with 50 µg SMS 201-995 twice (middle graph) and after 8 additional weeks of therapy with 100 µg of the compound twice daily (lower graph).

with pure GH-containing adenomas. Mean plasma GH levels decreased significantly in the patients with mixed GH/PRL-containing tumors between 2 and
10 hours after the oral administration of 2.5 mg bromocriptine compared to
those with pure GH-containing pituitary adenomas; 39 ± 4% and 68 ± 4% of
basal values, respectively ($P < 0.01$; Fig. 6). In the right part of Figure
6, the sensitivity of GH secretion to bromocriptine in individual patients
is shown. It is clear from these data that there is a considerable
overlap between both groups of patients. However, in general it can be
concluded that the simultaneous presence of PRL within a GH-secreting
tumor increases the sensitivity of GH to bromocriptine. Individual plasma
PRL levels, however, are of marginal value in predicting which acromegalic
patients are likely to respond to bromocriptine with a considerable
inhibition of GH secretion.

We compared the acute GH-inhibitory effects of 50 μg SMS 201-995 and
of 2.5 mg bromocriptine in 17 acromegalic patients (15). SMS 201-995
suppressed plasma GH levels after 2-6 hours to 5 μg/1 or less in 10 of
these 17 patients, while bromocriptine produced similar results in only 5
patients (Fig. 7). There was no homogeneity in the responsiveness to both
drugs in the patients studied, but the GH-lowering effect of 50 μg SMS
201-995 was significantly greater than that elicited by 2.5 mg bromocriptine (Fig. 8). SMS 201-995 and bromocriptine together significantly
suppressed plasma GH levels in 2 of 3 acromegalic patients who were
insensitive to both compounds tested separately. Most acromegalic
patients in this study responded better to SMS 201-995, while a few

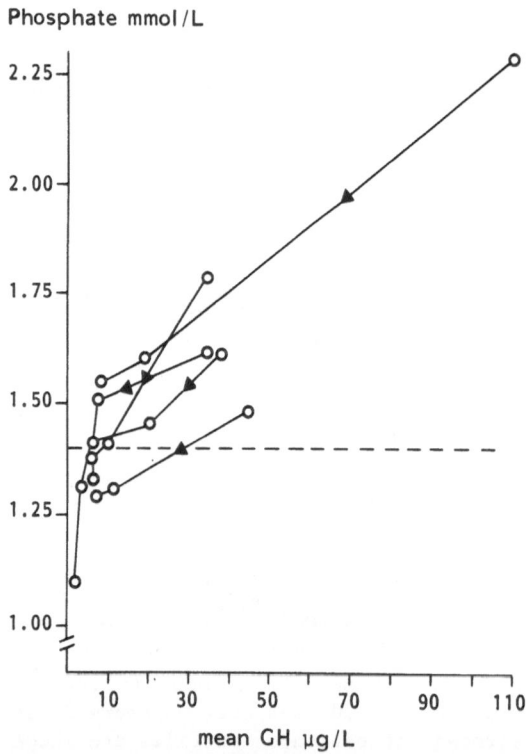

Fig. 4. The course of serum phosphate
and GH levels (mean of 20 samples
collected over a 24-hour period) during
therapy with 200-300 μg SMS 201-995 for
6-24 weeks in 5 acromegalic patients.

patients were more sensitive to the GH-lowering effect of bromocriptine. The combination of both SMS 201-995 and bromocriptine can be of value in a few acromegalic patients which do not respond to either of these drugs separately (15).

As mentioned above, we have reported that the variability in the sensitivity of GH release to bromocriptine was, to a certain degree, dependent on the presence of PRL within the GH-secreting tumors, thereby making GH release from mixed GH/PRL-secreting adenomas more sensitive to bromocriptine (12-14). We therefore also investigated whether the immuno-histochemical picture of the GH-secreting pituitary tumor, or the circula-ting PRL level, might play a role in the sensitivity of GH as well as PRL secretion, to SMS 201-995 in patients with acromegaly. We found that 11 of 18 patients had pure GH-containing tumors while 7 subjects had mixed GH/PRL-containing tumors (16). In two of these "mixed" tumor patients, there was evidence for GH and PRL being secreted by the same tumor cells. The sensitivity of GH secretion to SMS 201-995 was not different in the patients with pure GH or mixed GH/PRL-containing adenomas. Plasma PRL levels were not affected by SMS 201-995 in the patients with pure GH-secreting tumors, but were significantly suppressed in 4 of the 7 patients with mixed GH/PRL-containing tumors.

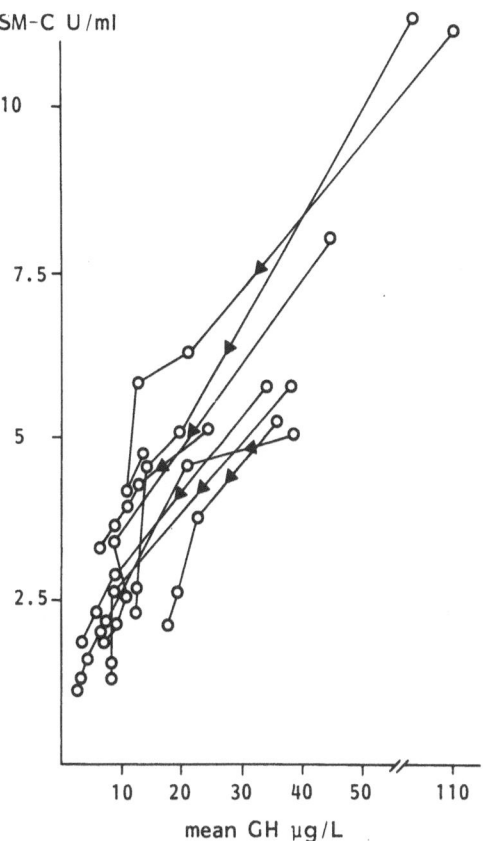

Fig. 5. The course of serum somato-medin-C and GH levels (mean of 20 samples collected over a 24-hour period) during therapy with 200-300 μg SMS 201-995 for 14-78 weeks in 8 acromegalic patients.

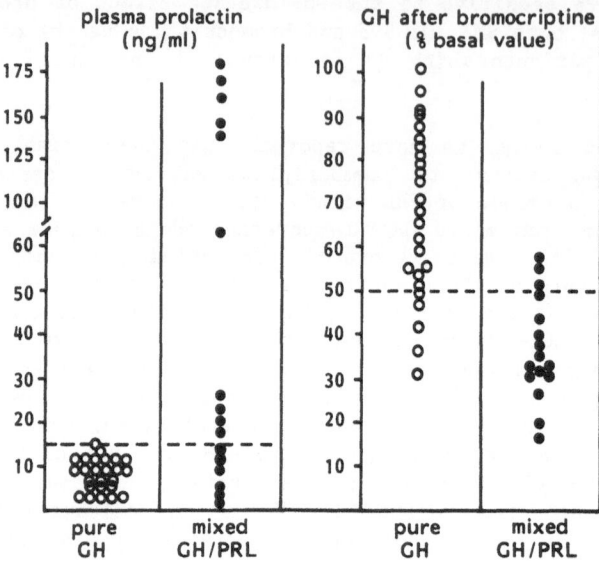

Fig. 6. The circulating PRL concentrations
(left) and the mean GH levels from 2-10 hours
after 2.5 mg bromocriptine as a percentage of
basal levels (right) in 25 acromegalic
patients with immunohistochemically pure
GH-containing (o) and in 16 acromegalics with
mixed GH/PRL-containing (•) pituitary tumors.

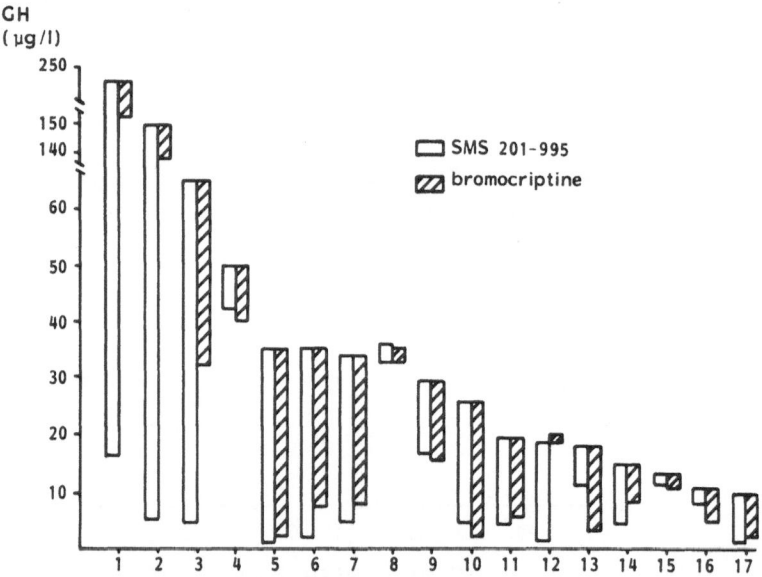

Fig. 7. A comparison between the effects of the subcutaneous administration of 50 μg SMS 201-995 and of the oral
administration of 2.5 mg bromocriptine on plasma GH levels
in 17 acromegalic patients. Plasma GH concentrations on a
control day were compared with those from 2-6 hours after
drug administration (from reference 15).

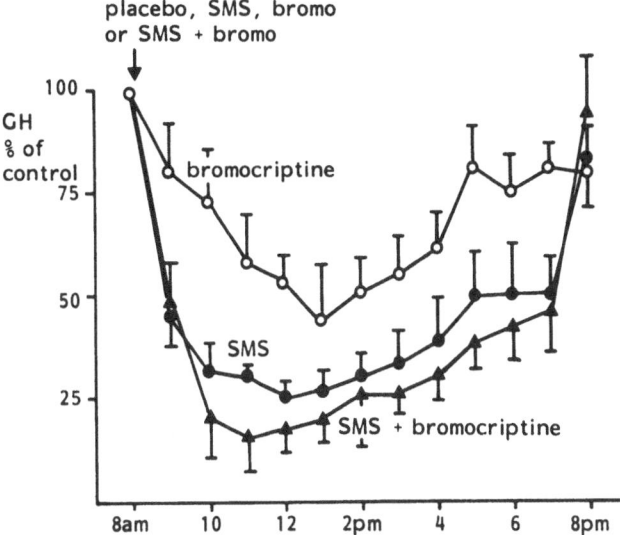

Fig. 8. The effects of SMS 201-995 (50 μg sc), bromocriptine (2.5 mg orally) and the combination of both compounds on plasma GH levels as a percentage of the GH levels on a control day in 7 acromegalic patients (mean ± SEM; from reference 15).

An example of the acute inhibitory effect of 50 μg SMS 201-995 on circulating GH and PRL levels in comparison with those on a control day in one patient is shown in Figure 9. In this patient, immunohistochemical analysis demonstrated a mixed GH/PRL-containing tumor consisting of one tumor cell type which secreted both GH and PRL. This patient was treated for 16 weeks with 300 μg SMS 201-995 daily. The mean GH levels decreased from 34.2 ± 3.0 to 2.6 ± 0.3 μg/l, respectively (mean of 20 samples ± SEM), and plasma PRL levels also normalized from 79.4 ± 4.0 to 13.6 ± 0.2 μg/l during therapy. In comparison, hyperprolactinemia in four patients with PRL-secreting tumors was not affected by SMS 201-995 administration.

CONCLUSIONS

GH secretion by the pituitary adenomas of acromegalic patients retained a variable but often significant sensitivity to somatostatin.

Treatment of 8 acromegalic patients for up to 78 weeks with the long-acting somatostatin analog, SMS 201-995, resulted in a rapid amelioration of the clinical signs and symptoms of the disease, and a (near) normalization of mean plasma GH and somatomedin-C concentrations. There was evidence of slight tumor shrinkage in some of these patients. No significant side effect was recorded throughout the treatment period. SMS 201-995 is an important and hopeful new addition to the medical management of acromegaly. Moreover, patients who do not benefit sufficiently from surgery or radiotherapy are candidates for therapy with SMS 201-995.

The simultaneous presence of PRL and GH within a GH-secreting pituitary adenoma determines, to some extent, whether GH release by this tumor is sensitive to the dopamine agonist bromocriptine. It seems as if the GH-secreting pituitary tumor cells of mixed GH/PRL-containing adenomas have adopted the normal characteristics of PRL secretion with regard to their sensitivity to dopamine. On the other hand, however, PRL secretion by GH/PRL-containing adenomas has adopted the normal characteristics of the tumorous GH-secreting tumor cells with regard to their sensitivity to somatostatin.

GH-secretion of acromegalic patients is in most cases more sensitive to SMS 201-995 than to bromocriptine. In a few cases a combination therapy with both drugs seems of benefit.

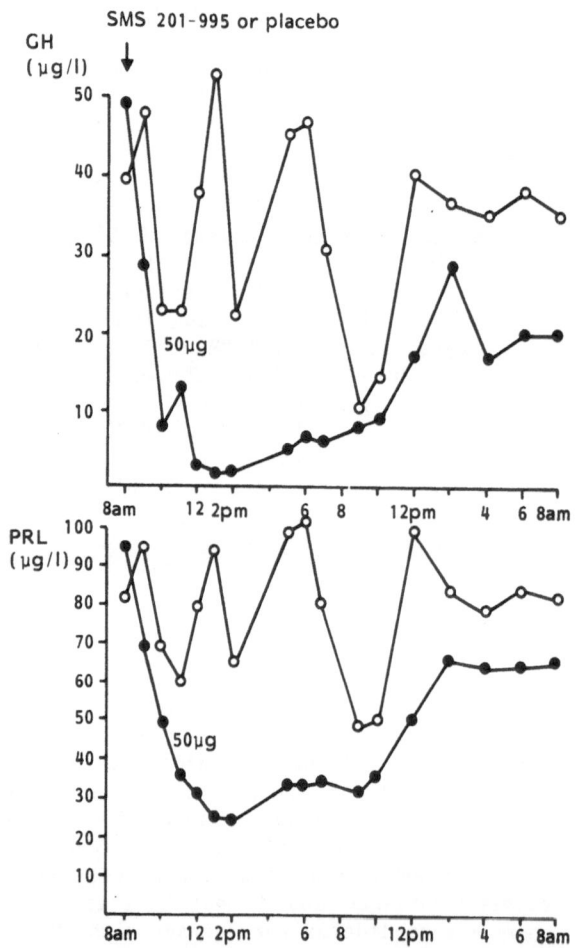

Fig. 9. The effect of the subcutaneous administration of 50 µg SMS 201-995 on plasma GH and PRL levels (●——●) in comparison with those on a control day (○——○) in an acromegalic patient with a mixed GH/PRL-containing pituitary adenoma (from reference 16).

REFERENCES

1. Lamberts SWJ, Verleun T, Oosterom R. The interrelationship between the effects of somatostatin and human pancreatic growth hormone-releasing factor on growth hormone release by cultured pituitary tumor cells from patients with acromegaly. J Clin Endocrinol Metab 1984; 58:250.
2. Besser GM, Mortimer CH, Carr D, et al. Growth hormone release inhibiting hormone in acromegaly. Br Med J 1974; 1:352.
3. Yen SSC, Siler TM, DeVane GW. Effect of somatostatin in patients with acromegaly: suppression of growth hormone, prolactin, insulin and glucose levels. N Engl J Med 1974; 290:935.
4. Dunn PJ, Donald RA, Espiner EA. A comparison of the effect of levodopa and somatostatin on the plasma levels of growth hormone, insulin, glucagon and prolactin in acromegaly. Clin Endocrinol (Oxf) 1976; 5:167.
5. Bauer W, Briner U, Doepfner W, et al. SMS 201-995: a very potent and selective octapeptide analogue of somatostatin with prolonged action. Life Sci 1982; 31:1133.
6. del Pozo E, Neufeld M, Schluter K, et al. Endocrine profile of a long-acting somatostatin derivative SMS 201-995. Study in normal volunteers following subcutaneous administration. Acta Endocrinol (Copenh) 1986; 111:433.
7. Lamberts SWJ, Oosterom R, Neufeld M, del Pozo E. The somatostatin analog SMS 201-995 induces long-acting inhibition of growth hormone secretion without rebound hypersecretion in acromegalic patients. J Clin Endocrinol Metab 1985; 60:1161.
8. Lamberts SWJ, Uitterlinden P, Verschoor L, van Dongen KJ, del Pozo E. Long-term treatment of acromegaly with the somatostatin analogue SMS 201-995. N Engl J Med 1985; 313:1576.
9. Wass JAM, Thorner MO, Morris DV, et al. Long-term treatment of acromegaly with bromocriptine. J Clin Endocrinol Metab 1975; 40:904.
10. Sachdev Y, Gopal K, Garg VK. Bromocriptine therapy in acromegaly: a long-term review of 35 cases. Postgrad Med J 1981; 57:210.
11. Oppizzi G, Liuzzi A, Chiodini P, et al. Dopaminergic treatment of acromegaly: different effects on hormone secretion and tumor size. J Clin Endocrinol Metab 1984; 58:988.
12. Lamberts SWJ, Klijn JGM, van Vroonhoven CCJ, Stefanko SZ, Liuzzi A. The role of prolactin in the inhibitory action of bromocriptine on growth hormone secretion in acromegaly. Acta Endocrinol (Copenh) 1983; 193:446.
13. Lamberts SWJ, Liuzzi A, Chiodini PG, Verde S, Klijn JGM. The value of plasma prolactin levels in the prediction of the responsiveness of growth hormone secretion to bromocriptine and TRH in acromegaly. Eur J Clin Invest 1982; 12:151.
14. Lamberts SWJ, Klijn JGM, van Vroonhoven CCJ, Stefanko SZ. Different responses of growth hormone secretion to guanfacine, bromocriptine, and thyrotropin-releasing hormone in acromegalic patients with pure growth hormone (GH)-containing and mixed GH/prolactin-containing pituitary adenomas. J Clin Endocrinol Metab 1985; 60:1148.
15. Lamberts SWJ, Zweens M, Verschoor L, del Pozo E. A comparison between the growth hormone lowering effects in acromegaly of the somatostatin analog SMS 201-995, bromocriptine and the combination of both drugs. J Clin Endocrinol Metab 1986; 63:16.
16. Lamberts SWJ, Zweens M, Klijn JGM, van Vroonhoven CCJ, Stefanko SZ, del Pozo E. The sensitivity of growth hormone and prolactin secretion to the somatostatin analog SMS 201-995 in patients with prolactinomas and acromegaly. Clin Endocrinol (Oxf) 1986 (in press).

25

THE USE OF DOPAMINE AGONISTS IN THE MANAGEMENT OF

ACROMEGALY

G. M. Besser and J. A. H. Wass

Department of Endocrinology
St. Bartholomew's Hospital
London EC1A 7BE UK

INTRODUCTION

Acromegaly, when untreated, is a chronic and debilitating disease which approximately halves life expectancy. Clearly all physical and biochemical evidence of acromegaly should be eradicated, but this is difficult to achieve by currently available therapeutic modalities. In most cases a combination of ablative and medical treatments are required.

Ideally, the aims of treatment should be long-term control or destruction of the tumor with preservation of normal anterior and posterior pituitary function. Somatic changes should be restored to normal without side effects or the induction of hypopituitarism, and cured acromegalics should have normal growth hormone levels. Normal subjects have undetectable growth hormone concentrations in the blood (less than 0.5 ng/ml or 1 mU/1) for more than 75% of the day. In addition, normal dynamics from growth hormone secretion must be demonstrated, particularly suppressibility of circulating growth hormone to undetectable levels after an oral glucose load and no rise in growth hormone after intravenous TRH. Furthermore, there should be a rise rather than a fall in serum growth hormone during a dopamine infusion. Circulating somatomedin-C levels should be in the normal range.

ABLATIVE THERAPY DIRECTED AT THE PITUITARY

It is generally agreed that it is very difficult to reduce circulating growth hormone levels to normal, as defined above, using surgical approaches including transsphenoidal hypophysectomy. Most acromegalic patients have tumors which are bigger than 10 mm in diameter, that is, they are macroadenomas. In contrast, smaller tumors, or microadenomas, may indeed be cured by expert transsphenoidal hypophysectomy, at least in the short term, in over 75% of cases. Most of these patients probably remain clinically normal although long-term follow-up data are still sparse. However, the majority of patients who have macroadenomas have tumors which infiltrate bone making these cases difficult to cure. Thus, after surgical ablative therapy, the majority of these patients are left with abnormal circulating growth hormone levels. These patients should have external pituitary irradiation, preferably using 4 or 15 MeV linear accelerators, to develop a lesion dose of 4,500 cGy (rads) in 25 fractions over 35 days. The treatment must be individually planned using the smallest target volume compatible with uniform irradiation of the lesion as shown radiologically, with immobilization of the whole head in an individually made plastic shell. This technique is safe and devoid of serious complications.

Growth hormone levels fall slowly after this treatment, and in 87 of our patients treated between 1970 and 1982, three years after radiotherapy mean growth hormone levels through the day were below 10 mU/l in 11% and below 20 mU/l in 43%. Seven years after radiotherapy they were below 10 mU/l in 86% of patients studied. These figures are similar to those reported by Eastman et al. (1). Our figures, and those of others, show that growth hormone values continue to fall for at least 10 years after treatment. It is clear, however, that radiotherapy, while safe and effective, produces normal growth hormone levels only slowly. Therefore, some interim therapy to lower growth hormone levels towards the normal range is necessary. Furthermore, with radiotherapy, hypopituitarism gradually and progressively appears. Thus, in our series, at the end of the mean of 5.7 years follow-up, 25% of patients who had not required replacement therapy prior to radiotherapy were now candidates for such treatment.

The place of dopamine agonist therapy and alternative medical treatments lies predominantly in patients who have had incomplete responses to surgery or radiotherapy or the combination, and still have elevated circulating growth hormone levels indicative of active acromegaly.

DOPAMINE AGONIST TREATMENT OF ACROMEGALY

Medical treatment of acromegaly has been effectively possible since 1973. It was shown that dopamine and dopamine agonists cause a rise in circulating growth hormone levels in normal subjects but a paradoxical fall in growth hormone levels in the majority of patients with acromegaly. Liuzzi et al. (2) showed that bromocriptine, a dopamine agonist, given as a single dose, lowered growth hormone levels in acromegalic patients.

We have treated a total of 161 patients with bromocriptine between July 1974 and January 1985. We have classified the patients arbitrarily into "responders" and "nonresponders," if the growth hormone levels did or did not fall by greater than a mean of 14 mU/l on long-term treatment, respectively (this value being twice the SD of the GH assay at a level of serum growth hormone of 60 mU/l). Seventy-five percent of patients on therapy have responded to bromocriptine in a daily dose of 10-60 mg (total) per day, given in 4 doses. Of these, 14% have a mean growth hormone level of less than 10 mU/l on treatment and a further 16% had mean serum growth hormone levels between 11 and 20 mU/l. Upon increasing the dose incrementally, we observed a fall in growth hormone levels in some patients with improving responses up to 60 mg/day. However, in the majority of patients no further fall in growth hormone was seen after 30 mg/day total dose.

No escape of growth hormone suppression, once obtained, has been seen during prolonged follow-up. If, in these patients, bromocriptine treatment is stopped, growth hormone levels rise again. Initially, there is a rebound to levels higher than those seen before treatment, but these return, within 3 or 4 weeks, to levels seen prior to commencement of therapy. For this reason it is our normal practice to combine bromocriptine therapy with radiotherapy. The radiotherapy produces a gradual fall in circulating growth hormone while the growth hormone levels are maintained suppressed at least in part with bromocriptine. Bromocriptine therapy is stopped every 12 months for reassessment of circulating growth hormone levels to establish whether or not medical treatment is still indicated.

Although bromocriptine has provided a major advance in the medical management of acromegaly, it is clear that growth hormone levels fall to normal only rarely.

THE SITE OF ACTION OF BROMOCRIPTINE IN ACROMEGALY

Bromocriptine has been shown to inhibit in vitro growth hormone release from human pituitaries of acromegalic patients suggesting a direct action of the dopamine agonist on the pituitary gland itself (3). In normal subjects it appears that dopamine acts on the median eminence to cause growth hormone secretion. Thus, in acromegalic patients, dopamine receptors which suppress growth hormone become manifest on the pituitary gland. It should be pointed out that when growth hormone levels are elevated in other circumstances, such as renal failure or liver disease, bromocriptine may then show the same paradoxical suppression of growth hormone as is seen in acromegalic patients. Thus, the paradoxical response is one related to elevated growth hormone levels rather than the acromegalic syndrome itself.

It is not possible to predict by any available test whether a new patient with acromegaly will or will not respond to bromocriptine. Even the response to an initial small test dose of bromocriptine is unreliable since it may be necessary to build up to high doses of the drug before suppression of growth hormone is seen. In our patients testing with TRH or LH-RH, and acute suppression test with bromocriptine, we have found that the determination of whether hyperprolactinemia is present or absent, does not predict the response to subsequent therapy. Similarly, the initial pretreatment growth hormone levels are poor predictors of the response to therapy.

SYMPTOMATIC RESPONSES

Clinical improvement is seen more frequently (over 90%) than the fall in circulating growth hormone level (75%) would suggest. Excessive sweating and headache improve rapidly with shrinking of the thickened skin, improvement of facial features and decrease in hand, foot and tongue size. Elevated blood pressure falls towards normal. Potency improves, and when amenorrhea is present due to hyperprolactinemia, this too improves. Clearly there is discrepancy between the clinical response and the response to the total immunoreactive growth hormone in the blood (4).

The reason for this discrepancy has been evaluated by assessment of a chromatographic profile of circulating growth hormone and measurement of somatomedin-C levels (4). It would appear that the monomeric form of growth hormone is preferentially suppressed by bromocriptine leaving in the circulation the polymeric form of growth hormone which is immunoreactive but of reduced biological activity. Furthermore, immunoreactive somatomedin-C levels may be suppressed even in the absence of suppression of growth hormone. These effects are difficult to reconcile; however, this observation may be accounted for, at least in part, by the preferential suppression of monomeric growth hormone and the dominance of immunoreactive but biologically inactive, polymeric growth hormone in the circulation. This would be expected to preferentially suppress somatomedin-C levels; however, there may be a specific effect on production of somatomedin-C which is quite separate from any effect on growth hormone.

CARBOHYDRATE TOLERANCE

The incidence of diabetes mellitus in our patients is 35%. On treatment this improved so that carbohydrate tolerance became normal in 70% of those in whom carbohydrate intolerance was present before treatment. Occasionally, significant improvement in carbohydrate tolerance occurred even though no significant fall in circulating growth hormone levels had been seen.

TUMOR SIZE AND BROMOCRIPTINE

It is well established that bromocriptine shrinks over 80% of prolactin secreting pituitary tumors. Mixed growth hormone and prolactin secreting tumors also decrease in size. In acromegaly shrinkage of pituitary tumor size is seen less often than in prolactinomas. It has been claimed by some that only those acromegalic tumors that also are associated with hyperprolactinemia shrink and that it is the prolactin secreting element of these tumors which respond. We have, therefore, specifically investigated acromegalic patients who have normal serum prolactin at presentation. We have found that these are generally smaller tumors than those associated with hyperprolactinemia since macroadenomas are usually associated with elevated circulating prolactin levels either due to simultaneous secretion of growth hormone and prolactin by the tumor or to pituitary stalk compression by the tumor. In our patients with normal prolactin levels, we have seen reduction in pituitary tumor size at 3 months in 47% of our subjects, thus demonstrating that bromocriptine can decrease the size of pure growth hormone secreting tumors.

METHOD OF BROMOCRIPTINE ADMINISTRATION

Growth hormone suppression by bromocriptine often lasts for only 6 hours after the dose. Therefore, the bromocriptine frequently has to be given in split doses 3 or 4 times a day. The optimum dose is reached by assessing patients clinically and biochemically on incremental doses of between 10 and 60 mg per day. Ideally increments of 10 mg/day should be given and then a "day-curve" for circulating growth hormone should be obtained. An indwelling needle is inserted in the acromegalic patient who is ambulant during the study, so that blood samples may be obtained 4-6 times during a single day. This allows the "mean growth hormone" for that day to be calculated. To avoid initiating side effects, dose increments should be slow and small. We increase the dose by a half to 1 tablet (1.25-2.5 mg) each day until the required dose is reached. Initially the treatment should be taken at night to avoid postural hypotension and bromocriptine must always be taken in the middle of food. Thus, our patients start the treatment at bedtime. Prior to retiring they have a snack in the middle of which they take their first dose. Once their dose regime is established, they take their doses in the middle of breakfast, lunch, and evening meal and often a dose on retiring in the middle of a snack.

SIDE EFFECTS

Side effects of dopamine agonist therapy have not been a major problem in our series if the precautions advised above are taken. The reported initiating side effects of nausea and hypotension are minimized by slow incremental introduction of the dose and administration during a bulk meal. In the long term, especially in patients on the higher doses, constipation has been noted and occasional patients complain of digital vasospasm introduced by cold weather. This is dose-responsive and in these patients we may reduce the dose in cold weather. Occasional patients (less than 1%) have developed acute depressive or psychotic illness. This must be watched for and responds to drug withdrawal.

OTHER DOPAMINE AGONISTS

Bromocriptine has been widely used throughout the world for the medical management of acromegaly. Other dopaminergic agonists, including lisuride, pergolide, mesulergine and lergotrile, have been tried but they have all presented problems, particularly with side effects or toxicological problems and they are not currently used.

ALTERNATIVE MEDICAL TREATMENT WITH SOMATOSTATIN OCTAPEPTIDE IN ACROMEGALY

Since the response to bromocriptine is usually only partial, other forms of medical treatment have been sought. Native somatostatin does lower growth hormone levels but the effect is only transient (5). The development of the somatostatin octapeptide (SMS 201-995) by Sandoz promises to be a major new therapeutic tool. It is currently given subcutaneously 2-3 times a day. In our series we have found excellent growth hormone suppression usually to undetectable levels in patients treated with 100 μg sc, 3 times a day. Growth hormone levels recover to low normal levels between injections but this provides a near normal profile of growth hormone secretion. We have attempted to establish whether addition of somatostatin to bromocriptine therapy is of any therapeutic benefit. It would appear that on somatostatin octapeptide, growth hormone levels are suppressed equally whether or not the patient is also treated with bromocriptine. Therefore, there is no indication to add bromocriptine to somatostatin in order to lower growth hormone levels. However, somatostatin octapeptide therapy only very rarely shrinks pituitary tumors and it may well be that bromocriptine may be added to somatostatin to increase the likelihood of tumor shrinkage. There is no doubt that the best medical treatment currently available is somatostatin octapeptide although some side effects of steatorrhea in particular may be encountered. The alternative treatment of bromocriptine has had much longer and more widespread use.

CONCLUSIONS

It is clear that medical treatment with bromocriptine, or somatostatin octapeptide, considerably alleviates the symptoms and signs of acromegaly and lowers growth hormone levels. Medical treatment of this sort should be used to augment ablative therapy, either surgical or radiotherapeutic or the combination where this treatment has failed to completely normalize (rendered undetectable for the majority of the day) circulating growth hormone levels. In the small proportion of elderly patients in whom ablative therapy is contraindicated, medical treatment may be used alone.

REFERENCES

1. Eastman RC, Gorden P, Roth J. Conventional supervoltage irradiation is an effective treatment for acromegaly. J Clin Endocrinol Metab 1979; 48:931-40.
2. Liuzzi A, Chiodini PG, Botalla L, Cremascoli G, Muller EE,

Silvestrini F. Decreased plasma growth hormone (GH) levels in acromegalics following CB 154 (2-Br-a-ergocryptine) administration. J Clin Endocrinol Metab 1974; 38:910-2.

3. Ishibashi M, Yamaji T, Kosaka K. Effect of bromocriptine on TRH-induced growth hormone and prolactin release in acromegalic patients. J Clin Endocrinol Metab 1977; 45:275-9.

4. Wass JAH, Clemmons DR, Underwood LE, Barrow I, Besser GM, Van Wyk JJ. Changes in circulating somatomedin-C levels in bromocriptine-treated acromegaly. Clin Endocrinol (Oxf) 1982; 17:369-77.

5. Besser GM, Mortimer CH, Carr D, et al. Growth hormone release inhibiting hormone in acromegaly. Br Med J 1974; 1:352-5.

26

DECISION ANALYSIS OF TREATMENT OPTIONS IN ACROMEGALY

K. von Werder, R. Fahlbusch, M. Losa, R. Oeckler, J. Pichl,
and J. Schopohl

Departments of Medicine and Neurosurgery
University of Munich, and
University of Erlangen, FRG

Acromegaly, although it is a slowly-progressing disease, leads to significant morbidity and mortality (1). Although microsurgical techniques and the introduction of more effective medical therapy have led to considerable improvement of therapeutical results, acromegaly is still a "stubborn therapeutic challenge" as Daughaday pointed out 16 years ago (2). The aim of treating patients suffering from acromegaly is normalizing elevated growth hormone (GH) and somatomedin-C (SM-C) levels while preserving normal anterior pituitary function. Furthermore, treatment has to be directed also against a possibly expanding tumor which may lead to destruction of the sella turcica, visual disturbances, and other neurological complications (3). The decision about the form of treatment is influenced not only by age, clinical situation, and operability but also by the size of the GH-producing pituitary tumor, height of the GH level and the underlying pathophysiology of GH hypersecretion.

Endocrine diagnostic workup has become more sophisticated allowing the differentiation between distinct types of acromegaly (4). This is exemplified by the more frequently discovered growth hormone releasing hormone (GHRH)-producing tumors, admittedly a rare cause of acromegaly (3). Furthermore, in patients in whom GH hypersecretion is independent of an ectopic GHRH source, distinct features of the GH secretion pattern can also be observed. An inappropriate rise of GH after TRH administration is observed in about 60% of patients (3-5). A majority of these patients exhibit a GH suppression after administration of dopamine (DA) agonists (6). Recently, it has been demonstrated that this prolactin (PRL)-like behavior of GH responsiveness to TRH and suppression after administration of DA agonists, correlates with the GH-like behavior of PRL, i.e., responsiveness of PRL levels to the administration of GHRH, suggesting the presence of a somatomammotrophic cell tumor (7). Patients with these tumors may respond differently to therapy compared to acromegalics who do not exhibit this GH and PRL secretion pattern (6).

There are several therapeutic approaches for treating acromegalics (Table 1) but their benefits and risks are still a matter of discussion. In the following, our personal experience in treating patients with acromegaly will be presented and discussed, together with the published literature, with the aim of proposing a rational strategy for the treatment of acromegaly.

Table 1. Therapy of acromegaly.

Operative therapy
    Transsphenoidal surgery
    Transfrontal surgery
    Combination of both
    Cryohypophysectomy
    Removal of GHRH-producing tumor

Radiotherapy
    Conventional external radiation (50 Gy)
    90 Yttrium implantation
    Heavy particles

Medical therapy
    Dopamine agonists
    Somatostatin analogs

OPERATIVE TREATMENT

The early efforts of surgical treatment of pituitary tumors date back to the end of the last century when Richard Caton and Frank Thomas Paul in 1893 performed a cranial operation in a 33-year-old woman with acromegaly in order to relieve cranial pressure (8). However, it was Herman Schloffer who first successfully operated on a pituitary tumor by the nasal route in 1906 (9). This technique was taken up and improved by Oskar Hirsch, reducing the initial mortality of 35% to 10% (10). Harvey Cushing operated on his first patient with acromegaly in 1909, removing about one-third of the anterior pituitary lobe (11). Due to the considerable mortality of the procedure, transsphenoidal surgery was abandoned in the late 1920s and only reintroduced in the late 1960s after microsurgical techniques had been developed allowing selective adenomectomy in encapsulated intra- and also suprasellar-extending tumors under televised radiofluoroscopic control (12). The transsphenoidal procedure can be combined with transfrontal surgery in cases with invasive tumors extending into the supra- and parasellar area (13,14).

In our institution between 1974 and 1982, 182 acromegalic patients with preoperative GH levels ranging from 5 to 500 ng/ml were subjected to transsphenoidal and occasionally transfrontal surgery. When it was (arbitrarily) decided that normalization of GH levels had occurred if GH levels had fallen below 5 ng/ml, 103 patients could be considered to be cured (Fig. 1). Of these normalized patients, 82 had preoperative GH levels below 50 ng/ml and 21 had levels above 50 ng/ml. Forty-six patients of the 182 with large pituitary adenomas and/or highly elevated GH levels, showed a fall of GH levels after surgery compared to pretreatment, though GH levels below 5 ng/ml were never encountered. Of the normalized acromegalics, only 2 recurrences were seen during later follow-up, whereas in 8 of the non-normalized patients, a further increase of the postoperatively-elevated GH levels was encountered (Fig. 1). The only parameters that were predictive for the outcome of surgery were tumor size and the preoperative GH level. Inappropriate stimulation by TRH/GHRH was not predictive of the outcome of surgery, nor did the persistence of this abnormality indicate later recurrence of GH hypersecretion. Of the surgically-normalized patients, 31 had inappropriate stimulation of GH by TRH/GHRH (200 µg/100 µg IV) 100% above basal level, which persisted in 20 patients after surgery. In patients with clinical improvement and a fall, but not normalization of GH levels, inappropriate stimulation of GH secretion occurred in 29 before, and 22 after surgery. In patients in whom the

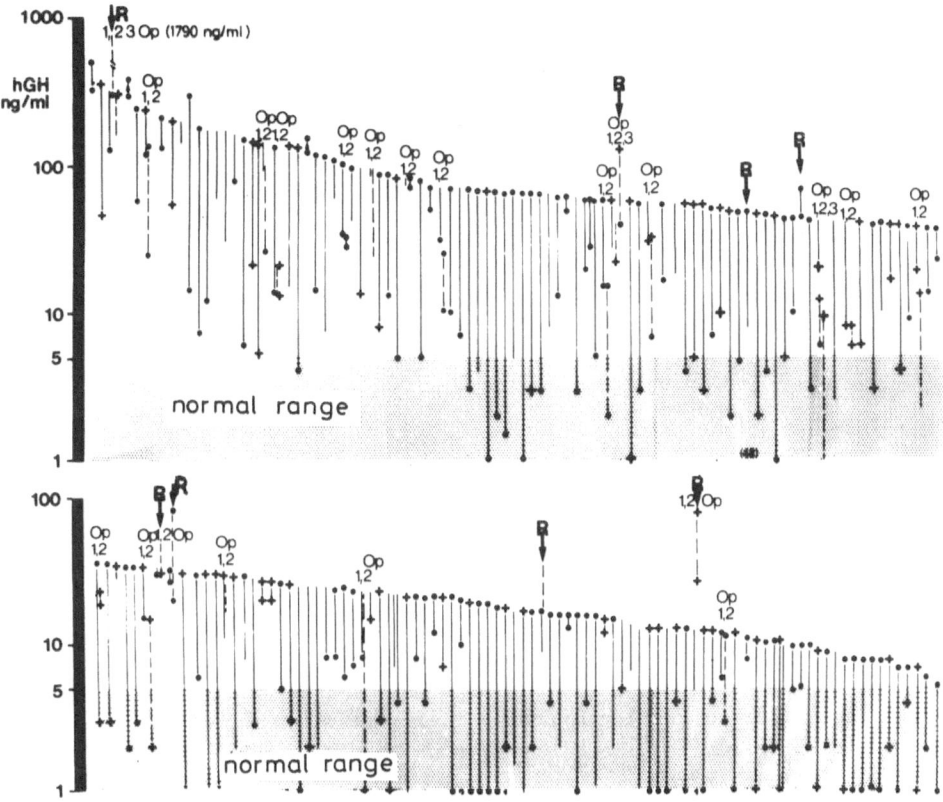

Fig. 1. Pre- and postoperative GH levels in 182 acromegalics.
The pre- and the postoperative GH levels represent the mean of 3
basal GH levels (1 to 3 months after surgery). TRH stimulation
was regarded as positive (+) if the basal level had increased by
at least 100%. Lack of response to TRH is depicted by a closed
circle (●). If there is only a single line without symbols at
the top (preop), or at the bottom (postop), the TRH test was not
performed. Op 1, 2, 3 represents first, second, and third
operation, respectively; R depicts later recurrences.

surgical procedure had no or little effect on basal GH levels, inappropriate stimulation by releasing hormones also persisted after surgery. Of
the 10 patients who had adenoma recurrence after surgery, 5 had inappropriate TRH/GHRH stimulation of GH secretion before, and 3 after surgery.
The presence of hyperprolactinemia (20%) did not influence the surgical
results. These findings, which were published two years ago (14), are in
good agreement with the neurosurgical literature (Table 2).

Complete clinical and biochemical resolution, a so-called cure of
acromegaly (i.e., GH levels below 5 ng/ml) and normalization of SM-C
levels has been reported in up to 90% of the patients with noninvasive
microadenomas and preoperative GH levels below 50 ng/ml (3,15,16). Surgical therapy is considerably less effective in invasive tumors in which
an overall normalization rate between 20 and 30% has been reported (17).
Whether intraoperative GH measurements, to search for tumor residue when
the GH levels have not fallen adequately, will improve the operative
results, is still debated (15). Cryohypophysectomy, either as a stereo-
taxic procedure or in combination with transsphenoidal surgery, has been
abandoned. The efficacy of this procedure is not better than microsurgery

269

Table 2. Effect of transsphenoidal microsurgery
on basal GH levels in patients with
acromegaly in a large series.

Authors (references)	No. of cases	GH levels below 5 ng/ml (%)	
Hardy (12)	160	123	(77)
Balagura et al. (13)	132	76	(58)
Quabbe (16)	152	83	(57)
Laws et al. (37)	140	82	(58)
Giovanelli et al. (38)	107	61	(57)
Ludecke et al. (17)	200	169	(85)
Von Werder (14)	182	106	(59)

but anterior pituitary failure is more common (18). The criteria for "cure" of acromegaly are poorly defined. Measurement of SM-C seems to be useful since it fluctuates little and seems to correlate well to the clinical situation (19). However, this definition has not been totally agreed upon (20). Ever since qualitative abnormalities in GH secretion have been demonstrated, it has been recognized that cure may imply complete normalization of GH secretion dynamic in the postoperative period (5,19). In some cases, clinical activity, postoperative GH levels, and SM-C levels may be completely normalized, but a pathological response to TRH, a lack of regular GH responsiveness to insulin-induced hypoglycemia, or exogenous GHRH administration may persist, thereby suggesting persistent abnormal GH secretion (14). Another qualitative abnormality in the GH secretion pattern of acromegalic patients is the persisting GH response during pulsatile GHRH stimulation. Whereas in normal subjects the GH response to the second GHRH pulse is blunted, acromegalics show a normal rise to the second and third pulse, if given in 2-hour intervals (21). Furthermore, this abnormality seems to persist in those postoperative patients who have normal basal GH and SM-C levels (Fig. 2). Therefore, although only complete normalization of all abnormalities of GH secretion may, in fact, prove "cure" of acromegaly, GH levels lower than 5 ng/ml may be considered as satisfactory results. Our data suggest that the qualitative abnormalities in GH secretion do not indicate a greater likelihood of recurrence, and should therefore not be regarded as an indication for further therapy, i.e., second surgery, radiotherapy or medical treatment.

RADIOTHERAPY

External radiation treatment was performed as early as 1909 (22). Many investigators have used radiotherapy as primary treatment of acromegaly (23) because it has been demonstrated to be highly effective in lowering GH levels though it often takes years before the latter reach the normal range (23,24). Whereas less than 20% of those patients treated by radiotherapy have normal GH levels within one year, 80% become normal within 5 or 6 years after irradiation. The most important side effect of radiotherapy is late partial or complete anterior pituitary failure. This complication is observed in up to half of all cases and occurs within 10 years after treatment (24). Major complications of radiotherapy, such as visual failure and cerebral radionecrosis, occur rarely if the total dosage of 5000 rads, given in a fractionated manner (e.g., 200 rads/day), is not exceeded. However, the latter complication has also been reported in cases irradiated adequately (25). The fact that pituitary failure occurs in patients who still show a normal GH response to direct stimulation with GHRH, is evidence for hypothalamic radiation involvement (26).

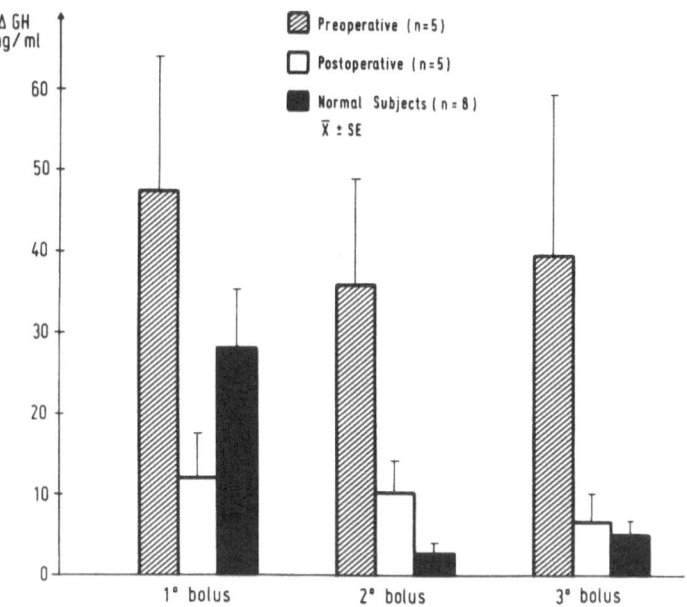

Fig. 2. Increase of GH levels (Δ GH = maximum level after GHRH) after 3 injections of 100 μg GHRH given in 2-hour intervals to 5 acromegalics before, and 2 months after transsphenoidal surgery (basal GH, 4.0 ng/ml) and 8 normal subjects. Whereas repetitive GHRH stimulation leads to blunting of the GH response in normal subjects, the latter is sustained in patients with acromegaly. After successful transsphenoidal surgery the GHRH-induced GH rise has diminished; however, in contrast to normals, no decrease of the GH response to the second GHRH pulse is observed.

We have not used radiotherapy as primary treatment of acromegaly. Thus, with one exception, we have irradiated only 27 patients as of 1984 (5000 rads from a high-voltage source) who had been operated on previously. GH levels before radiotherapy ranged from 5 to 498 ng/ml. The observation period after completion of radiotherapy ranged from 1 month to 4 years. Normalization of GH had occurred in 7 patients, while improvement was observed in 6; no effect was seen in 10 acromegalics, presumably due to the short follow-up period. In 4 patients, an increase of the GH levels was seen after radiotherapy (14).

Experience with heavy particle or proton beam irradiation has been limited to two centers in the United States. Although high radiation doses can be administered with this technique leading to clinical improvement within 6 months, and GH levels below 5 ng in more than half of the patients after 5 years, the incidence of hypopituitarism seems to be greater with this procedure (27). Furthermore, this treatment is contraindicated in patients with suprasellar adenoma extension because of the high risk of permanent oculomotor nerve damage.

Interstitial irradiation with 90 Yttrium has been performed only in few centers. Although the treatment is practically without any side effects, hypopituitarism typically occurs and the results seem to be less satisfactory than those obtained with microsurgery (28).

MEDICAL TREATMENT

In the past, several pharmacological agents have been proposed for the treatment of acromegaly. Thus, estrogens, high doses of progestins, chlorpromazine, and other dopamine antagonists have been examined. However, none of these drugs was shown to be effective in lowering GH levels sufficiently.

Liuzzi et al. (29) first reported that L-dopa led to a paradoxical reduction of GH levels in more than 50% of acromegalic patients. Subsequently, it has been shown that chronic administration of long-acting dopamine agonists such as bromocriptine and lisuride is able to lead to permanent reduction of GH levels in patients with acromegaly (30,31). Administration of these drugs has become an established form of medical treatment of acromegaly.

Bromocriptine

2-Br-alpha-ergocriptine, which has been proven to be highly effective in treatment of hyperprolactinemia, has also been widely used for the treatment of acromegaly (3). Some authors have proposed the administration of very high dosages, up to 40 and 60 mg/day (30), while others feel that an increase of the bromocriptine dosage above 20 mg/day does not result in a greater benefit with respect to lowering GH levels (16,32). Besser et al. (30), who reported the largest series, observed GH levels below 5 ng in 19%, and GH levels below 10 ng/ml in 78%, of their patients receiving bromocriptine treatment; clinical improvement was observed in 94% of all patients. The discrepancy between clinical and biochemical effects of bromocriptine are not clear, though evidence has been presented that bromocriptine lowers, preferentially, the "little" component of GH which is more biologically active (30,34). In contrast to prolactinomas, the effect of bromocriptine on tumor size is certainly less pronounced (35).

We have treated 46 patients with bromocriptine, 41 for persisting GH hypersecretion after surgery, and 5 who received primary bromocriptine treatment. The GH levels before treatment ranged from 5 to 798 ng/ml (Fig. 3). The bromocriptine dosage ranged from 1.25 to 90 mg per day and the duration of treatment was from 1 month to 8 years. In 17 patients, normal GH levels were achieved while administering bromocriptine. In 9 patients, there was a significant but incomplete fall of the elevated GH levels under bromocriptine treatment, whereas, in 15 patients, no significant effect was seen. Recurrences, with increases in GH levels, were seen in 4 patients during bromocriptine medication; 3 developed overt clinical acromegaly. We also observed a striking reduction of clinical activity in those patients in whom GH levels were not normalized completely.

In addition, 12 patients with acromegaly and hyperprolactinemia (PRL levels ranging from 600 to 50000 µU/ml) received bromocriptine in a dosage of 2.5 to 60 mg/day. Eleven had been operated on previously, and 4 of them had received additional radiotherapy with 4000 rads from a high-voltage source. Whereas bromocriptine led to normalization of prolactin levels in all 12 patients, GH levels normalized in only 5 subjects, a reduction in GH secretion was seen in 3, and no effect upon GH levels was observed in 4 patients. There was no significant increase in the responsiveness of GH levels to dopaminergic suppression in hyperprolactinemic acromegalics as compared to acromegalics with normal PRL levels. There was also no predictive value of the TRH/GHRH-stimulated GH secretion for the outcome of long-term dopaminergic therapy, which is in contrast to results obtained by Lamberts et al. (6) who found a good correlation of GH stimulation by TRH with acute GH suppression by dopaminergic agents. In 16 patients, bromocriptine was withdrawn after a mean treatment period of one year. In all patients GH levels returned to pretherapy values after the drug had been withdrawn (Fig. 4). Although lisuride (31) does not offer advantages over bromocriptine, the former can be tried in cases of bromocriptine intolerance and vice versa.

Somatostatin Analogs

Since long-acting somatostatin preparations have become available, these preparations have been used for the treatment of acromegaly with great success (36). The greatest experience has been obtained with the octapeptide analog, which, at a dosage of 50 μg sc, leads to a significant depression of GH levels lasting for up to 8 hours. Dosages of 3x50 to 3x10 μg SMS 201-995 sc were shown to normalize GH secretion in 90% of the acromegalics without serious side effects on carbohydrate metabolism or the gastrointestinal tract (36). We have treated 6 selected patients with

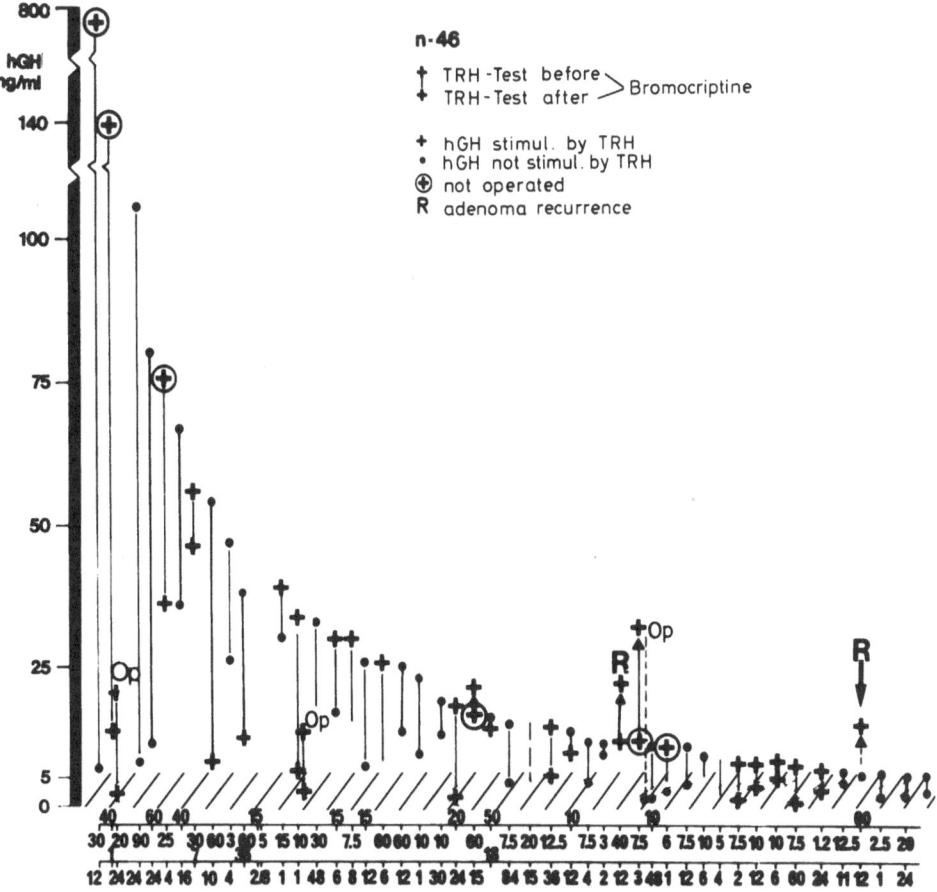

Fig. 3. Growth hormone levels (GH) before and during bromo-criptine therapy (mean of 3 basal levels) in 46 acromegalic patients. The daily bromocriptine dosage and duration of treatment are shown at the bottom of the figure. The first line of numbers represents the dosage of bromocriptine (mg/day), the bottom line the duration of therapy (months). TRH stimulation of GH secretion (100% increase) is depicted by +. The broken line represents patients who later received additional therapy; R signals recurrence of active acromegaly.

SMS 201-995 (Table 3). Of these, 2 patients had metastatic GHRH-producing tumors with acromegaly. In these patients, SMS 201-995 not only suppressed circulating GH levels but also GHRH concentrations (Fig. 5). One patient has been treated for more than two years with an impressive shrinkage of liver metastases, though the SMS 201-995 dosage had to be increased to 700 μg per day to insure complete suppression of GH and GHRH levels (Fig. 6). The 4 other patients had large invasive somatotrophic tumors, one of them being inoperable because of a suprasellar extension leading to foramen Monroi blockade. The other 3 patients had been operated on by transsphenoidal approach twice and had also received postoperative radiotherapy and dopaminergic agents without success. In all 4 patients, treatment with the somatostatin analog led to further decrease of the GH levels. Three patients received daily dosages of SMS 201-995 exceeding 500 μg/day (one patient up to 1200 μg SMS 201-995 daily), which could only be administered without side effects by using a portable pump for continuous sc infusion of the octapeptide.

CONCLUSIONS

Data in the literature, as well as our own experience, demonstrate that transsphenoidal microsurgery is the most effective form of primary treatment in patients with a radiologically-detectable pituitary tumor. Since patients with large invasive adenomas are rarely cured by surgery alone, even if transsphenoidal and transfrontal surgery is performed, postoperative radiotherapy seems to be indicated (Fig. 7).

In patients with noninvasive adenomas who have persisting acromegaly after surgery due to minor elevations of GH levels, postoperative dopamine agonist treatment is suggested. The latter may be tried as a primary therapy in the rare patients in whom no tumor is detectable by the most

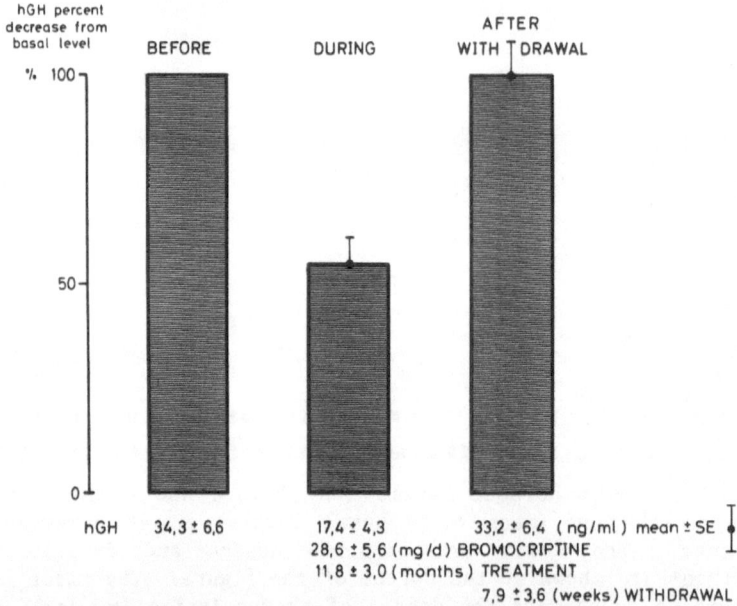

Fig. 4. Effect of bromocriptine treatment and withdrawal on GH levels in 16 acromegalics. The calculation is based on the mean of 3 basal levels before, during, and after bromocriptine treatment.

Table 3. SMS 201-995 therapy in selected cases of acromegaly.

Pt	Sex	Age	Pathology	Previous treatment	SMS 201-995 dosage (µg/ml)	Duration of treatment	GH-level (ng/ml) Initial	before SMS	during SMS
AS	f	24	Suprasellar extending macroadenoma	2 ts operations bromocriptine	200	2	100	60	<5
MS	f	25	Macroadenoma	3 ts operations, radiotherapy, bromocriptine	350* cscí	2	180	110	70*
HA	f	46	Macroadenoma	3 ts operations, radiotherapy, DA agonists	200	10	140	25	<5
MM	f	30	Giant adenoma with Foramen Monroi block-ade, Albright syndrome	Bromocriptine, ventriculo peri-toneal shunt	600-1200 cscí	3	560	350	50
BM	f	50	GHRH-producing carcinoid of breast with mediastinal metastasis, normal sella	Breast surgery thoracotomy	100	1/2	10	10	<1
BS	f	17	GHRH-producing jejunal tumor with liver metastasis; suprasella extending somatotroph hyperplasia	ts surgery, laparotomy, bromocriptine	700 cscí	27	450	25	<1

cscí = continuous subcutaneous infusion by portable pump; ts = transsphenoidal
*The dosage will be increased.

275

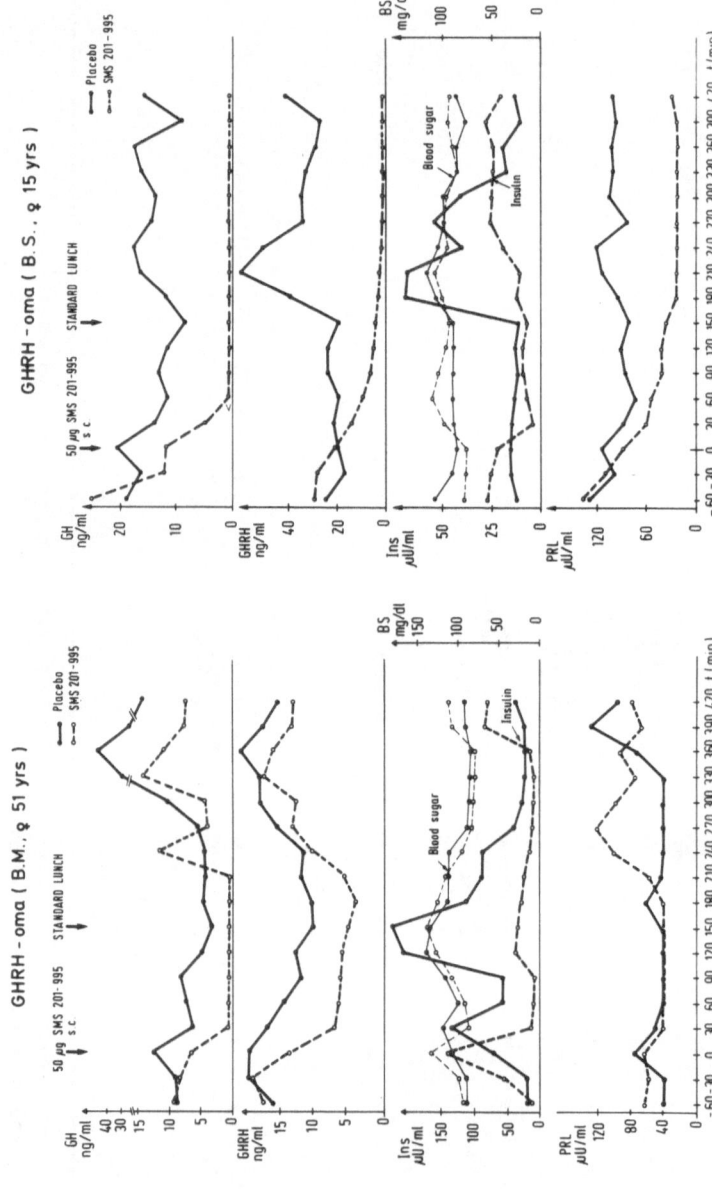

Fig. 5. GH, GHRH, insulin and blood sugar, and prolactin levels after sc injection of 50 µg SMS 201-995 compared to a control day in 2 patients with GHRH-omas. Within 1 hour after SMS injection, GH levels became undetectable and GHRH-levels had fallen. Postprandial insulin was also suppressed 3 hours after SMS 201-995 injection, although blood sugar remained normal because the insulin antagonist, GH, was suppressed at the same time. PRL levels decreased after SMS 201-995 administration compared to the control day only in patient BS.

sophisticated radiological investigation, or who are inoperable because of clinical reasons. Somatostatin analog treatment, which may be less acceptable because it needs several injections per day, should be reserved for those patients who fail to respond to surgery, radiotherapy, dopamine agonists, or who have metastatic GHRH-producing tumors (Fig. 7). With the exception of the latter situation, it is our experience that prediction of the efficacy of the various forms of long-term medical therapy cannot be made even when the most thorough biochemical evaluation has been performed.

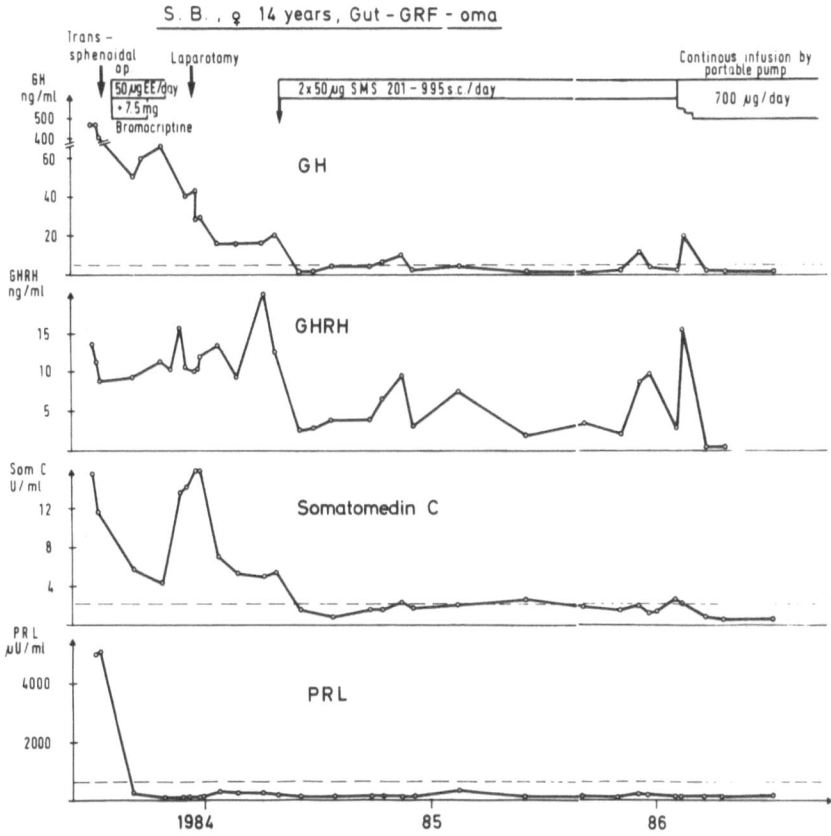

Fig. 6. GH, GHRH, somatomedin-C, and PRL levels before and after transsphenoidal surgery, laparotomy and during chronic SMS 201-995 treatment. GH levels fell from above 400 to 50 ng/ml after surgery and showed a further decrease after laparotomy although GHRH levels were not influenced. Only after starting SMS 201-995 treatment, GH levels were suppressed and GHRH levels fell by 75%. Somatomedin-C levels, which were already suppressed during a short period of estrogen treatment, were normalized during treatment with the octapeptide. However, the dosage had to be increased up to 700 µg/day to achieve and maintain complete GH and GHRH suppression. The initially-elevated PRL levels became normal after removal of the pituitary hyperplasia.

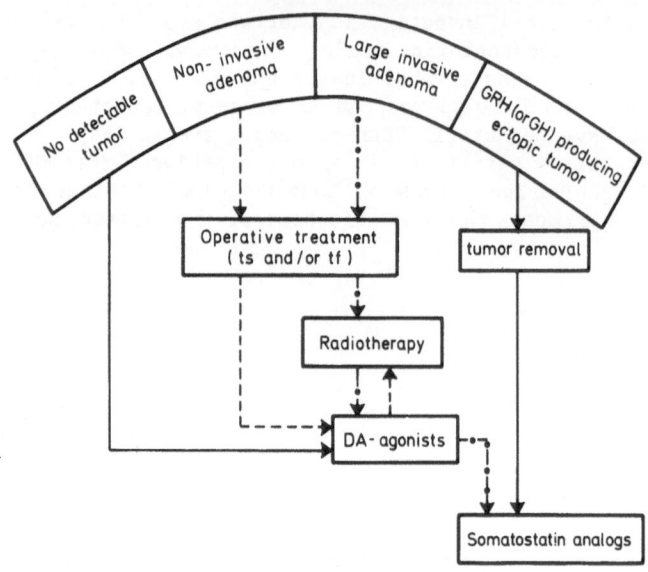

Fig. 7. Therapeutic strategy in acromegaly.

REFERENCES

1. Alexander L, Appleton D, Hall R, Ross WM, Wilkinson R. Epidemiology of acromegaly in the Newcastle region. Clin Endocrinol (Oxf) 1980; 12:71-9.
2. Daughaday WH. Acromegaly—a stubborn therapeutic challenge. N Engl J Med 1970; 282:1430.
3. Faglia G, Arosio M, Ambrosi B. Recent advances in diagnosis and treatment of acromegaly. In: Imura H, ed. The pituitary gland. New York: Raven Press, 1985:363-404.
4. Melmed S, Braunstein GD, Horvath E, Ezrin C, Kovacs K. Pathophysiology of acromegaly. Endocr Rev 1983; 4:271.
5. Faglia G, Paracchi A, Ferrari C, Beck-Peccoz P. Evaluation of the results of trans-sphenoidal surgery in acromegaly by assessment of the growth hormone response to thyrotrophin-releasing hormone. Clin Endocrinol (Oxf) 1978; 8:373.
6. Lamberts SWJ, Liuzzi A, Chiodini PG, Verde S, Klijn JGM, Birkenhager JC. The value of plasma prolactin levels in prediction of the responsiveness of growth hormone secretion to bromocriptine and TRH in acromegaly. Eur J Clin Invest 1982; 12:151-5.
7. Losa M, Schopohl J, Muller OA, von Werder K. Growth hormone releasing factor induces prolactin secretion in acromegalic patients but not in normal subjects. Acta Endocrinol (Copenh) 1985; 109:467.
8. Caton R, Paul FT. Notes on a case of acromegaly treated by operation. Br Med J 1893; 2:1421.
9. Schloffer H. Erfolgreiche operation eines hypophysentu-mors auf nasalem wege. Wien Klin Wochenschr 1907; 20:622.
10. Hirsch O. Eine neue methode der endonasalen operation von hypophysentumoren. Wien Med Wochenschr 1909; 59:636.
11. Cushing H. Partial hypophysectomy for acromegaly, with remarks on the function of the hypophysis. Ann Surg 1909; 1:1002.
12. Hardy J. Transsphenoidal microsurgical treatment of hypersecreting pituitary adenomas. In: Cumming IA, Funder JW, Mendelsohn FAO, eds. Endocrinology 1980. Proceedings of the 4th International Congress of Endocrinology. Canberra: Australian Academy of Science, 1980:715-8.
13. Balagura S, Derome P, Guiot G. Acromegaly: analysis of 132 cases treated surgically. Neurosurgery 1981; 8:413.

14. von Werder K, Eversmann T, Fahlbusch R, Muller OA, Rjosk H-K. Endocrine-active pituitary adenomas: long-term results of medical and surgical treatment. In: Camanni F, Muller EE, eds. Pituitary hyperfunction: physiopathology and clinical aspects. New York: Raven Press, 1984.

15. Ludecke DK. Recent development in the treatment of acromegaly. Neurosurg Rev 1985; 8:167.

16. Quabbe H-J. Treatment of acromegaly by transsphenoidal operation, 90-Yttrium implantation and bromocriptine: results in 230 patients. Clin Endocrinol (Oxf) 1982; 16:107.

17. Ludecke DK, William TH, Breustedt HJ, et al. Effectiveness of microsurgery in acromegaly—study of 200 cases [Abstract 383]. 6th International Congress of Endocrinology, Melbourne. Canberra: Union Offset, 1980.

18. Teasdale GM, Hay ID, Beasttall GH, et al. Cryosurgery or microsurgery in the management of acromegaly. JAMA 1982; 247:1289.

19. Schaison G, Couzinet B, Moatti N, Pertuiset B. Critical study of the growth hormone response to dynamic tests and the insulin growth factor assay in acromegaly after microsurgery. Clin Endocrinol (Oxf) 1983; 18:541.

20. Stonesifer LD, Jordan RM, Kohler PO. Somatomedin C in treated acromegaly: poor correlation with growth hormone and clinical response. J Clin Endocrinol Metab 1981; 53:931.

21. Losa M, Schopohl J, Konig A, Muller OA, von Werder K. Growth hormone and prolactin response to repetitive administration of growth hormone releasing hormone (GHRH) in acromegaly. J Clin Endocrinol Metab 1986; 63:475-80.

22. Gramegna A. Un cas d'acromegalie traite par la radiotherapie. Rev Neurol (Paris) 1909; 17:15.

23. Eastman RC, Gorden P, Roth J. Conventional supervoltage irradiation is an effective treatment for acromegaly. J Clin Endocrinol Metab 1979; 48:931.

24. Feek CM, McLelland J, Seth J, et al. How effective is external pituitary irradiation for growth hormone-secreting pituitary tumours? Clin Endocrinol (Oxf) 1984; 20:401.

25. Landolt AM. Hazards of radiotherapy in patients with pituitary adenomas. In: Derome PJ, Jedynak CP, Peillon F, eds. Pituitary adenomas. Paris: Ascelpios Pub, 1980:227-32.

26. Grossman A, Lytras N, Savage MO, et al. Growth hormone releasing factor: comparison of two analogues and demonstration of hypothalamic defect in growth hormone release after radiotherapy. Br Med J 1984; 288:1785.

27. Kjellberg RN, Kliman B, Swisher BJ. Radiosurgery for pituitary adenoma with bragg peak proton beam. In: Derome PJ, Jedynak CP, Peillon F, eds. Pituitary adenomas. Paris: Asclepois Pub, 1980:209-17.

28. Joplin GF, Banks L, Child DF, et al. Treatment of acromegaly by pituitary implantation of 90-Y. In: Fahlbusch R, von Werder W, eds. Treatment of pituitary adenomas. Stuttgart: G. Thieme, 1978.

29. Liuzzi A, Chiodini PG, Botalla L, Cremascoli G, Silvestrini F. Inhibitory effect of L-Dopa on GH-release in acromegalic patients. J Clin Endocrinol Metab 1972; 35:941.

30. Besser GM, Wass JAH, Thorner MO. Bromocriptine in the medical management of acromegaly. In: Goldstein M, Calne DB, Lieberman A, Thorner MO, eds. Ergot compounds and brain functions. New York: Raven Press, 1980:191-8.

31. Verde G, Chiodini PG, Liuzzi A, et al. Effectiveness of the dopamine agonist lisuride in the treatment of acromegaly and pathological hyperprolactinemic states. J Endocrinol Invest 1980; 4:405-14.

32. Chiodini PG, Liuzzi A, Botalla L, Oppizzi G, Muller EE, Silvestrini F. Stable reduction of plasma growth hormone (hGH) levels during

chronic administration of 2-Br-ergocryptine (CB-154) in acromegalic patients. J Clin Endocrinol Metab 1975; 40:705.

33. Eversmann T, Dietz A, Schopohl J, Gottsmann M, von Werder K. Human growth hormone in acromegaly: radioimmunoassay, radioreceptor assay, dextran gel filtration [Abstract 380]. 6th International Congress of Endocrinology, 1980.

34. Wass JAM, Clemmons DR, Underwood LE, Barrow I, Besser GM, Van Wyk JJ. Changes in circulating somatomedin-C levels in bromocriptine-treated acromegaly. Clin Endocrinol (Oxf) 1982; 17:369.

35. Wass JAM, Moult PJA, Thorner MO, et al. Reduction in pituitary tumour size in patients with prolactinomas and acromegaly treated with bromocriptine with or without radiotherapy. Lancet 1979; 2:66.

36. Lamberts SWJ, Uitterlinden P, Verschoor L, van Dongen KJ, del Pozo E. Long-term treatment of acromegaly with the somatostatin analogue SMS 201-995. N Engl J Med 1985; 313:1576.

37. Laws ER, Randall RV, Abboud CF. Surgical treatment of acromegaly: results in 140 patients. In: Givens JR, ed. Hormone-secreting pituitary tumours. Chicago: Year Book Medical Pubs., Inc., 1982: 225-8.

38. Giovanelli MA, Gaini SM, Tomei G, et al. Transsphenoidal micro-surgical treatment of acromegaly. In: Lamberts SWJ, Tilders FJH, van der Veen EA, Assies J, eds. Proceedings of the 3rd European Workshop on Pituitary Adenomas. Amsterdam: Free University Press, 1984:215-24.

AUTHOR INDEX

SUBJECT INDEX